ORTHOPAEDIC MANAGEMENT OF NEUROMUSCULAR DISORDERS

ORTHOPAEDIC MANAGEMENT OF NEUROMUSCULAR DISORDERS

James C. Drennan, M.D.

Director of Orthopaedics
Newington Children's Hospital
Newington, Connecticut

J. B. Lippincott Company
Philadelphia • Toronto

Sponsoring Editor: Darlene D. Pedersen
Manuscript Editor: Randi Boyette
Indexer: Marianna Nelson
Designer: Rita Vaughton

Production Supervisor: N. Carol Kerr
Production Assistant: Charlene Catlett Squibb
Compositor: Waldman Graphics, Inc.
Printer/Binder: Halliday Lithograph

1   3   5   6   4   2

Library of Congress Cataloging in Publication Data

Drennan, James C. (James Cyril), DATE
  Orthopaedic management of neuromuscular disorders.

  Includes index.
  1. Musculoskeletal   system—Surgery.   2. Neuromuscular   diseases—Surgery.
3. Neuromuscular diseases.   I. Title. [DNLM: 1. Neuromuscular diseases—Therapy.
2. Neuromuscular diseases—Rehabilitation.   WE 550 D772o]
RD680.D73   616.7'406   82-18
ISBN 0-397-50469-1   AACR2

The author and publisher have exerted every effort to ensure that drug selection and dosage set forth in this text are in accord with current recommendations and practice at the time of publication. However, in view of ongoing research, changes in government regulations, and the constant flow of information relating to drug therapy and drug reactions, the reader is urged to check the package insert for each drug for any change in indications and dosage and for added warnings and precautions. This is particularly important when the recommended agent is a new or infrequently employed drug.

Printed in the United States of America

To Jimmy,
        the inspiration for all my work

Preface

The past decade has seen a marked increase in the medical under-standing of neuromuscular disorders. Biochemical and electro-physiologic studies, as well as muscle biopsy evaluation by enzyme histochemistry and electron microscopy, have led to the identifica-tion of new disease entities and classifications associated with mus-cle weakness, wasting, and other types of neuromuscular dysfunction.

This expanded medical knowledge should create the climate for improving the quality of life for patients affected by neuromuscular disorders. Regrettably, however, during the past decade there has been decreasing emphasis and interest in rehabilitation on the part of the practicing physician and in resident training programs. A variety of more acute care advances, such as total joint replacement, have gained prominence at the expense of rehabilitation. This book is aimed at bridging the growing gap between medical understanding and the increasing inadequacies of medicine to deliver the appropriate quality of care to patients with neuromuscular disorders.

Orthopaedic Management of Neuromuscular Disorders is di-rected to the orthopaedist, neurologist, pediatrician, and family prac-titioner, as well as to the allied medical personnel who are involved in this care system. It presents a comprehensive rehabilitation pro-gram and philosophy for patients with spinal dysrhaphism and motor unit disease, including those with involvement of anterior-horn cell, peripheral nerve, and voluntary muscle, as well as of the spinal cerebellar tract. Lesions at each of these neurologic levels may be considered when there is a differential diagnosis of disease involving muscles. The similarities and differences of each pathologic process are discussed in regard to diagnosis and clinical management.

Many of the patients affected by a neuromuscular disorder are most appropriately managed in a multidiscipline clinic where the talents of several different medical personnel can be used. The orthopaedist involved in this type of ongoing care must realize that each specific problem forms only an isolated segment of total care and that the individual problem must be put into proper perspective with regard to both the immediate and long-term needs of the patient. Recognition of the real needs of the total child and the ability to listen and communicate actively as a member of the team are prerequisites to this rehabilitation philosophy.

Several of the neuromuscular disorders discussed have had recent dramatic changes in their prognoses and treatments. Levels of activity and life prognosis have both been improved, creating a need for increased excellence in the delivery of multidiscipline care. The responsible physician must be aware that, unlike static neuromuscular disorders such as polio and cerebral palsy, many of the conditions can be expected to progress and, therefore, the goals and objectives of the individual patient may change with time. Several of these syndromes include a broad spectrum of severity of disease, making it necessary to have individual approaches to the developing problems. This book offers a variety of surgical and nonsurgical approaches to specific problems. It is emphasized that while surgery forms only one element of the total treatment program in these disorders, its timing and postoperative rehabilitation are critical in developing carefully planned, long-term goals for the individual patient.

I wish to acknowledge the invaluable help and technical assistance of Marianna Nelson, the patience and understanding of Irene Coté, the typing proficiency of Lorraine Bergstrom, the secretarial assistance of Alice Patz, and the photographic assistance of Raymond Martin, Richard Brown, and Donald Gale. And finally, I express my gratitude to my wife; without her continuing support and understanding this book would not have been written.

James C. Drennan, M.D.

Contents

ORTHOPAEDIC MANAGEMENT OF NEUROMUSCULAR DISORDERS

Chapter 1

Evaluation of Neuromuscular Disorders

An established diagnosis, the cornerstone that determines the structure of care for the patient with neuromuscular disease, permits the physician and the rehabilitation team to set realistic short- and long-term goals. The diagnosis is based upon a thorough history, physical examination, and results of appropriate laboratory studies. The patient's age and personal and social environment and the long-term prognosis of the disease are other factors that may influence specific treatment recommendations.

One of the essential components of establishing and carrying out goals is to include the patient's family in the rehabilitation team. In this capacity, family members make a positive commitment. They assume an active role in the child's treatment, for example, by finding a practical application or need for a motor skill acquired in therapy so that the patient can maintain the skill for a long period of time.

THE PATIENT'S MEDICAL HISTORY

A child's medical history is based upon the parents' observations. Children have not developed adequate memories or concepts of time and cannot be considered reliable reporters until they approach 6 years of age.

Because many neuromuscular conditions

are determined genetically, the physician must obtain a thorough family history. This history should include the mother's complete obstetric history, including number of miscarriages, activity of the fetus *in utero*, the child's birth weight, and problems in the neonatal period; any delay in the child's motor development or loss of a previously learned activity; the child's age at onset of the complaint; and systemic symptoms including weight loss, rash, elevated temperature, or seizures. Members of the family should be examined for more subtle expressions of the disease. Individual members may need to have additional laboratory studies done, such as serum enzyme evaluation or muscle biopsy.

The physician must be familiar with motor and social milestones in children (Table 1-1). This enables him to ascertain that the child with a neuromuscular disease has reached a functional plateau at an age when his peers are learning more sophisticated skills. During this time the rate of motor maturation temporarily exceeds the clinical progression of the disease. In Duchenne muscular dystrophy the well-known "golden period," which is the time

span between the age at diagnosis and the time when decreasing motor function is recognized, serves as an example.

Serial photographs may be helpful in demonstrating subtle physical alterations.

PHYSICAL EXAMINATION

Infant

Patience and gentleness are required for adequate physical assessment of the small child. Many of these patients are aware of their physical differences and have developed the ability to control adult activity and responses adroitly. The physician should establish rapport with the child and observe his motor activities before beginning the examination. The normal infant moves the extremities vigorously and at random. The examiner should note the absence or decrease in spontaneous movement and posturing, possible head lag, and paradoxical respiration. In lower motorneuron disease the lower extremities hang limply when the child is suspended vertically by the axillae. When the infant is held in ven-

TABLE 1-1. Selected Developmental Milestones

GROSS MOTOR SKILLS	FINE MOTOR SKILLS
1 MONTH	
Has incomplete head control	Follows to midline
Has tonic neck reflex	Fixes both eyes on light
4 MONTHS	
Turns from back to side	Brings object to mouth
Rolls over	Follows 180 degrees visually
6 MONTHS	
Sits without support	Transfers object
Has reciprocal leg pattern	Picks up spoon
9 MONTHS	
Crawls freely	Shakes bell
Pulls self to stand	Develops pincer grip
12 MONTHS	
Walks with assistance	Can release object voluntarily
Climbs	Follows simple commands
15 MONTHS	
Lets self down from standing to sitting	
Attains standing position unaided	
18 MONTHS	
Throws and catches ball	
Creeps backward down stairs	
21 MONTHS	
Squats	Turns knob
Walks up and down stairs	Begins hand preference
24 MONTHS	
Alternates feet walking upstairs	Turns pages singly
Runs	Likes to take things apart

tral suspension, head and trunk position and control can be determined. Associated anomalies, such as clubfeet or ectodermal dysplasia overlying the spine, should be noted.

The patient should be examined for a rash on the face and extremities. The typical facies of a patient with infantile spinal muscular atrophy and myotonia dystrophica should be familiar to the examiner. The tongue should be well illuminated on examination to detect fasciculation suggestive of lower motor-neuron disease. Excessive drooling is noted in both hypotonic cerebral palsy and myotonia dystrophica. In the latter, nasal speech may be apparent. A thorough ophthalmologic examination may be warranted.

The physician begins the examination while the mother holds the fully clothed infant on her lap. After gaining the child's confidence, the examiner can continue the evaluation of the child, who can now be undressed and placed on the examining table. By noting the distribution of muscle weakness, the physician can differentiate between neuropathy and myopathy. Although it is difficult to assess muscle strength accurately in infants, the physician can describe it as being either weak or against gravity as he observes the infant during motor activity.

Palpation may reveal an increased rubbery consistency of specific muscles of the extremities, suggesting either a dystrophic or infiltrative process. Range of motion of joints should be recorded at each visit and any changes should be noted. Sensory examination is limited to visible responses to pinpricks.

THE "FLOPPY BABY"

The hypotonic infant has decreased muscle tone and may suffer early pulmonary compromise.[3,6] Decreased resistance to passive movement leads to abnormal posturing, such as the frog position. The physician can also detect hypotonia by watching for head lag and observing head and trunk control when the infant is held in dorsal suspension (Fig. 1-1). The differential diagnosis includes hypotonic cerebral palsy, infantile spinal muscular atrophy, benign congenital myopathies, fiber-type disproportion, infantile myotonia dystrophica, myasthenia gravis, myopathic arthrogryposis multiplex congenita, Guillain–Barré

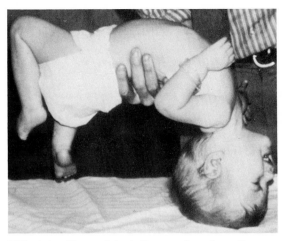

FIG. 1-1. Floppy infant. Suspension allows the hypotonic limbs to flop about. Diagnosis permits the establishment of appropriate long-term management.

syndrome, Down's syndrome, systemic illness, and Pompe's disease.[8,9] This latter disease, which is caused by infantile acid maltase deficiency, leads to increased glycogen storage. Death usually occurs within 2 years. The clinical characteristics distinguishing each of the other disease entities will be discussed in subsequent chapters.

Young Child

A more detailed musculoskeletal examination is possible when the child is able to stand. The physician observes posture for excessive lordosis or wide-based stance. The physician analyzes the gait, noting not only how the child transfers weight through the lower extremities but also if there is associated movement of the upper extremities and trunk. Gait analysis in the older child may reveal a decreased arm swing, subtle leg circumduction, scissorlike movement, or shuffling. Motor activities, such as running or crouching, magnify the subtle physical signs.

Older Child

Children are able to communicate accurately with the physician when they reach the age of 6 years. It then becomes possible for the orthopaedist to assess the motor power of individual muscles. Sensory examination also becomes reliable at approximately the same age. The Jendrassik maneuver, in which the child clasps his hands and squeezes them together, can amplify the presence of deep-tendon reflexes. Performance of simple motor tasks augments the "soft signs."[2] When the patient rises from the floor or does deep knee bends, pelvic girdle or quadriceps weakness may be evident. Weakness of the tibialis anterior may be apparent when the patient attempts to heel-walk. Running may reveal an increase in muscle tone or ataxia.

The distribution of muscle weakness is important. Generally, in myopathic diseases proximal muscles, which are affected before distal muscles, demonstrate much greater weakness early in the disease than the degree of atrophy would indicate. The converse is true in neuropathies. The physician should palpate muscles for consistency, enlargement, and tenderness and determine the strength of individual muscles. A prolonged period of contraction following voluntary stimulation should be sought. The examiner should determine range of motion of major joints so that he can evaluate any acquired condition, such as a dislocated hip.

Careful neurologic examination is mandatory and sensory responses must be checked individually. Decreased vibratory sensation of the toes may be present long before there is clinical evidence of Charcot–Marie–Tooth disease. The deep-tendon reflexes, absent in infantile spinal muscular atrophy, are increased in hypotonic cerebral palsy. A positive Babinski sign confirms upper motor-neuron disease. Abnormalities in the Romberg and rapid-alternating-eye-movement tests indicate cerebellar involvement. Evaluation of mental function is necessary because organic mental deterioration is an integral part of some of these symptoms. Evaluation can be accomplished to some extent during physical examination through normal conversation. However, formal testing may be required in some cases.

EVALUATION OF INVESTIGATIVE STUDIES

Laboratory Data

Serum creatine phosphokinase (CPK) is the most sensitive test for demonstrating abnormalities in striated muscle function. The increased level of this enzyme is due to a malfunction of the sarcolemmal membrane of the muscle. Rapid and extensive damage to this membrane allows greater egress of the enzymes into the serum. The sensitivity of this test is demonstrated by the fact that even the introduction of an electromyographic needle can cause an increase. Therefore, it is necessary to obtain serum enzyme determinations before an electromyogram is done. The level of elevation parallels the rate and amount of muscle necrosis and decreases with time as the muscle mass shrinks. Marked elevations are associated with fulminant muscle breakdown. Values greater than 10 times normal reflect a myopathic disorder of the dystrophic, myositic, or necrotic type. The most spectacular levels are seen in early stages of the Duchenne type of muscular dystrophy in which increases of 200 to 300 times the normal may be found. Cord-blood CPK levels should be obtained in all males who are at risk for carrying Duchenne dystrophy.[7] Also, serum CPK may be elevated in limb-girdle dystrophy, dermatomyositis, acid maltase deficiency, and spinal muscular atrophy. Aldolase and serum glutamic-oxaloacetic transaminase (SGOT) are other important serum enzymes in the study of striated muscle function. Marked elevation of the SGOT level may occur in polymyositis.

Electromyography

An electromyogram (EMG) is a record of electrical changes occurring in muscle when electrodes are placed either on the skin over the muscle or are inserted into the muscle. The latter technique has more clinical applications. It records the electrical activity produced by needle insertion, spontaneous activity in the relaxed resting muscle, interference patterns in full forceful contraction against resistance, and the character of individual muscle action potentials during weak or submaximal contracture.

An EMG differentiates a myopathic process from a denervation disorder but rarely helps in establishing a definitive diagnosis. Characteristically, lower motor-neuron disorders show the presence of fibrillation potentials rather than the normal interference pattern. The fibrillation potential represents spontaneous firings of individual muscle groups. In spinal muscular atrophy both fibrillation and fasciculation are present with a decreased number of recordings due to the diminished number of total motor units. The potentials are brief, biphasic, and of low voltage in the early stages of the denervation process but become prolonged, polyphasic, and of high voltage during the chronic phase.

Electromyography in myopathic disorders is characterized by polyphasic action potentials of low voltage. Myopathies rarely demonstrate electromyographic changes characteristic of a neuropathy, whereas a denervation process may show neuropathic or myopathic mixed patterns. The characteristic "dive bomber" sound of myotonia dystrophica, which is caused by rapid repetitive discharges of the stimulated fibers, is perhaps the best known aural finding. Also in myotonia dystrophica, the EMG demonstrates an abnormally long contraction followed by decreased ability of the muscle to relax. The repetitive waxing and waning, high-frequency discharges of myotonia can also be found in Pompe's disease.

Nerve-Conduction Studies

Studies of nerve conduction help the physician to establish the diagnosis of peripheral neuropathy. Most commonly the tests are performed on the median, ulnar, peroneal, and posterior tibial nerves. Normal values in the child over 5 years of age are 50 m to 60 m per second distal to the elbow and 60 m to 80 m per second between the shoulder and elbow. Measurements in the lower extremity are 40 m to 50 m per second. In infants, conduction velocities are approximately 40% of the adult measurement. The small neural fibers complete myelination by the end of the third year when conduction becomes essentially adult.

The velocity of motor-nerve conduction is determined by stimulating a nerve at two points along its course and recording in each case the time of contracture of peripheral muscle supplied by the nerve. Muscle contractions are commonly recorded in the upper extremity following wrist (distal) and elbow (proximal) stimulation. Conduction velocity is determined by measuring the distance between the distal and proximal stimulation points and applying the formula $\dfrac{D}{L2-L1}$.[1] In

order to ensure that all nerve fibers are appropriately excited, the intensity of the stimuli should be supramaximal, that is, 50% more than the amount necessary to produce a maximum muscle response.

Velocities of nerve conduction are normal in anterior-horn-cell disease, nerve-root disease, and myopathies. In Charcot–Marie–Tooth disease, the velocity of motor conduction may be lower than normal before clinical deficits are apparent. This study helps the physician to determine whether the peripheral neuropathy involves an isolated nerve or if it represents a disseminated process. Conduction of sensory nerves is determined by using a ring electrode on a finger or toe, applying electrical stimulation, and recording over the more proximal nerve (orthodromic). The value of conduction studies will be discussed in the section on specific forms of spinocerebellar disease.

Muscle Biopsy

Muscle biopsy is fundamental in determining a diagnosis of neuromuscular disease.[5] Biopsy material can be examined with both histologic and histochemical stains, as well as with electron microscopy.

The criterion for selecting a patient for biopsy is clinical evidence of neuromuscular disease, such as muscle weakness. The distribution of muscle weakness is established by physical examination, and the site for muscle biopsy is determined. Muscles with relatively little involvement are selected in chronic diseases, such as Duchenne dystrophy, because they demonstrate the greatest diagnostic changes. A more severely involved muscle is chosen in an acute illness, since the process will not have had sufficient time to progress to extensive destruction. The rectus femoris, vastus lateralis, and biceps brachii are the muscles most commonly biopsied. The position of the extremity during the procedure is important for histologic assessment of the size of muscle fibers. The biceps brachii should always be biopsied with the arm in extension. If the vastus lateralis is biopsied with the knee in extension, the muscle is shortened, resulting in an unsatisfactory histologic interpretation. Muscle clamps are not recommended if electron microscopic studies are necessary. Use of clamps may also result in loss of correct orientation of the muscle fibers for subsequent processing.

DUBOWITZ AND BROOKE PROCEDURE

Local anesthesia without epinephrine is used for skin infiltration for the Dubowitz and Brooke procedure.[4] Infiltration of muscles should be avoided, since it distorts the tissue. A 1½-in skin incision is made, the fascia incised longitudinally, and the direction of the fibers of the muscle belly determined. A 1-in × 1-in strip of muscle is bluntly isolated, and a black silk suture is passed at either end. A cylinder of muscle is excised, including the sutures. The specimen must be stretched over a broken tongue blade to maintain the muscles in a stretched position when electron microscopic studies are performed.

The specimen is frozen rapidly with liquid nitrogen ($-160°C$) to prevent loss of soluble enzymes and development of artifacts. The tragacanth–isopenthane method is preferable for enzyme histochemistry. On a standard microtome chuck, the specimen is sectioned in both the longitudinal and transverse planes.

NOMENCLATURE OF FIBER TYPES

The difference in histochemical staining properties establishes the basis for the division of skeletal muscle into Type-1 and Type-2 fibers.[4] Type-1 fiber is high in oxidative activity and low in glycolytic and adenosine triphosphatase (ATPase) activity. Type-2 fiber is just the opposite. Type-3 fiber, rich in both oxidative and glycolytic enzymes, is sometimes referred to as an *intermediate* type. In skeletal muscle fiber Types 1 and 2, the normal ratio is 1:2.

CHARACTERISTIC MYOPATHIC CHANGES

A random distribution of enlarged or small fibers is common in myopathy. The typical Type-1 predominance in myopathy is noted when greater than 50% of Type-1 fiber occurs in a microscopic field. Phagocytosis is another characteristic of myopathy, as well as inflammatory cellular reaction in an inflammatory myopathy. Routine hematoxylin and eosin preparation may demonstrate baso-

philic staining in regenerating muscle fiber and pale staining in necrotic fiber.

CHARACTERISTIC NEUROPATHIC CHANGES

Small-group atrophy, in which a small cluster of fibers is surrounded by fibers of relatively normal size, is typical of neuropathic disease. Small angular fibers may also be noted in groups or scattered among normal fibers. Fiber-type grouping in which fibers of one histochemical type are grouped together, instead of presenting in the usual interdigitative pattern, is also common. A Type-2 predominance, typical of lower motor-neuron disease, is present when greater than 80% of Type-2 fiber is in the field.

Electrocardiography

Some of the neuromuscular diseases demonstrate a consistent electrocardiographic abnormality. Duchenne muscular dystrophy, Friedreich's ataxia, and myotonia dystrophica exemplify disease processes with abnormal electrocardiograms.

Radiologic Evaluation

Diagnosis may be further clarified by appropriate use of radiography. In infancy particular attention is focused on the spine for evidence of spinal dysrhaphism or the presence and type of scoliosis. Congenital dislocated hips in the newborn are associated with a variety of benign myopathies as well as myotonia dystrophica. As the child matures, roentgenograms demonstrate the windblown position of the hips, including an adducted "hip at risk." Secondary adaptive increases in coxa valga and anteversion may contribute to the precariousness of the hip stability. Weight-bearing roentgenograms allow the physician to analyze the bony structure in a cavus foot deformity and to determine whether corrective efforts should be concentrated on the hindfoot or forefoot. The physician may modify his corrective efforts when he detects the development of posterior tibial subluxation on a roentgenogram in a patient who has serial wedging plaster casts for knee flexion contractures. Soft-tissue studies may show a loss of soft-tissue planes early in the inflammatory process and also demonstrate the subcutaneous nodules of calcinosis universalis and dermatomyositis. In the patient with Duchenne muscular dystrophy, soft-tissue radiography discloses muscle wasting with fat replacement.

Ophthalmologic Evaluation

Ophthalmologic examination may reveal optic atrophy, retinitis pigmentosa, nystagmus, and extraocular motor paresis. Lenticular opacity may require use of a slit lamp to establish the diagnosis of myotonia dystrophica.

Amniocentesis

Amniocentesis, a relatively new diagnostic procedure, may be used at 14 wk to 16 wk of gestation. A modest increase in CPK levels has been associated with Duchenne muscular dystrophy. In Pompe's disease (testing for α-1,4-glucosidase) and in myelomeningocele (testing for α-fetoprotein), diagnosis can be determined by amniocentesis.

REFERENCES

1. Bradley WG: Disorders of Peripheral Nerves. London, Blackwell Scientific Publications, 1974
2. Brooke MH: A Clinician's View of Neuromuscular Diseases. Baltimore, Williams & Wilkins, 1977
3. Dubowitz V: The Floppy Infant. In Clinics in Developmental Medicine, No. 31. Lavenham, Suffolk, Lavenham Press, 1969
4. Dubowitz V, Brooke MH: Muscle Biopsy: A Modern Approach. London, Saunders, 1973
5. Greenfield JG, Cornman T, Shy GM: The prognostic value of the muscle biopsy in the "floppy infant." Brain 81:461, 1958
6. Walton JN: The "floppy" infant. Cerebral Palsy Bulletin 2:10, 1960
7. Zellweger H, Antonik A: Newborn screening for Duchenne muscular dystrophy. Pediatrics 5, No. 1:30, 1975
8. Zellweger H, Ionasescu V: Early onset of myotonic dystrophy in infants. Am J Dis Child 125:601, 1973
9. Zellweger H, Afifi A, McCormick WF, Mergner W: Benign congenital muscular dystrophy: a special form of congenital hypotonia. Clin Pediatr (Phila) 6:655, 1967

Chapter 2

Progressive Muscular Dystrophy

The muscular dystrophies are a group of non-inflammatory inherited disorders with progressive degeneration and weakness of the skeletal muscle, without apparent cause in the peripheral or central nervous system.

Progressive muscular dystrophy in humans has been classified by Walton into the following categories[52]:

1. The "pure" muscular dystrophies
   A. Sex-linked muscular dystrophy
       Severe (Duchenne type)
       Benign (Becker type)
   B. Autosomal recessive muscular dystrophy

   Limb-girdle types
   Childhood muscular dystrophy
       (except Duchenne)
   Congenital muscular dystrophies
   C. Autosomal dominant
       Facioscapulohumeral muscular
       dystrophy
   D. Distal muscular dystrophy
   E. Ocular muscular dystrophy
   F. Oculopharyngeal muscular dystrophy

2. Cases with myotonia
   A. Myotonia congenita
   B. Dystrophia myotonica
   C. Paramyotonia congenita

The muscular dystrophies have been subdivided on the basis of clinical distribution, severity of muscle weakness, and patterns of genetic inheritance. An established accurate diagnosis is important both for prognosis and management of the individual case and for identification of the genetic pattern, which may be of critical importance to the family at risk.

No single factor has been identified as the cause of muscular dystrophy.[2] It is recognized as a hereditary disease. A recent study demonstrated that the impairment of verbal intelligence in patients with Duchenne muscular dystrophy is early and nonprogressive.[35] This impairment is independent of performance quotient, which varies with the level of physical activity and general motor control. Other recent studies demonstrated abnormalities in the red-blood-cell membranes, suggesting possible systemic disease.[39,42] The variety of studies being carried out emphasizes the renewed interest in establishing the site of the primary defect.[4,30]

Sex-Linked Muscular Dystrophy

DUCHENNE TYPE

Meryon first described this disease in 1852.[36] Duchenne de Boulogne in 1868 noted the pseudohypertrophic enlargement of the calf muscles which were, nonetheless, abnormal and weak.[17]

This disease has worldwide distribution; it occurs only in males except in rare cases when it is associated with Turner's syndrome. Generally, it is transmitted by a sex-linked, recessive gene. There is a positive maternal family history in greater than 60% of the cases. One third of the cases represents a spontaneous mutation. This form of dystrophy occurs in 1 in 3000 live births.

Initially the patient has selective, symmetrical weakness of the pelvic-girdle muscles. Three to 5 years later shoulder-girdle muscles become involved. The weakness is progressive; patients who are managed ineffectively frequently are unable to ambulate within 4 years of recognition of the disease.

Clinical Features

Although the infant with Duchenne muscular dystrophy achieves motor milestones appropriately, motor deficiencies generally become evident between 18 and 36 months of age. The parents may notice that the child is late in achieving independent ambulation or that he walks on his toes. When the child presents after the age of 3 years, he may stumble and fall and be unable to hop, jump, or run normally. Children with this disease have difficulty climbing stairs and accomplish this feat by climbing one stair at a time and by leading with the dominant foot. Leg pains, which may develop early, especially in the calf, occur abruptly and may last 2 to 3 days.[15]

Clinically, the child may appear to improve between the ages of 3 and 7. During this period, developmental gains outstrip the rate of progression of the disorder because of natural growth and the development of newly acquired motor skills. Loss of function or definitive regression usually does not occur until age 7. As the weakness progresses, the child develops compensatory changes in gait and stance, and walking becomes more difficult.

The hip extensors become affected first. Initially the patient compensates for this by carrying the head and shoulders behind the pelvis to maintain the weight-line posterior to the hip joint (Fig. 2-1). Progressive weakness of the trunk and pelvic girdle causes a more exaggerated, compensatory, lordotic posture which helps to maintain the center of gravity posterior to the hip. The patient is faced with the dual problem of maintaining both the hip and knee of the stance-phase limb in full extension while simultaneously attempting to advance himself in space (Fig. 2-2). The strong iliofemoral ligament resists hyperextension and the hip can be maintained in the extended weight-bearing position with little or no muscle effort. In the erect position the center of gravity normally passes anterior

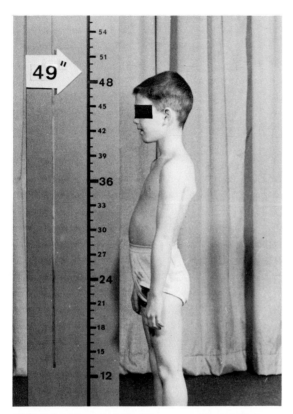

FIG. 2-1. Dorsal shift of the upper trunk initially compensates for the gluteus maximus weakness. (Courtesy of Newington Children's Hospital)

pelvis rotates forward. Iliotibial contraction of the swing-phase limb prevents that limb from adducting with resultant loss of the wide-based equilibrium. The iliotibial band acts as a passive stabilizing force for the knee of the weight-bearing limb.

Eventually toe-walking is required to compensate for increasing quadriceps weakness. This posture enables the weight-line to continue to pass in front of the knee joint (Fig. 2-4). As plantar flexion becomes fixed, the patient's upright position becomes even more precarious. Forefoot and hindfoot inversion develops as peroneal strength diminishes (Fig. 2-5). The chin is drawn back because of the need to maintain balance and because of early involvement of the anterior neck flexors (Fig. 2-6).

Although weakness in the shoulder girdle may not be noticed for several years after onset, it usually can be found on examination. This weakness precludes crutch-assisted am-

to the center of motion of the knee joint. Body weight tends to keep the joint extended once it has been extended by the quadriceps. With weight on one limb, the knee is further extended and stabilized by medial rotation of the femur on the tibial condyles and by the compensatory tibial external rotation that develops (Fig. 2-3). The excessive trunk lordosis places abdominal weight anterior to the knee joint, which further stabilizes the knee extension.

To walk, the patient must now adapt his gait by combining lateral trunk rotation and oscillation. He does this by swinging the pelvis and the entire upper body over the weight-bearing femoral head. This allows him to elevate and propel the opposite limb forward. Lateral flexion in the lumbar spine is also necessary to develop this side-to-side sway. The patient must adopt a delicate gait pattern in which swaying transfers the weight to the hyperextended hip while the contralateral

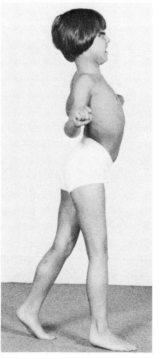

FIG. 2-2. Lordosis and upper-trunk displacement become more exaggerated as the pelvic girdle becomes more involved. The upper extremities can no longer function in the reciprocal gait pattern because the patient uses them to help transfer weight and maintain balance.

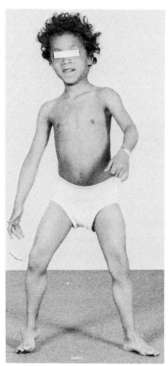

FIG. 2-3. Severely involved 5-year-old patient whose wide-based gait includes external tibial rotation.

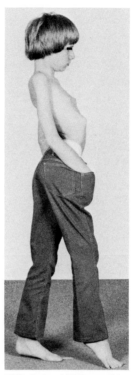

FIG. 2-4. While walking, this 13-year-old boy requires manual stabilization, as well as plantar flexion and excessive trunk lordosis, to ensure extension of his weight-bearing hip during midstance.

bulation. Ultimately all muscles are involved including the facial, oculopharyngeal, and respiratory muscles, although these groups usually are spared until late in the course of the disease.

The disease progresses slowly but unremittingly. Periods of rapid clinical deterioration may be noted following immobilization in bed for respiratory infections, fractures, or following orthopaedic surgery. Skeletal muscle must lose 30% to 50% of its bulk before clinical signs are present. It is estimated that with total recumbency there is a 3% loss of muscle strength per day. Objective testing of muscles against gravity and manual resistance demonstrates a striking correlation between the rate of loss of strength and increasing age for any given patient.[60] This pattern does not change during growth spurts or bracing. Variability in the severity of the disease can be documented clearly by 7 years of age and appears to be related to earlier age at the onset of symptoms.

The patient may experience difficulty with perceptual and visual concepts. Also, depression is first noted at age 5 years when the child, who realizes something is wrong, becomes withdrawn and shy. It again becomes evident at age 10 years when the untreated patient begins to use a wheelchair and later in adolescence when the patient is confined to bed.

Physical Examination

Clinical diagnosis is based upon analysis of gait, evidence of specific muscle weakness, and the absence of any sensory deficit. Gait must be observed from the front and rear of the patient as well as from the side so that the clinician can analyze compensatory movement of the trunk and extremities. This compensatory posture in the young child gradually becomes fixed as the disease progresses.

A valuable clinical test is Gowers' maneuver (Fig. 2-7).[25] The patient is placed on

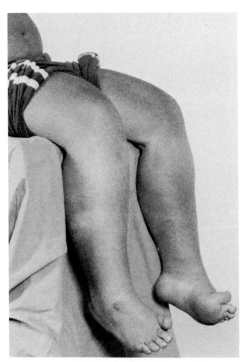

FIG. 2-5. Retained unopposed strength in posterior tibial muscle causes dynamic equinovarus. Ambulation is made precarious by limiting weight-bearing to the lateral aspect of the forefoot.

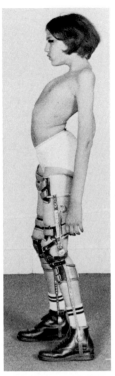

FIG. 2-6. This adolescent is still able to stand but is unable to walk, having exhausted his compensatory trunk and head adaptations.

the floor in the prone position and asked to rise. Initially, he can do this without much difficulty. However, as the disease progresses, he performs this maneuver more slowly and uses a chair for support. He assumes a quadriped position, grasps the legs with the hands, and because of quadriceps weakness he gradually walks the hands up proximally to the knees before being able to extend the back. Patients with congenital myopathies also show a positive Gowers' test.

Meryon's sign, an indication of shoulder-girdle weakness, is demonstrated by lifting the child under the arms and noting how he slides through the examiner's hands (Fig. 2-8).

The Ober test is used to detect a fixed deformity of the iliotibial band.[37] It is traditionally performed with the patient placed in a lateral position. The table-side limb is flexed at the hip and knee. In the normal person this locks the pelvis for the remainder of the test. The examiner places one hand on the patient's pelvis and the other on the patient's foot. The ipsilateral hip is flexed, abducted,

and extended while the knee is kept flexed at 90°. The extremity should drop well below a horizontal line parallel to the table. The angle that the thigh makes with the horizontal line represents the degree of abduction contracture.

The Thomas test demonstrates flexion contracture of the hip. The patient is examined in the supine position and both thighs are placed on the abdomen in complete passive flexion, thus locking the pelvis. Then one limb is extended and its flexion contracture is measured.

Generalized weakness of the trunk musculature limits the value of the Ober and Thomas tests. Patients with dystrophy are unable to stabilize the pelvis and an increased pelvic obliquity develops with unilateral hip passive extension. An effective way of determining actual hip flexion and abduction contractures is to examine the patient in the supine position, flex both thighs on the abdomen, and then extend one limb in maximum internal rotation and adduction (Fig. 2-

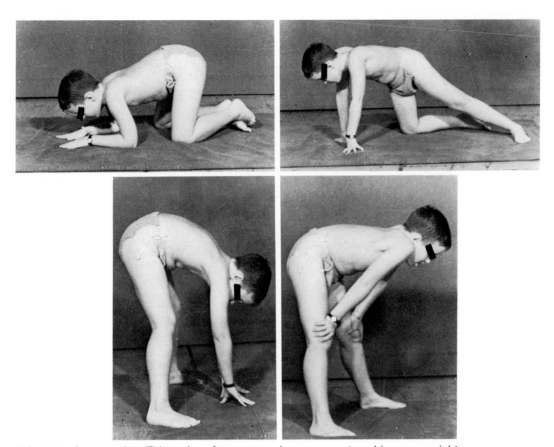

FIG. 2-7. Gowers' sign. This series of maneuvers is necessary to achieve an upright posture. It occurs with all types of pelvic girdle weakness. The child "climbs up his legs" when rising from the floor. (Courtesy of Newington Children's Hospital)

9). This places the fascia lata and hip flexion contractures under maximum tension. A second examiner may be needed to stabilize the pelvis during this part of the examination.

Straight-leg raising demonstrates contracture of the hamstrings. The ipsilateral knee must be maintained in full extension and the contralateral limb must be extended on the examining table in order to control the pelvis. When the child's muscle control decreases and the weight of his extremity increases, the examiner may use his shoulder to elevate the ipsilateral limb. Knee flexion should be measured with a goniometer since deformity above 15° is likely to jeopardize ambulatory potential. To rule out subtalar motion, heel-cord tightness must be measured with the heel inverted.

Contractures are noted in the pelvic-girdle region first. The patient tends to assume a frog-leg posture in recumbency. This contributes to contracture of the iliotibial band, which results in loss of internal hip rotation, genu valgum, and external rotation of the tibia. The calves generally appear enlarged and when palpated have the consistency of hard rubber balls (Fig. 2-10). Forefoot equinus, noted in young children who are toe walkers, will evolve into the more characteristic equinovarus foot deformity. When examining the shoulder girdle, it is noted that the sternal part of the pectoralis major is more involved than the clavicular head. The serratus anterior and neck flexors become involved in the later stages of the disease. Subsequently, the biceps brachii and brachioradialis are involved. This weakness precludes crutch-assisted ambulation. Eventually loss of elbow and shoulder stability markedly interferes with hand function. The compensatory lordosis may

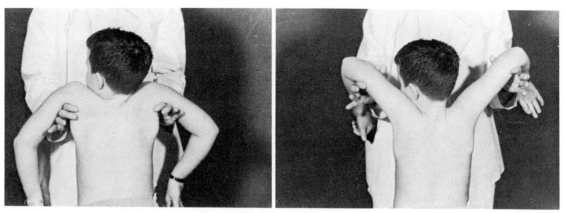

FIG. 2-8. Meryon's sign. Shoulder-girdle weakness allows the child to slip through the examiner's grasp and precludes future use of crutches. (Courtesy of Newington Children's Hospital)

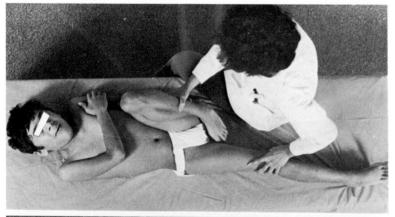

FIG. 2-9. Only by intentionally adducting and internally rotating the extended limb can adaptive shortening of the anterior fascia lata be demonstrated (bottom). The pelvis is stabilized by rotating the flexed contralateral limb into external rotation.

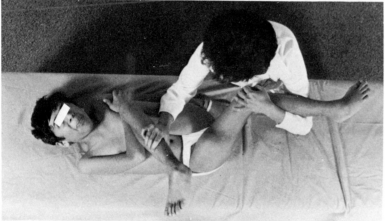

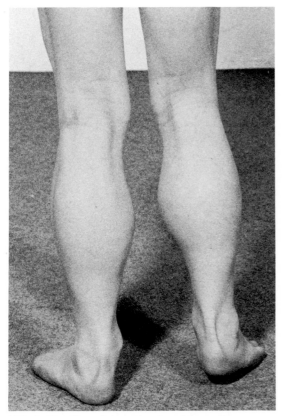

FIG. 2-10. Pseudohypertrophy of the calf.

become fixed as the disease progresses. Body habitus is generally either short and stocky or tall and very slender.

Laboratory Data

The creatine phosphokinase (CPK) level is markedly increased in the early stages of Duchenne dystrophy.[48] The normal CPK level of 60 U to 70 U/liter may rise above 1000 U/liter in the young dystrophic patient. As the disease progresses, the muscle bulk diminishes and the CPK level falls into the hundreds but never returns to normal even in the severely handicapped patient who is in a wheelchair.

CPK testing should be carried out on newborns with suspected muscular dystrophy. CPK levels may be elevated briefly in normal newborns because compression of the skeletal muscle during delivery can affect the permeability of the cell membranes, thereby allowing CPK to leak into the bloodstream. When neonatal levels are high, a second CPK test should be performed several months later to confirm the elevation.[58] The serum glutamic oxaloacetic transaminase (SGOT), lactic dehydrogenase (LDH), and aldolase levels are less significant because they are not unique to striated-muscle disease.[49]

CPK testing can also be used to identify 80% of female dystrophic carriers who are between 1 and 20 years of age. Because the CPK level of a carrier varies widely from time to time, the serum must be drawn at least three times with a minimum of 1 week between tests. Elevations may be only 2 to 3 times above normal. The highest level is selected. The woman to be tested should avoid undue physical exertion one week before the study because the CPK level increases after strenuous exercise. It may decrease during pregnancy and falls throughout adult life.

ELECTROMYOGRAM

Characteristically, the electromyographic pattern is of low-amplitude, short-duration, polyphasic motor-unit action potentials.

ELECTROCARDIOGRAM

Myocardial degeneration is a constant finding and electrocardiographic changes are present in more than 90% of patients. The characteristic electrocardiogram (ECG) shows tall R waves in the right precordial leads. Persistent tachycardia is common, and sudden chronic cardiac failure is rare. If an ECG demonstrates progression of cardiomyopathy, a pediatric cardiology consultation is necessary. Consideration may be given to performing echocardiography as well as a multi-gaited acquisition (MUGA) scan to determine the strength of ventricular contraction.[40]

MUSCLE BIOPSY

Biopsy findings are those of a nonspecific myopathy.[28] Fibrosis, the most pronounced change in patients with Duchenne dystrophy, occurs early in the disease with a proliferation of endomesial and paramesial connective tissue.[16] There is degeneration and subsequent loss of fibers and variation in fiber size with abnormal enlargement or atrophy of fibers. These fibers are replaced by connective tissue and, subsequently, adipose tissue. Increased cellularity with occasional internal migration of sarcolemmal nuclei and proliferation of endomesial fibroblasts and variable inflammatory response are also noted. Small groups of basophilic fibers and persistence of undifferentiated Type-2C muscle fibers can also be seen. Moth-eaten and whorled fibers, which are common in other forms of dystrophy, are rarely seen in Duchenne dystrophy. Fiber-splitting, considered a hallmark of the myopathies, is rare in patients with Duchenne dystrophy. Histochemical studies performed for ATPase reaction demonstrate a poor differentiation of fiber types and a prevalence of Type-1 fibers.

Differential Diagnosis

Group-IV spinal muscular atrophy (Kugelberg–Welander disease), dermatomyositis, Pompe's disease (acid maltase glucosidase deficiency), and congenital myopathy are other neuromuscular diseases that present with girdle weakness in the first decade.

Patients with Group-IV spinal muscular atrophy walk independently before the disease becomes clinically evident. Their patterns of gait and stance may resemble those seen in muscular dystrophy. The age of onset determines whether this disease mimics the Duchenne or the limb-girdle types of muscular dystrophy. Shoulder-girdle involvement occurs a few years after onset. Physical examination may demonstrate fasciculations in the tongue or peripheral muscles. These fasciculations can be heard with a stethoscope. Laboratory investigations demonstrate that CPK levels may be normal or slightly elevated. The electromyogram (EMG) demonstrates high-amplitude, long-duration, polyphasic potential and fibrillation potential at rest.

Patients with polymyositis and dermatomyositis are initially lethargic and irritable. A violaceous discoloration over the major joints with a butterfly distribution on the face may be present. Muscle weakness accompanies muscle tenderness. Muscle weakness in polymyositis generally affects all muscle girdles, whereas muscular involvement is much more selective in Duchenne dystrophy. Polymyositis is more common in females. The erythrocyte sedimentation rate (ESR) is ele-vated and muscle biopsy reveals myopathic changes with inflammatory cell infiltration, especially in the perifascicular areas.

The age of onset and rate of progression vary in patients who have acid maltase (α-1,4-glucosidase) deficiency. Those who develop the condition late, especially adults, tend to be less severely affected. The disease is autosomal recessive. In the infantile form (Pompe's disease), the child develops normally for 2 to 4 months, but then significant weakness and hypotonia occur and are soon followed by respiratory distress and cardiac failure. Physical examination reveals an inactive infant lying in a frog-leg position with massive cardiomegaly and hepatomegaly secondary to cardiac failure. Macroglossia is noted. Deep-tendon reflexes are markedly diminished and weakness is diffuse. In the late infantile or early childhood form, patients are asymptomatic during the first year of life and the disease progresses slowly thereafter. Because symptoms mimic those of Duchenne dystrophy,[47] muscle biopsy and bioassay for missing enzymes are needed to help the physician make appropriate diagnosis. Myotonia is demonstrated on an electromyogram.

Congenital myopathies tend to be nonprogressive. The CPK is normal or slightly elevated. Accurate diagnosis is based on histochemical and electron-microscopic evaluation of the muscle biopsy. Diagnosis of carnitine myopathy, in which there is a weakness of the shoulders, hips, and neck, can be confirmed only by special stains.[17]

Management

The patient with suspected Duchenne dystrophy should have a prompt medical evaluation. The implication of this diagnosis is universally recognized and medical accuracy is vital. The evaluation can be accomplished most effectively through hospitalization for a thorough physical examination and laboratory studies. Formal evaluation of muscles and functional testing are an important part of the initial work-up. During this period the neurologist has the opportunity to discuss the results of the diagnostic tests privately with the parents so that they can respond openly and begin to adjust to the realization that their son has a progressive neuromuscular disease. Acceptance frequently is a slow process, particularly for the father. A skilled clinical psychologist or psychiatrist can help the family to express feelings about grief and dying.

Follow-Up Care

The team approach in a muscle disease clinic provides total rehabilitative care and social counseling.[43] Two physicians form an effective medical nucleus: the neurologist is responsible for establishing the diagnosis and giving genetic counseling and educational and social guidance; the orthopaedist performs surgery and directs the physical rehabilitation program by prescribing orthoses, instructing therapists, and making recommendations for activities of daily living. As the cornerstone of the team, the nurse coordinator creates a valuable communication link between the family and team members and acts as the medical ombudsman to schools and social agencies. The role of the physical therapist will be described in detail. The occupational therapist can be consulted by patients who have problems with assistive devices or orthoses for the upper extremities. A qualified orthotist helps to implement the orthopaedist's rehabilitation program. The psychologist combines a knowledge of neuromuscular diseases with an understanding of the processes of grief and dying. The social worker and representative of the Muscular Dystrophy Association also make valuable contributions.

It is important to create a positive and caring atmosphere and for team members to listen to the needs of the patient and family. Because of the severity of the disease, the ability to cope with ensuing medical crises requires trust and understanding on the part of both the family and the team. Although it is important that team members be available to assist the family in making major medical decisions, the family may refer minor, acute medical problems to the family physician. However, problems that are life-threatening, such as pneumonia, or activity-threatening, such as a fracture of the lower extremity, are most effectively managed by the team.

During a pre-clinic conference the team can discuss the scheduled patients and others in the community who have problems. This conference serves the same function for community patients as regular walk-rounds do for coordinating the care of inpatients.

Realistic scheduling of appointments is accomplished when the specialists to be seen and laboratory studies to be done are written in the last clinic note. Periodic tests, such as roentgenograms, pulmonary function studies, an electrocardiogram, and a physical therapy evaluation, should be done before the clinic begins.[9] Although families are encouraged to take advantage of the availability of the team during clinic hours, they may request additional appointments. A clinic that is held weekly allows the family to feel secure and facilitates the solution of many problems.

GENETIC COUNSELING

It is essential that the correct diagnosis be established before genetic counseling is undertaken.[18] The physician must interpret the clinical and family history, serum CPK levels, EMG findings, and the muscle biopsy report.

The definition of a female at risk includes (1) a definite carrier who has a son with the disease and a previous case on the female side of the family, (2) a probable carrier who has two or more affected sons but has no family history of the disease, and (3) a possible carrier who has one affected son but has no family history of the disease.

The sex of a fetus can be determined by amniocentesis as early as 14 to 16 weeks of gestation. The family must be made aware that 50% of newborn males will be normal and one half of the females will be carriers.

PHYSICAL THERAPY

Physical therapy is directed toward (1) preliminary and ongoing assessment of muscle strength and functional capacity, (2) prevention or correction of contractures by passive stretching, (3) preoperative assessment, (4) instruction in postoperative gait training with braces, (5) teaching transfer techniques to the patient and family, and (6) measurement of wheelchair and orthotic equipment.[10]

FUNCTIONAL TESTING. Through functional testing the therapist assesses the patient's ability to perform standard tasks in a measured time period. This type of evaluation can be performed even on a young child. As the substitute pattern necessary to perform the task becomes more complex, the time required for performing the task increases. Tests that can be carried out in the clinic setting include (1) standing from lying down (under 3 sec, normal) (2) climbing four stairs (under 8 sec), (3) running or walking 30 feet, (4) standing from a sitting position on the floor or in a chair (under 2 sec), and (5) putting on or taking off a T-shirt.[21] All major muscle groups are objectively tested for residual strength. Functional strength of the quadriceps is tested when the patient sits on an examining table with the knee flexed at 90° and with the thigh horizontal to the floor. The knee is then actively extended. If the patient is unable to achieve the last few degrees of full extension, muscle strength has decreased to a fair–minus grade, a level that correlates closely with the patient's difficulty in maintaining independent ambulation.

EARLY TREATMENT.   When the diagnosis has been established and before muscle strength has deteriorated, a program of maximum resistance exercises should be instituted. These should be performed several times daily for short periods with emphasis on the primary movers of the pelvic-girdle and the trunk musculature.[31,50,51] An overly vigorous program should be avoided because it may cause an increased rate of muscle destruction.

Contractures are more easily prevented than corrected.[26] Given the proper instruction and incentive, parents can perform pain-free, range-of-motion exercises to avoid the development of deformities. These exercises should be done twice daily on a firm surface and should include stretching of the fascia lata, proximal hamstrings, hip and knee flexors, and ankle plantar flexors. By flexing both hips and then extending one limb in maximum adduction and internal rotation, the hip flexors and the iliotibial band are stretched. Parents must learn the neutral position of motion in order to detect early correctable deformity. Reassessment is carried out each time the exercises are performed.

LATER TREATMENT.   The program of stretching and isometric exercises continues with emphasis on the borderline functional groups of muscles. Despite this, contractures of the hip flexors, proximal hamstrings, and iliotibial band may develop as progressive pelvic

and trunk weakness forces the patient to assume a lordotic, wide-based posture. Eventually a fixed equinovarus deformity may develop in an asymmetrical fashion as muscle imbalance is added to the static equinus position. Full knee extension and plantar flexion persist in the dominant weight-bearing limb.[6] The extremity used for balance during stance more rapidly acquires a heel-cord contracture that is accompanied by mild knee and hip flexion contractures. These further jeopardize ambulatory status and must be recognized by the therapist.

Patients who continue independent ambulation should be instructed in how to break a fall with their arms to prevent serious injury. This skill becomes important later when lower-extremity braces with locked knee joints are required.

Patients threatened with loss of ambulation become candidates for lower-extremity surgery and orthotic control. Before surgery, when there is no pain or discomfort, the therapist teaches the patient the skills he will need postoperatively. Also, at this time, the therapist establishes personal contact with the family, discusses potential physical barriers at home and in school, and establishes goals of the therapy program.

Following surgery, patients are placed on a Circ-o-lectric bed (Stryker). The therapist supervises nurses in using the bed for repetitive, short-duration tilting. This allows the patient with long leg casts to assume an upright position soon after surgery and thus avoids the discomfort associated with swelling that could be caused by prolonged lower-limb dependency.

Balance training is begun when the patient is able to tolerate tilting in the upright position. First the patient learns to stand by resting the buttocks on the posterior aspect of the long leg casts. Then he advances to walking in parallel bars. His casts are protected by fracture boots. Asymmetrical weakness of the pelvic musculature may require the use of a low lift under one boot to allow the boy to advance both limbs. An underlying perceptual problem may become apparent at this time. The patient wears a safety belt to prevent him from jack-knifing forward while learning the rudiments of lateral transfer of his weight. The therapist quickly recognizes that short, husky dystrophic patients have a greater problem in transferring weight from side to side than do tall, slender patients (Fig. 2-11).

Since involvement of shoulder-girdle muscles precludes the use of crutches, a rollator or reciprocal walker frequently adds stability to the insecure, postoperative patient. The goal is ambulation with the rollator at the time of discharge 3 to 10 days following surgery. A program is started that includes standing a minimum of 4 hours a day. The therapist communicates with the school nurse or therapist to ensure continuity of this program when the child returns to school (Fig. 2-12). Instruction in home care includes techniques of getting the child in and out of chairs safely and recommendations for clothing with velcro zippers or snaps to simplify dressing.

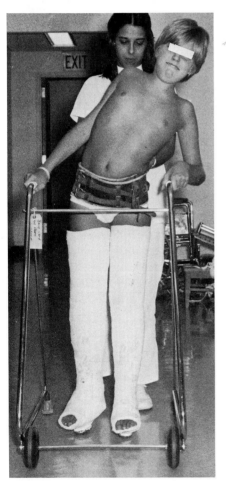

FIG. 2-11. The pendulum-like transference of trunk weight over the stance limb permits progression of the opposite limb in space.

Five weeks following surgery, the child is readmitted for delivery of orthoses and additional training. Initially, he receives hydrotherapy to relieve knee stiffness. The Circ-o-lectric bed is used again for tilting. The patient is fitted with polypropylene knee–ankle–foot orthoses that have spring-loaded, drop-lock knee joints (Fig. 2-13).[54] The proper size of oxford-style shoes cannot be obtained until after the braces have been fitted. A low heel wedge may be needed to compensate for a functional length discrepancy. The therapist teaches transfer and balance techniques, how to lock and unlock the knee joints, and how to rise from a chair (Fig. 2-14). At follow-up clinic visits, he or she reassesses the fit of the braces and reviews the techniques taught previously. Instruction for the nonambulator includes techniques to achieve proper positioning, both in a wheelchair and in recumbency, and recommendations for modifications of the wheelchair or trunk orthoses. A headrest may become necessary when neck muscles become weak and can no longer support the head (Fig. 2-15). The therapist evaluates the home to determine special needs. The unbraced patient confined to a wheelchair may develop contractures that may limit him to sleeping on his side. This results in trochanteric discomfort and requires frequent position changes during the night. The use of pillows or a Roho dry flotation system (Roho Research and Development Corporation) may dramatically lessen the need for these nocturnal position changes (Fig. 2-16). The physical therapist may work with a respiratory therapist to develop positions to enhance the pulmonary program.

WHEELCHAIR. A wheelchair is indicated for the patient who is no longer capable of independent ambulation. This change in mobility may cause a dramatic functional change and an increased body weight because physical stimulation is absent. The wheelchair should be of the folding variety, with brakes and extendable leg rests. A firm seat made of plywood is necessary to provide a stable, balanced support for both ischia.[23] The more seriously involved patient may require a seatbelt, an extended backrest, or a headrest (Figs. 2-17 and 2-18). The wheelchair also may be fitted with a balanced forearm orthosis for purposes of facilitating personal hygiene and feeding (Fig. 2-19). The dystrophic patient who is physi-

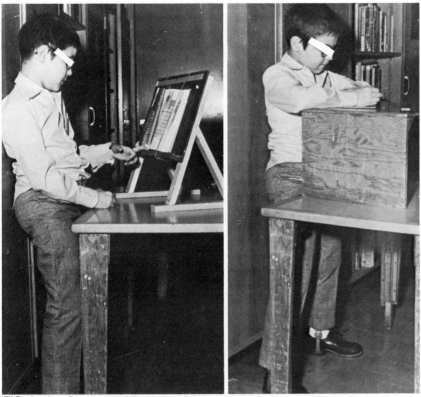

FIG. 2-12. Simple modifications of the regular classroom allow a braced patient to remain standing, thereby increasing his activity level and independence.

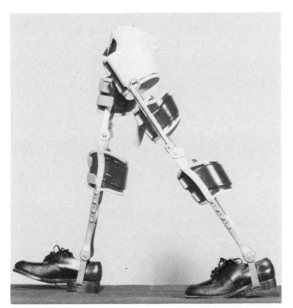

FIG. 2-13. This traditional type of spring-loaded, drop-lock, knee joint, long leg brace is now being replaced by plastic models. This orthosis can be lengthened but is far heavier than its plastic alternative.

cally unable to propel himself may benefit by an electrically powered chair. Spring-booster chairs also have limited application.[55]

TRANSFER TECHNIQUES. A Hoyer lift (Everest & Jennings, distributors) or a Lift-Aid portable lifter (Trans-Aid Lifter Corporation) can be used for most transfers (Fig. 2-20). Proper sling placement is essential for successful use of the lifters. The patient should be rolled toward the nurse or parent and with the sling properly positioned before the patient is returned to the supine position. A similar maneuver carried out on the opposite side of the bed allows the sling to be straightened out and the patient to be centered on the sling. Then the portable lifter is placed over the patient and he is raised to a sitting position or until the buttocks are clear of the bed. The patient's legs are grasped and he is turned to a dangle position. He is then raised slightly and moved from the bed. The procedure is reversed to return the patient to bed.

Nonambulatory patients need to wear long leg braces when making pivot transfers. This

FIG. 2-14. A therapist can perform a pivot transfer by moving the patient to the edge of the wheelchair seat, supporting him beneath his buttocks, and pivoting him while controlling one lower extremity with her knees. It is important to keep the patient's body weight close to the therapist during this transfer. She can position the patient properly against the wheelchair backrest by crossing the patient's arms to avoid his slipping through. This could occur because of shoulder girdle weakness.

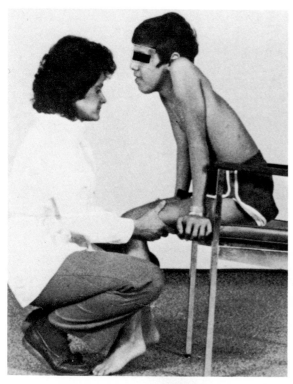
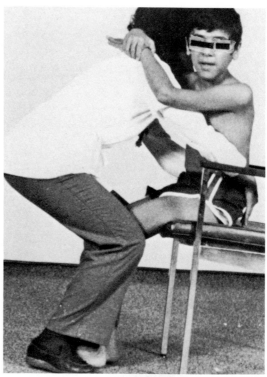
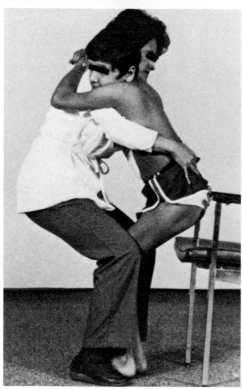
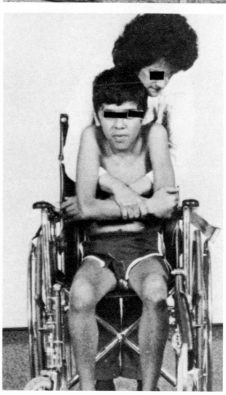

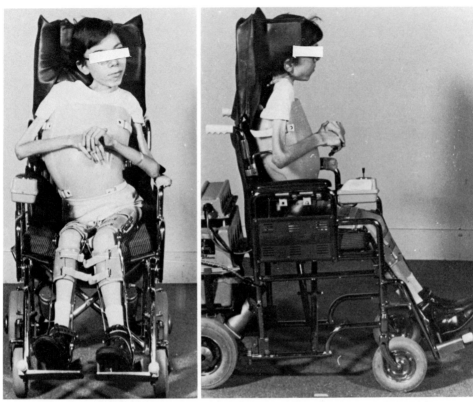

FIG. 2-15. Neck weakness can be accommodated by the addition of a quadriplegic headrest extension and a lateral head support.

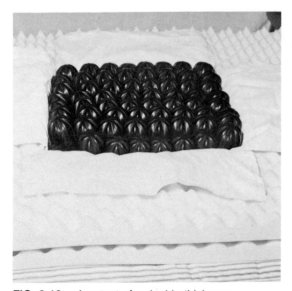

FIG. 2-16. A cutout of a double-thickness eggcrate mattress permits nocturnal use of the Roho dry flotation system. This air cushion can also be used in a wheelchair which has a solid seat.

method enables patients to help themselves, thus easing the strain on parents, especially older ones with low-back discomfort. The patient cannot be expected to assist actively in transfer because of a weak shoulder girdle. A transfer board is contraindicated in those who cannot use their pelvic girdle.

OCCUPATIONAL THERAPIST, SOCIAL WORKER, NURSE, AND PSYCHOLOGIST

The occupational therapist screens for activities of daily living and gives instruction in hygiene, dressing, grooming, feeding, and meal preparation. This therapist also is responsible for evaluating the patient's use of the upper extremities. The occupational therapist prescribes, and occasionally fabricates, adaptive equipment for dressing, feeding, writing, typing, and telephoning to help the patient perform tasks more efficiently (Fig. 2-21). A balanced forearm orthosis may assist in retaining independent feeding and writing

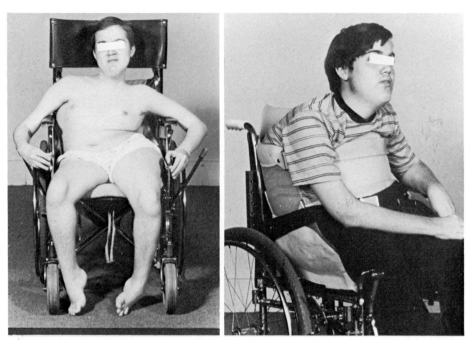

FIG. 2-17. Constant contact with the wheelchair in an upright position caused pain and skin irritation over this adolescent's convex rib cage. The use of a Vitrathene seat insert alleviated the problem.

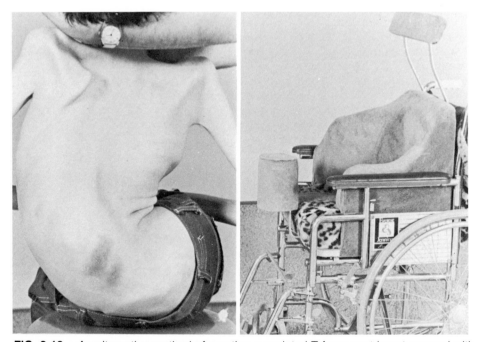

FIG. 2-18. An alternative method of creating a sculpted T-foam seat insert covered with velour afforded relief of low back pain in this cachectic patient with severe lumbar lordoscoliosis.

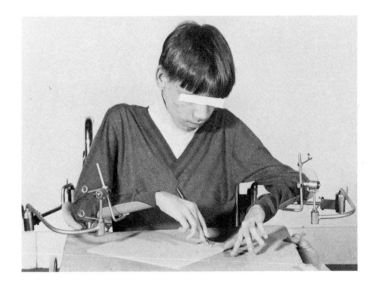

FIG. 2-19. This adolescent is able to participate in regular classroom activities by using a balanced forearm orthosis and an electric typewriter.

skills.[11] The therapist plans vocational rehabilitation programs and tests and trains and screens for simulated work activities and endurance.

The social worker coordinates the activities of health and welfare organizations in the community to ensure that the prescribed services are performed. He or she talks with families on a regular basis about financial assistance from state, health, and welfare agencies and maintains up-to-date school data.

The specialty clinic nurse acts as the patient's advocate. The nurse must be able to recognize and coordinate various physical and psychosocial needs of children with neuromuscular diseases.[22] He or she is responsible for coordinating these programs in the hospital, school system, and home environment so that total care can be delivered.

The role of the psychologist is to support the efforts of the orthopaedist and neurologist in the long-term treatment and medical management of the muscle-disease patient. This is done by consulting with team colleagues on the psychologic correlates of chronic and often fatal illness and by assisting the patient and family as they attempt to cope with the medical and psychologic effects of the disease.

Preoperative Evaluation

Preoperative gait analysis and photography form a baseline upon which to compare post-operative functional improvement and correction of deformity. The physical therapist evaluates the upper- and lower-extremity function and instructs the family in skills that will be needed postoperatively. Other rehabilitation goals are established as the social worker begins discharge planning.

The dystrophic patient undergoing general anesthesia should have pulmonary function studies.[29] The forced expiratory volume in the first second (FEV-1), or the ability to generate a cough, is the most important function after normal levels of gasses in the arterial blood have been demonstrated.[20] Chest roentgenograms and routine analyses of blood and urine are also obtained.

Anesthetics

Inhalation anesthetics, particularly halothane, have been used widely. Muscle relaxants rarely are indicated, even in patients requiring endotracheal intubation for spinal surgery. Cardiac arrest during induction of anesthesia has been reported with the use of succinylcholine chloride.[41] Patients with cardiopulmonary compromise need only local anesthetics when limited soft-tissue procedures are performed.

Surgical Procedures

Surgery of the lower extremities is indicated when independent walking becomes precar-

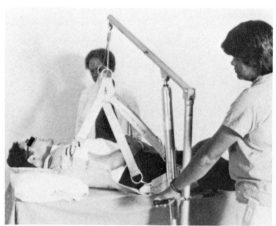
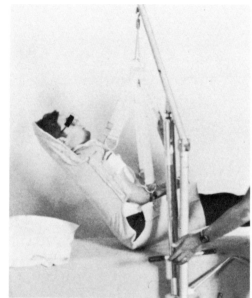
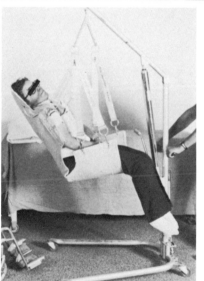
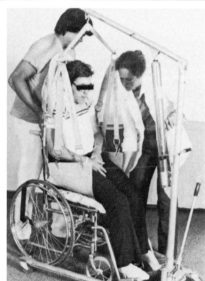

FIG. 2-20. A one-person transfer can be performed easily for a severely involved Duchenne adolescent.

ious and when contractures are painful or interfere with essential daily activities. Braces are required postoperatively and measurements for these are obtained before surgery.

EQUINUS CONTRACTURES

Equinus deformity of the forefoot may develop in the more severely involved young Duchenne patient. Tight plantar structures, particularly the medial fascia, can be palpated when the forefoot is forcibly dorsiflexed. Weight-bearing lateral roentgenograms demonstrate that a line drawn through the talar longitudinal axis passes through either the base or superior to the first metatarsal shaft and creates a measurable forefoot equinus.

Equinus contractures are corrected by a plantar release made through a lateral incision. The medial incision traditionally used for Steindler stripping has been abandoned because with this method there was considera-

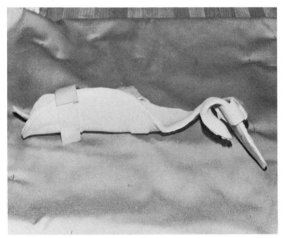

FIG. 2-21. Increasing forearm and hand muscle weakness may require special adaptive equipment if the patient is to retain any independent upper-extremity activity.

ble tension on the skin over the medial longitudinal arch after satisfactory correction had been achieved. This tension resulted in frequent dehiscence of the surgical incision.

This equinus deformity must be differentiated from the equinus occasionally found in Duchenne patients over the age of 10 years. In these older patients more hindfoot deformity is noted on roentgenograms, and management requires formal transfer of the posterior tibial tendon combined with heel-cord tenot-

omy. Forefoot equinus also may be noted in the Becker's dystrophy patient during the second or third decade of life.

LATERAL PLANTAR RELEASE. A longitudinal incision is made along the lateral aspect of the inferior calcaneal tuberosity and is carried distally to the calcaneal cuboid joint (Fig. 2-22A). The plantar fascia is identified at its origin and its entire breadth is separated from the plantar fat pad, which is carefully preserved. The plantar fascia is sharply incised at its origin. Extraperiosteal dissection is done to completely denude the os calcis of intrinsic musculature and plantar ligaments (Fig. 2-22B). The abductor digiti quinti is released to the level of the calcaneal cuboid joint to expose the long plantar ligament, which must be completely divided to flatten both the lateral and medial longitudinal arches of the foot. This ligament has dual insertions into the plantar aspect of the cuboid, while its more superficial fibers continue forward to the bases of the second, third, and fourth metatarsi. The ligament should be divided on the plantar aspect of the calcaneal cuboid joint carefully, so as not to violate the synovium. Release of the abductor hallucis requires sharp dissection and must be complete because the procedure is performed to lengthen the medial longitudinal arch. Mayo scissors may be needed to release isolated, recalcitrant aspects of this muscle. By dissecting close to bone, the plan-

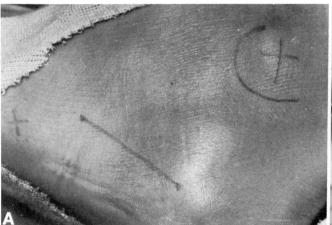
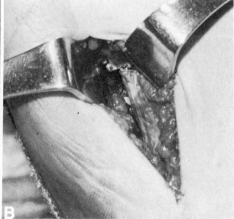

FIG. 2-22. (**A**) This demonstrates the lateral heel skin incision. The malleolus and the base of the fifth metatarsus are illustrated. (**B**) This shows division of the long and short plantar ligaments.

tar neurovascular structures are not injured. The wound is irrigated and closed with an interrupted, absorbable suture. A short leg cast without a molded arch is applied. A double-thickness felt pad is placed under the forefoot to ensure equal distribution of corrective forces. If postoperative lateral roentgenograms demonstrate the need for remanipulation, this can be done under general anesthesia 7 to 10 days later. The second cast may have a metatarsal bar that allows the patient to weight-bear while further correction is being gained. After the patient has been immobilized for 3 to 4 weeks, he can wear a plastic ankle–foot orthosis that extends to the metatarsal heads.

EQUINOVARUS CONTRACTURES

Generally equinus contractures are accompanied by varus deformity of the heel. The posterior tibial muscle retains good function despite the progression of muscle weakness in other areas. Its transfer to the dorsum of the foot prevents recurrence of equinovarus and actively contributes to dorsiflexion of the foot. This procedure is recommended for patients with equinovarus deformity who retain potential for ambulation with long leg braces.[45] It is most commonly performed between the ages of 8 to 12 years and results in an additional 3 to 5 years of independent ambulation.[6,13,45]

The initial recommendation for surgery is made when the patient demonstrates a loss of antigravity quadriceps strength (Fig. 2-23). This degree of weakness prevents the boy who stumbles from being able to regain an upright stance. This problem occurs approximately one year after the patient loses the ability to climb stairs. Generally, the initial discussion with the family precedes surgery by 3 to 6 months, and the family at that point is cautioned to be aware of changes in activity patterns and particularly to note an increasing incidence of falling. The procedure may also be indicated for the boy who has recently been confined to a wheelchair but who retains a strong desire to resume walking.

BILATERAL ANTERIOR TRANSFERS OF TIBIALIS POSTERIOR TENDONS. Four separate surgical incisions are required to perform bilateral anterior transfer of the tibialis posterior ten-

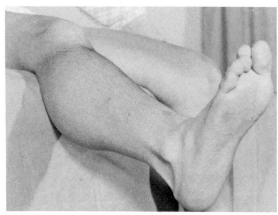

FIG. 2-23. Inability fully to extend the knee against gravity indicates that the quadriceps can maintain the knee in extension only under optimal conditions. Increasing falls and decreasing functional activity become evident at this point.

dons (Fig. 2-24A). The initial incision begins at the insertion of the tibialis posterior and extends proximally toward the medial malleolus. The surgeon frees the tendon from its insertion while preserving as much of its length as possible. Vincula in the tendon tunnel must be sharply divided. Additional length for the transfer, important particularly when there is fixed equinovarus, can be gained by including a short segment of the second head of the tendon. The circumference of the tendon is trimmed to allow passage through the posterior tibial tunnel.

A Kocher clamp is placed on the tip of the freed tendon and longitudinal traction is applied. By palpating the posterior calf, the muscle belly of the tibialis posterior can be located. This establishes the location for the second incision, which is made proximal to the superior crural retinaculum. The distal muscle belly is freed circumferentially by blunt dissection anterior to the flexor digitorum longus. An umbilical tape used for traction brings the tendon into the second operative field. An incidental heel-cord tenotomy is also performed through this incision.

A third incision, slightly more distal than the second, is made over the tibialis anterior tendon. The dissection is carried between the tendons of the tibialis anterior and the extensor hallucis longus, with care being taken to preserve the neurovascular structures. The interosseous membrane is exposed just prox-

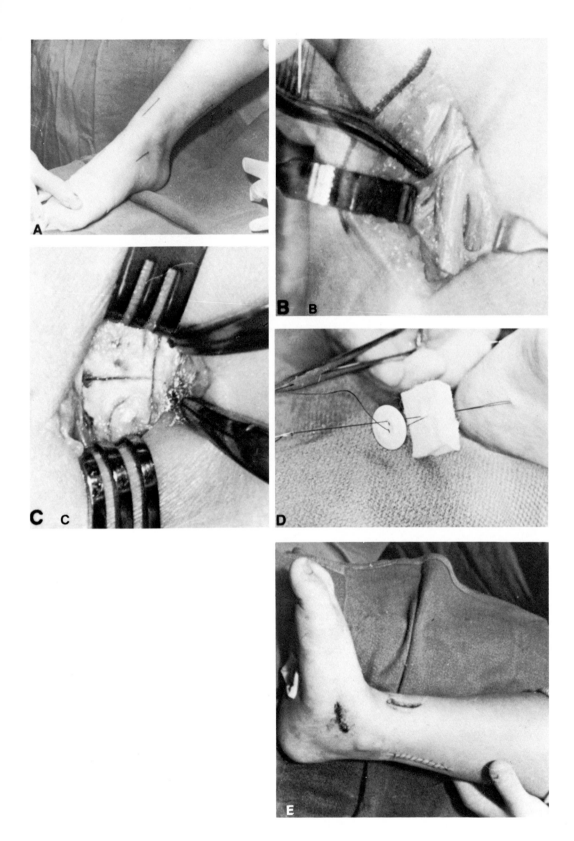

◀ **FIG. 2-24.** (**A**) This demonstrates surgical incisions. (**B**) A generous window must be cut through the interosseous membrane to permit tendon transfer. (**C**) Care must be taken in developing the periosteal flaps, or decortication of the soft cuneiform bone will inadvertently occur. (**D**) The tendon is fastened over a non-weight-bearing aspect of the medial longitudinal arch. Occasional skin breakdown noted in this area does not delay functional ambulation with braces. (**E**) The transfer should be under sufficient tension to hold the foot at a right angle relative to the tibia.

imal to the tibial fibular syndesmosis and a generous window in the interosseous membrane is cut with a No. 11 Parker scalpel (Fig. 2-24B). The periosteum should not be stripped from the tibia or fibula. The tibialis posterior is brought through the window with a tendon passer carefully so as not to kink, twist, or constrict it, or damage the neurovascular structures.

The first two incisions are closed and the fourth is made over the cuneiform in line with the third toe. The extensor tendons are retracted permitting creation of cuneiform osteoperiosteal flaps (Fig. 2-24C). Using Paton burrs, a tunnel, with its proximal edge beveled, is made through the bone in the direction of the medial longitudinal arch. This bone is extremely soft. The tendon is passed superficial to the crural ligament into the fourth field and a sturdy Bunnell woven suture is used. This suture is passed through the plantar skin into a felt pad and a button that is placed on the non-weight-bearing plantar surface of the medial longitudinal arch (Fig. 2-24D). After the tendon has been secured, the osteoperiosteal flaps are closed with enough tension so that the foot can be passively held at a right angle (Fig. 2-24E). The remaining incisions are closed and long leg casts are applied.

For the first 24 hours postoperatively the patient is placed on a Circ-o-lectric bed with his feet elevated. Then tilting is started for short periods and increased until the patient is able to assume an upright position. At this time he can begin to use parallel bars for gait training (Fig. 2-25A). Maximum standing with the Circ-o-lectric bed is continued throughout the hospitalization. The patient can be discharged after he has achieved satisfactory ambulation with the rollator (Fig. 2-25B), usually within 7 to 10 days. Five weeks following surgery, the patient is readmitted for appli-

cation of orthoses.[46] Physical therapy and Circ-o-lectric bed tilting programs are continued.

TENOTOMIES. Percutaneous heel-cord tenotomies have been reserved for the nonambulatory patient with a pure equinus contracture who cannot wear shoes. The nonambulatory patient with moderately severe equinovarus deformity experiences pain on the lateral border of the forefoot when it is in contact with the wheelchair footrest. Open tenotomies of the heel cord and posterior tibial and long toe flexors should be performed. When the foot is maximally dorsiflexed to ensure adequate correction, the toes must be evaluated for the development of hammer-toe flexion contractures. This new deformity would cause considerable postoperative discomfort for patients who cannot voluntarily move their toes. Open tenotomy performed through a plantar longitudinal incision beneath the first phalanx is recommended to render the toe flexors flail. The skin creases should not be violated by the incision. Although general anesthesia without intubation is preferred, surgery also can be performed under local anesthesia in the patient with severely restricted pulmonary function.

INGROWN TOENAILS. Ingrown toenails are most likely to occur in the nonambulatory patient who uses long leg braces for pivot transfers. High-top shoes are replaced infrequently, resulting in an accumulation of sweat in shoes that may, in addition, have a toe box too narrow for the forefoot. Also, excessive sweating may cause maceration of the nail groove. Foot soaks and absorbent powder help to decrease the amount of perspiration. A second pair of shoes is helpful. Oxford-style shoes with a roomy toe box and a straight inner last can be modified to accept orthotic attachment. Another prophylactic measure is a toe

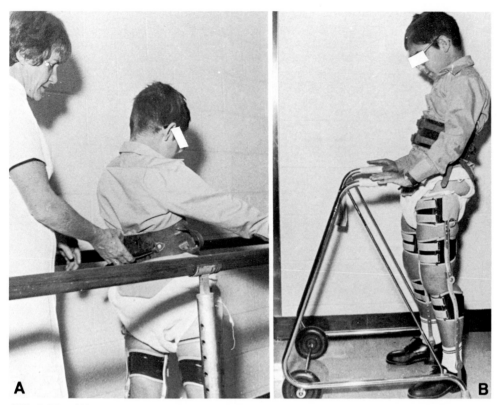

FIG. 2-25. (**A**) A safety walking belt is required while the child, in both long leg casts and braces, learns to transfer weight to the stance limb. (**B**) The rollator offers a greater standing base to patients mastering a new gait pattern.

spacer (Fig. 2-26). This simple plastic orthosis slips over the great toe and its C-shaped lateral extension separates the first and second toes.

Prophylactic management is very effective. Toenails should be trimmed straight across without trimming the corners. If one of the lateral nail margins becomes covered with the soft tissue of the nail groove, it should be gently elevated with a wisp of cotton or a blunt toothpick. If inflammation does occur, prompt conservative treatment should be instituted with warm soaks. After the inflammation has subsided, partial excision of the germinal matrix, the offending part of the nail, and the accompanying eponychium can be performed under local anesthesia.

KNEE FLEXION CONTRACTURES

In the independent ambulator, contractures generally develop asymmetrically as the pa-

tient's standing balance becomes more precarious. A knee flexion contracture of more than a few degrees combined with a hip flex-

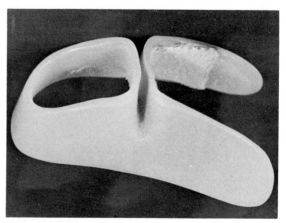

FIG. 2-26. A toe spacer separates the first and second toes and prevents excessive nail bed maceration.

ion contracture jeopardizes ambulation and renders the quadriceps increasingly insufficient. Using long leg plastic orthoses at night and stretching the hamstrings help to alleviate this problem.

Patients ambulating with long leg braces can tolerate up to 15° of knee flexion contracture in the limb that is used for partial weight-bearing during stance. Serial ambulatory casts that are wedged daily may be needed to reduce a contracture to this acceptable degree. However, those who suffer a transient loss of ambulation may rapidly develop a mild contracture which will respond to a brief course of hydrotherapy and skin traction. Therefore, if this program provides prompt correction, the cast wedging regimen need not be employed.

HIP AND KNEE FLEXION CONTRACTURES

The skeletally immature patient who can no longer stand is apt to develop flexion contractures of the hip and knee, particularly when he spends long periods of time in a wheelchair. Prevention consists of using long leg braces with the knees locked in extension during the day on at least a part-time basis. However, if long leg braces are used at night, short leg braces should be worn during the day to prevent ankle deformity.

Contractures of the lower extremities can make comfortable positioning difficult and may lead to the development of hamstring spasm with considerable discomfort when transfer is attempted. Patients who cannot voluntarily extend the knee also develop symptoms of chondromalacia patellae after they have been sitting for long periods (Fig. 2-27). Passive movement of the limb gives temporary relief whereas an open hamstring tenotomy provides more permanent relief. In fact, patients with marked flexion contractures will obtain symptomatic relief from a tenotomy even if it achieves only partial correction.

Because the iliotibial band is located anterior and lateral to the axis of the hip and posterior and lateral to the knee axis, the band can produce flexion deformities of both joints. Its contracture forces the hip into a fixed position of external rotation, abduction, and flexion while causing flexion, external rotation, and valgus of the knee.

The Yount fasciotomy corrects mild flexion deformities of the hip and knee by resection of a block of the iliotibial band and lateral intermuscular septum from the distal lateral femur.[56] The Ober procedure releases the fascia overlying the anterior and lateral musculature, which originates from the pelvis.[37] More pronounced joint deformities can be corrected by combining these two procedures.

SURGICAL TECHNIQUE (YOUNT). The patient is in the supine position and a tourniquet is used. The fascia lata is exposed through a longitudinal incision immediately proximal to the femoral condyle (Fig. 2-28). A Farabeuf rugine is used to expose the iliotibial band from the midline anteriorly to the biceps tendon. At least a 1-in section of the iliotibial band and lateral intermuscular septum should be resected. The exposed fascia is initially incised proximally and the fibrofatty replacement tissue is swept away from its inner aspect. This allows the surgeon to follow the plane of the lateral intermuscular septum to its insertion

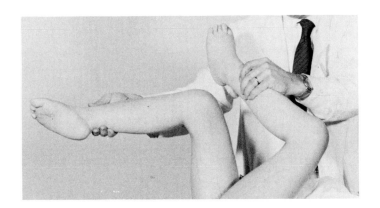

FIG. 2-27. Patients with severe fixed deformity cannot initiate active knee movement and may develop significant retropatellar discomfort.

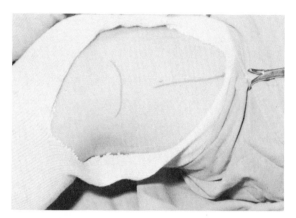

FIG. 2-28. The incision for Yount fasciotomy is outlined. The location of the lateral femoral condyle is indicated.

in the lateral femur. The proximal incision is then extended to the level of the biceps femoris tendon. A second incision is made parallel and distal to this and *en bloc* resection of the fascia lata and intermuscular septum is performed. After resection the limb must be adducted to be certain that the osseous attachment of the intermuscular septum has been completely resected. As the knee is extended, additional bands of the fascia lata should be sought anteriorly and posteriorly for division. The wound should be thoroughly irrigated and then closed with a subcuticular suture. Since the Yount fasciotomy is frequently done with a posterior iliotibial transfer, the limb is immobilized in a long leg cast for 5 weeks.

SURGICAL TECHNIQUE (OBER). The patient is placed in a supine position and the procedure is performed without endotracheal intubation. The incision is begun at the middle of the iliac crest and brought anteriorly parallel to the inguinal crease. The point at which the incision passes beneath the anterior superior iliac spine is determined by the amount of hip flexion contracture. As the flexion contracture is corrected, the incision tends to migrate proximally, but at the end of the procedure it should remain distal to the spine.

The presenting fascia lata is exposed with a rugine until the sacroiliac joint is palpated posteriorly. The iliotibial band is divided from the ilium by electrocautery. The sartorius is circumferentially freed up and its fatty re-

placement tissue also is divided by electrocautery. The rectus femoris may require division. By following the pubis medially to the area of the psoas bursa, the psoas tendon is identified and then, with the hip flexed, the exposed tendon is divided under direct vision. After determining the tension fo the neurovascular structures, the wound is irrigated and then closed with a subcuticular suture.

Some hip flexion may be required initially to accommodate the tension on the neurovascular structures. When the Ober release is performed at the same time as the Yount fasciotomy in nonambulatory patients, a Circ-o-lectric bed is used for several days postoperatively before comfortable extension of the hips is possible.

SURGICAL TECHNIQUE (HAMSTRING TENOTOMY). While using a tourniquet, two longitudinal incisions are made over the midcoronal aspect of the femoral condyles. The medial incision allows access to the gracilis and semitendinosus as well as the medial extension of the fascia lata. Through the lateral exposure the biceps femoris can be sectioned and a 1-in block of the iliotibial band, including the lateral intermuscular septum, is excised. Also the strong lateral fibers of the lower part of the vasti, which are attached to the iliotibial band, are divided. Contractures of the anterior extension of the fascia lata can be noted when the knee is gradually extended. In patients with a long-standing deformity, additional isolation and division of the popliteal extension of the fascia may be necessary. A utility dressing, including a posterior plaster splint, is applied to provide comfort during the immediate postoperative period.

SPINAL DEFORMITY

Lordosis in the ambulatory patient is exaggerated by the continuous weakening of the trunk musculature. Wilkins noted that the spinal extensor muscles, which retained voluntary contraction but which could no longer resist gravity, still permitted the patient with lumbar lordosis to sit erect with a level pelvis.[53] However, with further deterioration of the strength of these muscles, the sitting posture was converted to a functional kyphosis and the risk of developing scoliosis was increased.

Wilkins hypothesized that kyphotic posture unlocked the posterior facet joints and increased the tension on the posterior spinal ligaments, creating an unstable spine with risk of progression of the lateral curve. Thus he developed a radiologic kyphotic index (Fig. 2-29) as an objective method of determining the risk of an individual patient developing significant scoliosis. The index is obtained from a sitting lateral roentgenogram and represents the ratio of the distance between a line drawn from the anteroinferior angle of the body of the seventh cervical vertebra to the sacral promontory and the distance measured at a right angle from this line to the anteroinferior angle of the vertebral body at the apex of the curve.

He also identified a small group of patients who, early in the course of the disease, developed a position of spinal extension, which resulted in a stiff lordotic spine with little scoliosis. These patients were at an average age of nearly 20 years at the time of examination and may represent a subgroup in progressive muscular dystrophy.

Generally, scoliosis becomes apparent clinically either during the last 10 months of limited ambulation or after the boy becomes confined to a wheelchair.[8,38] In ambulatory patients who develop scoliosis, the curve can be expected to progress rapidly after the patients lose the upright position.[44] Untreated, the scoliosis may cause the patient to become bedridden. The curve usually develops in the paralytic long C pattern in the thoracolumbar areas (Fig. 2-30).[52] With increasing weakness, vertebrae are added to the curve, which eventually involves the pelvis. This leads to difficulty in sitting and causes discomfort and pressure in the trochanteric region. The patient uses his elbows as crutches to maintain an erect position, and this prevents him from using his arms for other functions.

TREATMENT OF SPINAL DEFORMITY

Observation only is recommended for patients with scoliotic curves that measure less than 25° (Fig. 2-31). Ambulatory patients with greater curves should wear spinal orthoses at night. Daytime use is contraindicated because with the resultant loss of the functional

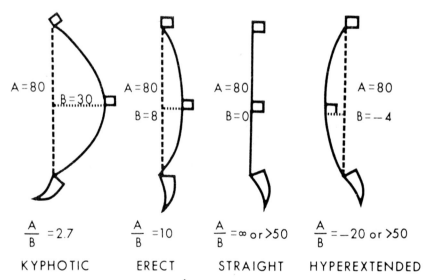

$$\frac{A}{B} = 2.7 \qquad \frac{A}{B} = 10 \qquad \frac{A}{B} = \infty \text{ or } > 50 \qquad \frac{A}{B} = -20 \text{ or } > 50$$

KYPHOTIC · · · · · ERECT · · · · · STRAIGHT · · · · · HYPEREXTENDED

FIG. 2-29. The kyphotic index ($\frac{A}{B}$ The kyphotic index) obtained from a sitting lateral spinal roentgenogram is a reliable guide in determining patients who will develop progressive scoliosis. The perpendicular line extends from the anterior aspect of C1 to S1. The short horizontal limb extends to the inferior aspect of the vertebral body farthest from the first line. The lower the kyphotic index, the greater the risk of progressive scoliosis. (Wilkins KE, Gibson DA: The patterns of spinal deformity in Duchenne muscular dystrophy. J Bone Joint Surg 58A:24, 1976)

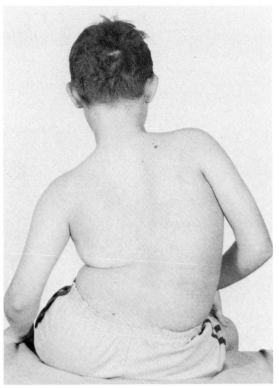

FIG. 2-30. Scoliosis generally follows a paralytic, long, C-shaped curve in nonambulatory patients.

lordosis the patient is unable to stand upright. Orthoses give passive support and thus can be effectively used for skeletally immature patients in whom a spinal fusion is not yet indicated.[14,20] Successful use of an orthosis is related to parental cooperation and lack of obesity in a patient (Fig. 2-32).

Spinal fusion is indicated when (1) an untreated curve progresses above 45° or (2) when there is significant progression in the degree or length of the curve in patients who have been temporarily controlled in a spinal orthosis. Posterior fusion to the sacrum can be accomplished by using either the Harrington system (Fig. 2-33) or segmental spinal stabilization. The goal is to achieve a stable spine so that the upper end of the corrected curve is centered over the body of the sacrum. If the Harrington method is chosen, more than one rod is used to provide greater stability. Bending the square-ended rods at the time of surgery, as well as using alar hooks, allows for retention of normal lordosis. One advantage of segmental spinal stabilization, my method of choice, is that an orthosis or plaster immobilization is not needed postoperatively.

Postoperatively the patient uses a Circ-o-lectric bed, and resistive exercises to both the

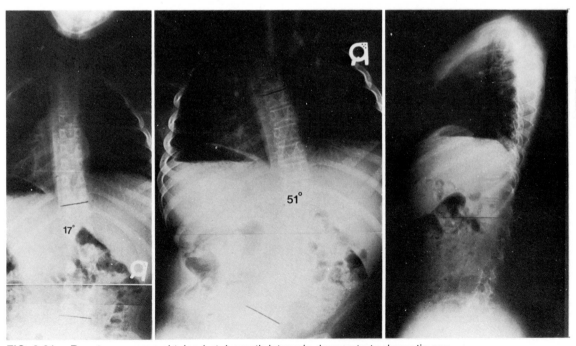

FIG. 2-31. Roentgenograms obtained at 4-month intervals demonstrate dramatic progression of scoliosis in an adolescent at the time he lost independent ambulatory ability. Lateral roentgenograms demonstrate a low kyphotic index.

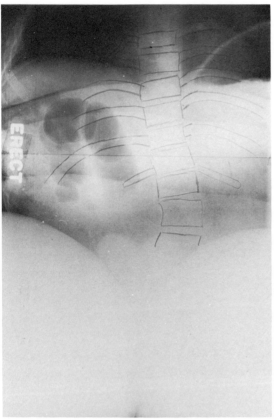

FIG. 2-32. Short, obese patients are poor orthotic candidates. The opaque areas at the bottom of the illustration represent the girth of the lower extremities in the seated patient. The massive thighs severely limit the potential length of the spinal brace.

upper extremities and the head and neck are begun the day after surgery. This early mobilization prevents significant loss of head control and function of the upper extremities. One week postoperatively patients with Harrington rods can wear a two-piece spinal orthosis (Fig. 2-34) and sit in a wheelchair. The wheelchair platform may need to be tilted so that the patient's head is aligned properly and his eyes are in a horizontal plane.

Some patients, either those who can stand or those who have to use a wheelchair, may have lumbar back pain from their excessive lordosis. Iliopsoas tenotomy may be required for relief of this pain.

Cardiopulmonary Measures

Respiratory infection is a constant threat and is the most common cause of death among patients with Duchenne type muscular dystrophy.[9] A decreased total lung capacity and an increased residual volume are associated with a decrease in intercostal muscle strength. A significant increase in the arterial carbon dioxide level in a patient without infection is a grim prognostic sign. Dyspnea, nightmares, and increased heart rate and blood pressure may be associated with hypercarbia. The development of scoliosis leads to further diminution in vital capacity. In the later stage of muscular dystrophy, an apparently innocuous respiratory infection may require hospitalization and treatment with antibiotics.[1] Alexander reports the successful home use of mechanical ventilation with late-stage Duchenne dystrophy patients.[3] Cardiac failure usually is acute, despite the use of digoxin and diuretics (Fig. 2-35).

Fractures

Adolescents whose quadriceps weakness requires knee–ankle–foot orthoses to stabilize the knee in the upright position are the most vulnerable to fractures. These injuries most commonly occur when the patient is not using braces and the paretic limb is subject to rotatory forces. Fractures may occur during times of personal hygiene or in a fall from a wheelchair. Aggressive, positive management is required so that the patient will retain standing or ambulatory abilities.

Undisplaced fractures occur in the distal femur or tibia. The patient is initially kept comfortable in a long leg splint and uses a Circ-o-lectric bed for weight-bearing on the uninvolved, braced limb. Also the patient starts a program of power-building exercises for upper-extremity and neck muscles. When swelling and discomfort have subsided, he resumes wearing the knee–ankle–foot orthosis on the injured limb. Then, when he is able to be tilted upright and can bear full weight without pain, he can start walking with a rollator.

Displaced lower-extremity fractures require prompt surgical stabilization (Fig. 2-36). Families must be cautioned that weight-bearing during the immediate rehabilitation period carries an increased risk of loss of fixation and subsequent delayed union. The day following surgery, tilting is initiated (Fig. 2-37). Later when swelling and discomfort have subsided, ambulation with a rollator is begun. If the family elects a nonsurgical approach, they

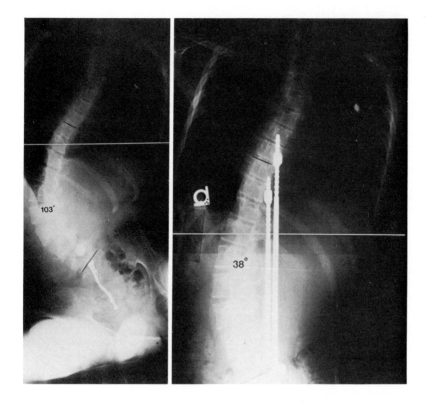

103°

38°

FIG. 2-33. Fusion with Harrington instrumentation stabilizes the spine. Note the use of the sacral alar hook.

must understand that the child will be recumbent for 6 to 8 weeks. When this course is chosen, a power-building program for neck and shoulder-girdle muscles is started.

Upper-extremity fractures occur when the patient in braces falls. Because he lacks adequate musculature, the force of the fall is transmitted directly to bone. Forearm fractures can be managed with a short arm cast, whereas use of a sling and swathe is an appropriate method for stabilizing humeral fractures.

BECKER'S MUSCULAR DYSTROPHY

Becker's muscular dystrophy is similar to Duchenne muscular dystrophy in clinical appearance and distribution of weakness. It is a slowly progressive, sex-linked recessive disease that eventually confines the patient to a wheelchair and causes premature death.[5]

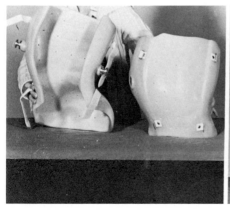

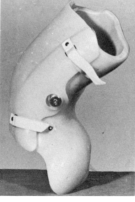

FIG. 2-34. A two-piece spinal orthosis is required after Harrington instrumentation to permit upright activities. Prolonged postoperative recumbency could result in loss of head control.

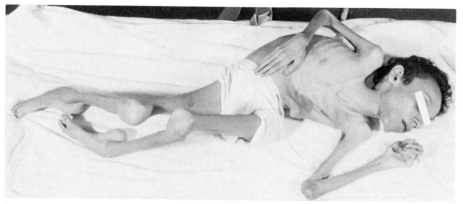

FIG. 2-35. Inanition and cardiac failure generally are responsible for death late in adolescence.

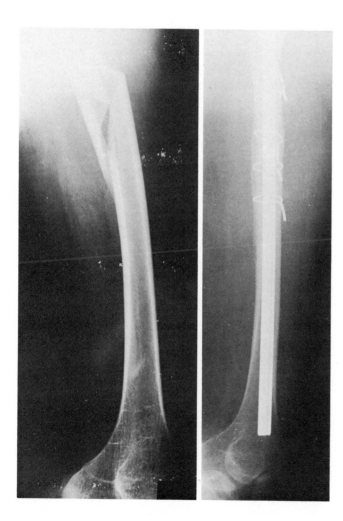

FIG. 2-36. Fractures in an ambulatory patient should be managed by prompt internal fixation so that the patient can regain an upright position.

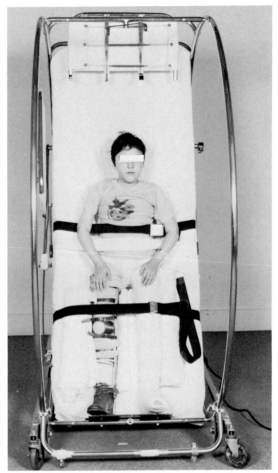

FIG. 2-37. Combining the Circ-o-lectric bed and weight-bearing in the braced limb is effective in the immediate management of both undisplaced and surgically stabilized lower-extremity fractures.

The onset is generally after age 7 and rarely occurs after age 25. Around the age of 10 the patient may walk on his toes or may waddle. The upper extremities become involved 2 to 10 years later.

The following factors confirm the diagnosis[7]: (1) sex-linked recessive inheritance; (2) ambulation maintained at least until age 16; (3) calf pseudohypertrophy, which usually is found early in the disease; (4) early contracture of the tendo Achillis with contractures of other muscles later; and (5) specific distribution of muscle wasting. Weakness affects the muscles that move the hip joints and the tibialis anterior as well as the supraspinatus, infraspinatus, serratus anterior, the pectorals, biceps, and brachioradialis. Other muscles are spared until late in the disease. As the dystrophy progresses, deep-tendon reflexes are lost, but the ankle jerks remain until late in the disease.

Generally these patients develop gait abnormalities by age 15, but few patients are confined to a wheelchair before age 25. The mean age of loss of ambulation is 30; mean life expectancy is 36. Family history may reveal that a maternal uncle has been diagnosed as having muscular dystrophy but has remained ambulatory into adult life.

Patients with Becker's dystrophy differ in several respects from those with Duchenne dystrophy. They rarely are mentally retarded. CPK levels are not as high as those in patients with Duchenne dystrophy. Fifty percent of Becker carriers have CPK elevations that, when present, are not as pronounced as those in the

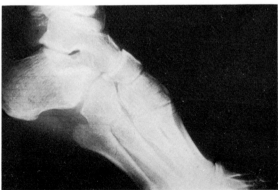
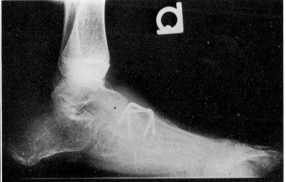

FIG. 2-38. By combining soft-tissue and bony procedures, the surgeon can obtain plantigrade feet in a patient who retains strong quadriceps. (Courtesy of Newington Children's Hospital)

Duchenne carrier. An electromyogram shows changes compatible with both a chronic myopathy and neuropathy. Muscle biopsy demonstrates changes of both denervation and myopathy, with fiber atrophy and hypertrophy as well as fiber splitting. Approximately one half have a normal electrocardiogram.

Orthopaedic problems are related primarily to the lower extremities. Early in the course of the disease, patients develop equinus of both the hindfoot and forefoot; both these deformities are progressive. An intrinsic release followed by a Cole midfoot wedge ostectomy and staged heel-cord lengthening helps younger patients (Fig. 2-38). Older patients with more precarious gait are better managed by an intrinsic release and staged heel-cord lengthening. The patient who is barely able to walk may benefit from a simple heel-cord tenotomy (Fig. 2-39). Unlike the Duchenne dystrophy patient, the patient with Becker's dystrophy rarely develops hindfoot varus in conjunction with the equinus. If equinovarus does occur, it can be managed by a simple tenotomy of the heel cord and posterior tibial tendons. Postoperatively, patients are treated with a Circ-o-lectric bed and long leg weight-bearing casts. These patients generally have asymmetrical development of foot deformities and muscle weakness. Following surgery, careful titration of heel and sole lifts may be necessary to make walking easier for the patient.

An ankle–foot orthosis may be required to maintain correction in the younger patient.

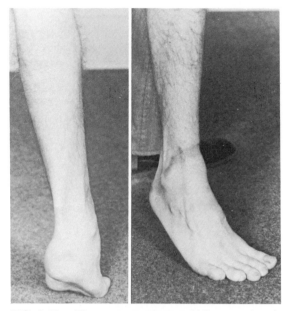

FIG. 2-39. The postoperative morbidity associated with osseous procedures precludes their use in the older patient with tenuous ambulation.

As weakness of the hip and knee becomes more pronounced, a long leg brace should be used.

Although increased lumbar lordosis may develop in the ambulatory patient, it rarely requires treatment. Scoliosis occurs only when the patient becomes confined to a wheelchair. Retention of upper extremity function allows the patient to use a rollator. Patients with weakness in the pelvic girdle may benefit by using an elevated toilet seat.

Autosomal Recessive Muscular Dystrophy

LIMB-GIRDLE TYPE

Limb-girdle type of muscular dystrophy is transmitted by an autosomal recessive trait. However, sporadic cases are not uncommon. Although the age at onset is extremely variable, the disease frequently begins in the second or third decade and occasionally in middle life. If it starts in the fourth decade or later, it progresses rapidly with the likely outcome that the patient will become confined to a wheelchair within 3 years of onset. All members of a family seem to have the same degree of severity of illness.

Initial weakness is noted in either the pelvic or the shoulder girdle. There is a variable but generally slow rate of progression. Severe disability and contractures are uncommon. By the time patients become wheelchair bound, they have reached skeletal maturation and the relative growth disproportion between muscle and bone has been avoided. However, many patients who remain borderline ambulators do develop severe and intractable low back pain because of excessive lordosis and lumbar degenerative arthritis.

Pelvic-Girdle Type

In 1876 Leyden[34] first described pelvic-girdle type of muscular dystrophy, which is more common than scapulohumeral dystrophy. Distribution of weakness and clinical presentation are similar to the Duchenne type. The iliopsoas, gluteus maximus, and quadriceps usually are affected early in the disease. Often a degree of shoulder-girdle involvement occurs early in the disease. The serrati, trapezius, rhomboids, latissimi, and the sternal portion of the pectoralis major are most often involved. The scapulae may wing but do not migrate upward and laterally as in facioscapulohumeral dystrophy (Fig. 2-40). There is preferential weakness and atrophy of the biceps, which are marked even in mild cases and prove to be important diagnostic findings. The disease spreads to involve the clavicular portion of the pectoralis major, and weakness

may later involve the extensors and flexors of the wrist and fingers. Deltoid involvement occurs late. Asymmetrical weakness and wasting of muscles may occur. If the disease remains limited predominantly to the hips and thighs, or to the shoulders and arms, a better prognosis usually can be expected. Differential diagnosis includes the Kugelberg–Welander syndrome as well as congenital and metabolic myopathies.

Shoulder-Girdle Type

The scapulohumeral form described by Erb in 1884 is rare.[19] It presents with weakness in the serratus anterior, trapezius, and rhomboids. Involvement of the pelvic-girdle muscles may not occur for many years. Both forms of limb-girdle dystrophy are distinguished from Duchenne dystrophy by the fact that approximately only 20% of patients develop pseudohypertrophy of the calf muscles. Cardiac involvement or intellectual impairment is uncommon. Muscle biopsy demonstrates considerable variation in the size of fibers and shows numerous internal nuclei and splitting of fibers. In addition, the fibers demonstrate a "moth-eaten" appearance, and whorled fi-

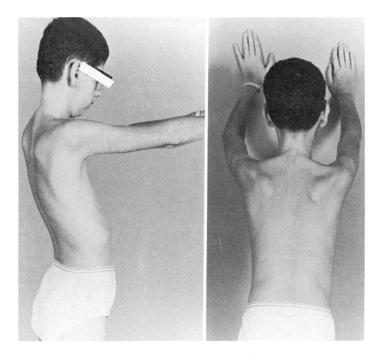

FIG. 2-40. Compare the position of this adolescent's scapulae with those of the patient in Figure 2-44.

bers may also be noted. The CPK is usually slightly or moderately elevated. Usually death occurs before age 40 from cardiopulmonary complications.

Autosomal Dominant Muscular Dystrophy

FACIOSCAPULOHUMERAL DYSTROPHY

Facioscapulohumeral dystrophy, considered the most benign form of muscular dystrophy, is transmitted as an autosomal dominant trait.[33] The degree of severity and age at onset are more variable than in almost any other neuromuscular disease. Within a family, mild and severe cases may be seen in both the same and different generations.

Onset occurs at any age from childhood to adult life. Typically the disease becomes evident at the end of the first or during the second decade of life. A child of an affected adult may show facial weakness in the first decade (Fig. 2-41). This may precede scapulohumeral muscle involvement or it may be noted concurrently. The progressive weakness continues for decades and is associated with periods of relatively rapid deterioration. Cardiopulmonary compromise may cause death in early adult life.

Facial weakness is evidenced by the patient's inability to purse the lips or drink through a straw, whistle, blow, or puff out the cheeks. During sleep the eyes may remain open slightly. Facial examination may demonstrate a small dimple on either side of the mouth. Wasting of the neck muscles allows the medial clavicles to jut forward forming a distinct step at the base of the neck (Fig. 2-42). The

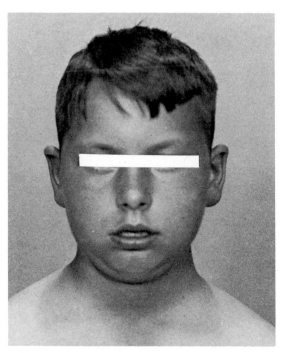

FIG. 2-41. Lack of forehead wrinkles and a transverse smile result from facial muscle weakness.

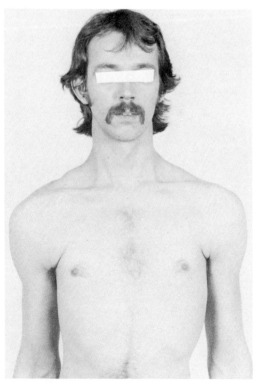

FIG. 2-42. The clavicles resume a horizontal position because of the weight of the upper extremities and weakness of the trapezius. A prominence at the sternoclavicular joint also can be seen.

clavicles lie horizontally and the shoulders droop. Involvement of the trapezius allows the scapulae to ride upward and forward.

Upper-Extremity Involvement

When the upper arm and shoulder muscles become involved, the patient is unable to lift objects above shoulder level. The serrati anterior, trapezius, rhomboids, and latissimus dorsi are generally involved. The deltoids may be surprisingly well preserved in many cases, creating a "Popeye" type of physical appearance (Fig. 2-43). Even in cases where the deltoids are not involved, the muscles lose their mechanical advantage because of lack of shoulder stability, which causes marked reduction in active abduction and flexion. With attempted abduction the scapulae ride farther forward and upward and the inferior angle wings (Fig. 2-44). The trapezius and biceps are involved early and may waste rapidly.

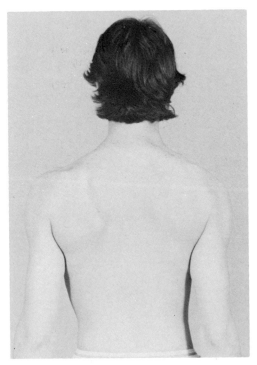

FIG. 2-43. Sparing of the deltoid is an important sign in determining patients who would benefit from scapular stabilization. This patient is able to abduct the upper extremities beyond 90° when the scapulae are stabilized manually.

TREATMENT

Copeland has found thoracoscapular fusion to be effective in managing patients who have symptomatic winging of the scapula but who retain a functional deltoid.[12] He noted that the ability to sustain flexion and abduction was important for the patient's function. He utilized tibial cortical grafts with screw fixation. For this procedure the patient is placed in the prone position with the upper extremities hanging over the side of the table. This places the scapula in the optimal position, with the scapular vertebral border 5 cm to 7 cm lateral to the spinous process. A surgical incision is made along the vertebral edge of the scapula. Approximately 2 cm on both the deep and superficial aspects of the scapula are denuded. The parietal pleura is separated from three ribs, usually the fourth, fifth, and sixth. A screw is passed through a drillhole made in both the scapula and tibial grafts and then through both cortices of the rib. Postoperative management is in a shoulder spica cast with the shoulder in 80° of abduction and 30° of flexion. The cast is bivalved at 3 months and the upper section is removed so that active abduction can be instituted. The procedure generally is done bilaterally, and Copeland reports excellent cosmetic results with an average range of abduction of 100° and flexion of 90°.

I have found thoracoscapular fusion to be beneficial for patients whose occupation requires the ability to sustain flexion and abduction. Preoperatively, the surgeon must assess the patient carefully to determine the optimal position for the scapula. I prefer the interposition of iliac bicortical grafts between the denuded scapula and the ribs.

Lower-Extremity Involvement

Later in the course of the disease, patients may develop footdrop because of paresis of the peroneal nerve musculature. The calf muscles become stronger than the tibialis anterior and the dorsiflexors. A polypropylene ankle–foot orthosis may be required for clinical management. Occasionally bilateral quadriceps weakness develops that requires the use of a unilateral knee–ankle–foot orthosis for the weaker limb. Fitting the patient with two long leg braces will seriously impede

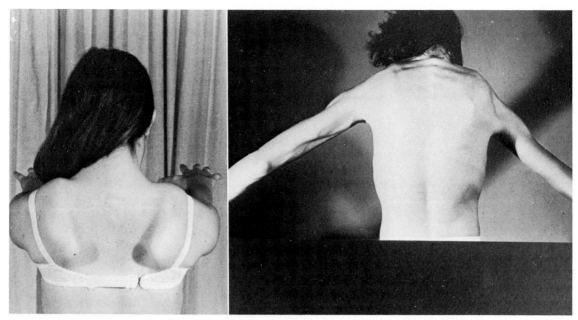

FIG. 2-44. Bilateral scapular winging and elevation demonstrate diffuse shoulder-girdle involvement. Scapular stabilization is not attempted when there is atrophy of the deltoids. (Courtesy of Newington Children's Hospital)

the patient's ability to rise from a chair. Hypertrophy of the extensor digitorum brevis occurs, a physical finding which is important in differentiating these patients from those with hereditary motor sensory disease. Deep-tendon reflexes, especially proximal reflexes, are lost early.

In the severely involved juvenile patient, there may be marked weakness of the wrist extensor, which leads to wristdrop. Wrist flexors maintain their normal strength. It may be necessary for the patient to use a functional upper-extremity orthosis since the hand itself remains functional.

Both scoliosis and lordosis may occur in these patients. They may have a functional lordosis that compensates for weakness in the pelvic girdle, but which may become structural and so severe that the sacrum assumes a horizontal plane (Fig. 2-45). Also the lordosis may extend into the thoracic area, particularly in skeletally immature patients who develop a paralytic pattern of scoliosis. Eventually the compensatory lordosis may lead to spondylosis and back pain, which seriously jeopardize the patient's ambulatory status. A flexible corset may relieve the back symptoms without nullifying the necessary func-

tional lordosis. Scoliosis without marked lordosis can be controlled by using a Milwaukee brace in the ambulatory skeletally immature patient. The thoracic suspension orthosis helps the nonambulatory patient by controlling both the lordosis and the scoliosis (Fig. 2-46). Posterior spinal fusion, either the Harrington or segmental stabilization method, may be required to control progressive curves.

Infantile Facioscapulohumeral Dystrophy

Infantile facioscapulohumeral dystrophy may present before the age of 1 year. One parent usually has mild facial weakness. An absence of smiling and drooling may be the presenting complaint. The eyes may remain open during sleep. The infantile form progresses more rapidly, resulting in total paralysis of the face and severe crippling and weakness of other major muscle groups. The patient is usually in a wheelchair by age 9. Since the upper extremities remain functional, the use of a motorized transporter may be important for activity (Fig. 2-47). A Möbius type of facial weakness may also be present and progress asymmetrically, at a relatively slow pace.[27]

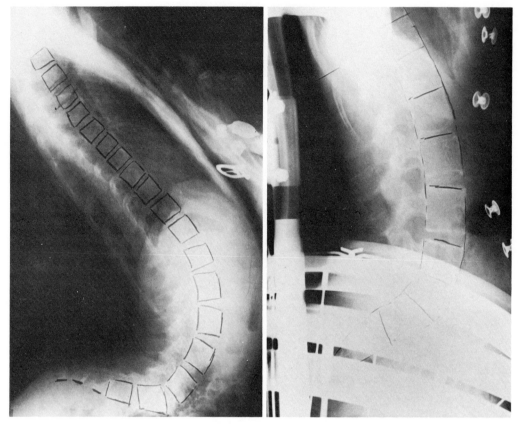

FIG. 2-45. The release of fixed hip-flexion contractures by Ober fasciotomies can reduce lumbar lordosis. The use of a thoracic suspension orthosis maintains the correction.

Scapuloperoneal Dystrophy

Scapuloperoneal dystrophy is a variant of facioscapulohumeral dystrophy. The peroneal and tibialis anterior muscles are involved early in the disease. Footdrop is an early complaint (Fig. 2-48), followed shortly by shoulder weakness, which is a typical symptom of facioscapulohumeral dystrophy. Approximately one half of these patients will develop facial weakness. Muscle biopsy is required for definitive diagnosis, because adults with nemaline myopathy may have the same progression of symptoms. The disease can be differentiated from the hereditary motor neuropathies by the presence of hypertrophy of the extensor digitorum brevis. Footdrop is managed primarily by orthoses.

A neuronal form of facioscapulohumeral distribution also has been identified. This disease progresses slowly. These patients can be clinically separated from dystrophy patients who are ambulatory by the presence of elbow flexion contractures which develop early in the disease (Fig. 2-49). This latter problem can be treated successfully with serial casts. Severe limitation of neck and trunk motion also may occur.

Ocular Dystrophy

Ocular dystrophy is a rare form of dystrophy the onset of which occurs in the teenage years.

Extraocular motor muscles are affected, resulting in diplopia and ptosis or strabismus, followed by limitation of ocular movements. Facial muscles, especially the frontalis and the orbicularis oculi, usually are involved. Approximately one half of these patients develop dysphagia. The disease progresses slowly and frequently involves the shoulder girdle; the pelvis may be involved later. Symptoms can be differentiated from those of myasthenia gravis because they are not related to fatigue and do not respond to edrophonium chloride (Tensilon). It should also be noted that these patients are extremely sensitive to curare.

Oculopharyngeal Dystrophy

Oculopharyngeal dystrophy is particularly common in French Canadians. Onset is in the third decade. Pharyngeal-muscle involvement results in dysarthria and dysphagia. Weakness of the hips and shoulder girdle is frequently noted.

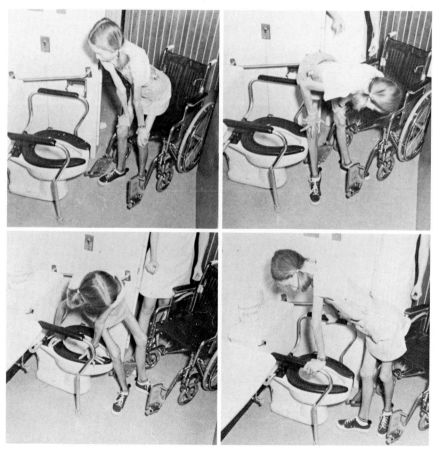

FIG. 2-46. Retained upper-extremity function permits independence with the thoracic suspension orthosis in many critical activities.

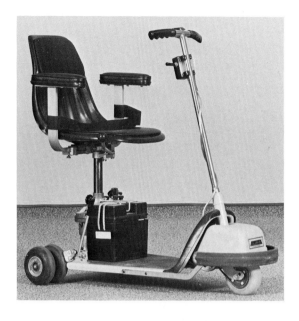

FIG. 2-47. A motorized transporter helps patients with neuromuscular disease retain functional upper extremities.

Distal Dystrophy

Distal dystrophy is transmitted as an autosomal dominant trait and is particularly common in Sweden. Onset of this rare disease[24] is after age 45. Initially the small hand muscles are involved; then clumsiness increases, and loss of fine-motor coordination is noted. The disease slowly spreads proximally. In the lower extremity, footdrop, which results from weakness of the tibialis anterior, as well as intrinsic wasting are noted. Physical examination demonstrates wasting of the intrinsic muscles of the hand, especially the thenar mass. Patients cannot fully extend their fingers and may develop wristdrop. Results from an electromyogram and muscle biopsy are compatible with those seen in a myopathy.

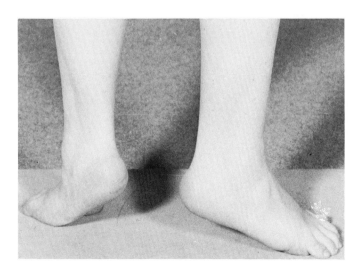

FIG. 2-48. Fixed equinus requires surgical correction before ankle-foot orthoses can be used.

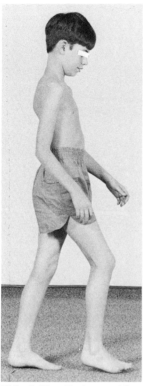

FIG. 2-49. Patients with a neuronal form may develop fixed contractures in the upper extremities. This is not found in other forms of facioscapulo-humeral dystrophy.

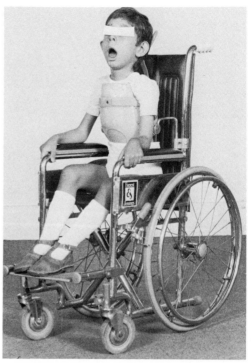

FIG. 2-50. Facial and neck muscle involvement is found in this 3-year-old with multiple fixed-extremity contractures.

Congenital Dystrophy

Congenital dystrophy is transmitted by an autosomal recessive pattern. The patient presents as a "floppy baby."[57,59] The mother may have noticed a decrease in fetal activity during the third trimester of pregnancy. There is generalized muscle weakness of the limbs and trunk that initially is greater proximally but later becomes generalized. Respiratory and facial muscles are involved (Fig. 2-50), and dysphagia may be noted in the newborn. Characteristic features include hypotonia and contractures at birth.

The most progressive and active phase of muscle degeneration takes place prior to birth. Motor milestones are delayed and there are long periods of clinical stability. Some functional improvement occurs during childhood, with little or no progression noted thereafter.

The contractures (Fig. 2-51) represent a "burnt-out" state in which cicatrix develops.[59] Initially deep-tendon reflexes are present but are lost later. Congenital contractures are amenable to nonsurgical treatment but will progress if they are not treated.[32] These contractures tend to recur during the second and third years. Extraocular motor muscles are spared and facial muscles may not be affected. Proximal and distal muscles are involved equally. Orthopaedic problems include bilateral clubfeet, torticollis, scoliosis (Fig. 2-52), and congenital dislocated hips.

The infant's CPK level may be as high as 1350 U/liter. Muscle biopsy may reveal extensive replacement of fat or collagen, or both, which is out of proportion to fiber necrosis or to the patient's strength.

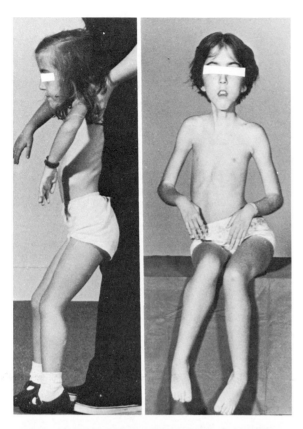

FIG. 2-51. Progression of contractures over a 4-year period during the first decade is shown.

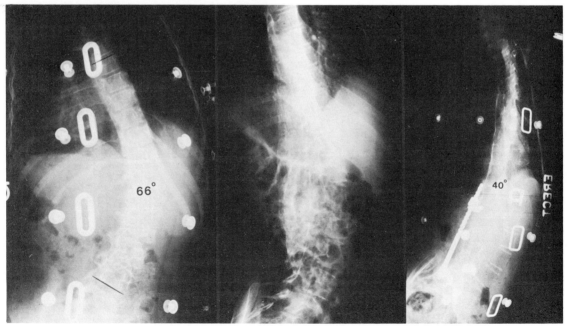

FIG. 2-52. Despite a solid fusion of a neuromuscular scoliosis to the mid-lumbar area, this dystrophic patient's sitting balance deteriorated because the initial fusion did not extend to the pelvis.

REFERENCES

1. Aberion G, Alba A, Lee MH, Solomon M: Pulmonary care of Duchenne type muscular dystrophy. NY State J Med 73:1206, May 15, 1973
2. Adams RD, Denny–Brown D, Pearson CM: Diseases of Muscle. A Study in Pathology, ed. 2. New York, Harper & Row, 1962
3. Alexander MA, Johnson EW, Petty J, Stauch D: Mechanical ventilation of patients with late stage Duchenne muscular dystrophy: Management in the home. Arch Phys Med Rehabil 60:289, 1979
4. Appenzeller O, Orgin G: Pathogenesis of muscular dystrophies. Arch Neurol 32:2, 1975
5. Becker PE: Two new families of benign sex-linked recessive muscular dystrophy. Rev Can Biol 21:551, 1962
6. Bowker JH, Halpin PJ: Factors determining success in reambulation of the child with progressive muscular dystrophy. Orthop Clin North Am 9(2):431, 1978
7. Bradley WG, Jones MZ, Mussini JM, Fawcett PR: Becker-type muscular dystrophy. Muscle Nerve 1:111, 1978
8. Bunch WH: Muscular dystrophy. In Hardy JH (ed): Spinal Deformity in Neurological and Muscular Disorders. St Louis, CV Mosby, 1974
9. Burke SS, Grove NM, Houser CR, Johnson DM: Respiratory aspects of pseudohypertrophic muscular dystrophy. Am J Dis Child 121:230, 1971
10. Cherry DB: Transfer technique for children with muscular dystrophy. Phys Ther 53:970, 1973
11. Chyatte SB, Long C, Vignos PJ: The balanced forearm orthosis in muscular dystrophy. Arch Phys Med Rehabil 46:633, 1965
12. Copeland SA, Howard RC: Thoracoscapular fusion for facioscapulohumeral dystrophy. J Bone Joint Surg 60B:547, 1978
13. Curtis BH: Orthopaedic management of muscular dystrophy and related disorders. Instruc Course Lect 19:78, 1970
14. Dorando C, Newman MK: Bracing for severe scoliosis of muscular dystrophy patients. Phys Ther Rev 37:230, 1957
15. Dubowitz V: Muscle Disorders in Childhood. Philadelphia, WB Saunders, 1978
16. Dubowitz V, Brooke MH: Muscle Biopsy: A Modern Approach. London, WB Saunders, 1973
17. Duchenne GB: Recherches sur la paralysie musculaire pseudo-hypertrophique ou paralysie myosclérosique. Archives Génerales de Médicine 11:5, 179, 305, 421, 552, 1868
18. Emery AE, Watt MS, Clack ER: The effects of genetic counselling in Duchenne muscular dystrophy. Clin Genet 3:147, 1972
19. Erb W: Über die 'juvenile form' der progressiven Muskelatrophie ihre Beziehunger zur sogennanten Pseudohypertrophie der Muskeln. Dtsch Arch Klin Med 34:467, 1884
20. Fisk JR, Bunch WH: Scoliosis in neuromuscular disease. Orthop Clin North Am 10(4):863, 1979
21. Florence JM, Brooke MH, Carroll JE: Evaluation of the child with muscular weakness. Orthop Clin North Am 9(2):49, 1978
22. Flynn I, Schwetz K, Williams D: Muscular dystrophy: Comprehensive nursing care. Nurs Clin North Am 14:123, 1979
23. Gibson DA, Wilkins KE: The management of spinal deformities in Duchenne muscular dystrophy. Clin Orthop 108:41, 1975
24. Gowers WR: A lecture on myopathy of a distal form. Br Med J 2:89, 1902
25. Gowers WR: Pseudohypertrophic Muscular Paralysis. London, J&A Churchill, 1879
26. Gucker T, III: The orthopaedic management of progressive muscular dystrophy. J Am Phys Ther Assoc 44:243, 1964
27. Hanson PA, Rowland LP: Möbius syndrome and facioscapulohumeral muscular dystrophy. Arch Neurol 24:31, 1971
28. Hudgson P, Pearce GW, Walton JN: Preclinical muscular dystrophy: Histopathological changes observed on muscle biopsy. Brain 90:565, 1967
29. Inkley SR, Oldenburg FC, Vignos PJ: Pulmonary function in Duchenne muscular dystrophy related to stage of disease. Am J Med 56:297, 1974
30. Jerusalem F, Engel AG, Gomez MR: Duchenne dystrophy. II. Morphometric study of the muscle microvasculature. Brain 97:115, 1974
31. Johnson EW, Kennedy JH: Comprehensive management of Duchenne muscular dystrophy. Arch Phys Med Rehabil 52:110, 1971
32. Jones R, Khan R, Hughes S, Dubowitz V: Congenital muscular dystrophy. The importance of early diagnosis and orthopaedic management in the long-term prognosis. J Bone Joint Surg 61B:13, 1979
33. Landouzy L, Déjérine J: De la myopathie atrophique progressive (myopathie héréditaire), débutant, dans l'enfance, par le face, sans altération du système nerveux. C R Acad Sci Paris, 98:53, 1884
34. Leyden E: Klinik der Ruckenmarks–Krankheiten, vol 2. Berlin, Hirschwalk, 1876
35. Marsh GG, Munsat TL: Evidence for early impairment of verbal intelligence in Duchenne muscular dystrophy. Arch Dis Child 49:118, 1974
36. Meryon E: On granular or fatty degeneration of the voluntary muscles. Trans Med Chir Soc Edin 35:72, 1852
37. Ober FR: The role of the iliotibial band and fascia lata as a factor in the causation of lowback disabilities and sciatica. J Bone Joint Surg 18:105, 1936
38. Robin GC, Brief LP: Scoliosis in childhood muscular dystrophy. J Bone Joint Surg 53A:466, 1971
39. Roses AD, Roses MJ, Miller SE, Hull KL, Appel SH: Carrier detection in Duchenne muscular dystrophy. N Engl J Med 294:193, 1976
40. Sanyal SK, Leung RK, Tierney RC, Gilmartin R, Pitner S: Mitral valve prolapse syndrome in children with Duchenne's progressive muscular dystrophy. Pediatrics 63:116, 1979
41. Seay AR, Ziter FA, Thompson JA: Cardiac arrest during induction of anesthesia in Duchenne muscular dystrophy. J Pediatr 93:88, 1978
42. Shohet SB, Layzer RB: The "muscle" of the red cell. N Engl J Med 294:221, 1976
43. Siegel IM: The management of muscular dystrophy. A clinical review. Muscle Nerve 1:453, 1978
44. Siegel IM: Scoliosis in muscular dystrophy. Clin Orthop 93:235, 1973
45. Spencer GE Jr: Orthopaedic care of progressive muscular dystrophy. J Bone Joint Surg 49A:1201, 1967
46. Spencer GE Jr, Vignos PJ Jr: Bracing for ambulation

in childhood progressive muscular dystrophy. J Bone Joint Surg 44A:234, 1962

47. Tanaka K, Shimazu S, Oya N, Tomisawa M, Kusunoki T, Soyama K, Ono E: Muscular form of glycogenosis Type II (Pompe's disease). Pediatrics 63:124, 1979

48. Thomson WH, Leyburn P, Walton JN: Serum enzyme activity in muscular dystrophy. Br Med J 2(5208):1276, 1960

49. Vignos PJ Jr: Diagnosis of progressive muscular dystrophy. J Bone Joint Surg 49A:1212, 1967

50. Vignos PJ Jr, Spencer GE Jr, Archibald KC: Management of progressive muscular dystrophy in childhood. JAMA 184:89, 1963

51. Vignos PJ Jr, Watkins MP: The effect of exercise in muscular dystrophy. JAMA 197:843, 1966

52. Walton JN: Disorders of Voluntary Muscle. Boston, Little, Brown & Co, 1964

53. Wilkins KE, Gibson DA: The patterns of spinal deformity in Duchenne muscular dystrophy. J Bone Joint Surg 58A:24, 1976

54. Yates G: Molded plastics in bracing. Clin Orthop 102:46, 1974

55. Young PT: Spring-booster chairs for patients with muscular dystrophy. Phys Ther 52:1286, 1972

56. Yount CC: The role of the tensor fasciae femoris in certain deformities of the lower extremities. J Bone Joint Surg 8:171, 1926

57. Zellweger H, Afifi A, McCormick WF, Mergner W: Benign congenital muscular dystrophy: A special form of congenital hypotonia. Clin Pediatr 6:655, 1967

58. Zellweger H, Antonik A: Newborn screening for Duchenne muscular dystrophy. Pediatrics 5(1):30, 1975

59. Zellweger H, McCormick WF, Mergner W: Severe congenital muscular dystrophy. Am J Dis Child 114:591, 1967

60. Ziter FA, Allsop KG, Tyler FH: Assessment of muscle strength in Duchenne muscular dystrophy. Neurology 27:981, 1977

3

Myotonia and Other Disorders

MYOTONIC DISORDERS

Myotonic syndromes are characterized by the inability of skeletal muscle to relax after a strong contraction that results either from voluntary movement or mechanical stimulation.[17] Gradual relaxation may be prolonged over several seconds. This is demonstrated clinically by slow relaxation of a clenched fist or by persistent dimpling after a blow of the reflex hammer on a muscle belly, such as the thenar eminence (Fig. 3-1) or the tongue. With repetition of the same movement, myotonia decreases or disappears. An electromyogram demonstrates spontaneous myotonic bursts when the patient voluntarily contracts a muscle. There is a prolonged series of rhythmic activity that is of high frequency and high amplitude initially, but later gradually wanes in amplitude and slows down.

Myotonia Dystrophica (Steinert's Disease)

Myotonic dystrophy is a steadily progressive, diffuse, systemic disease in which myotonia and muscular atrophy are accompanied by gonadal atrophy, cataracts, frontal baldness (Fig. 3-2), heart disease, and mental deficiency. The disease is transmitted as an autosomal dominant trait and usually occurs in

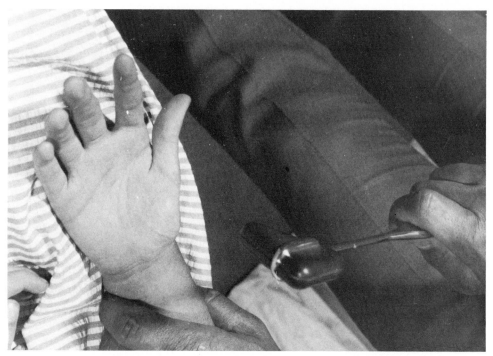

FIG. 3-1. Dimpling and prolonged adduction contracture of the thumb follow a blow of the reflex hammer on the thenar eminence.

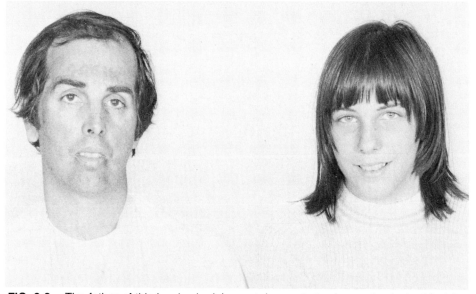

FIG. 3-2. The father of this involved adolescent demonstrates increasing lack of facial expression and frontal baldness.

late adolescence or early adult life. Marked variability in severity may be noted within an individual family. A slowly progressive weakness affects distal muscles more than the hips or shoulders. As the disease spreads slowly proximally, it involves the quadriceps and hamstrings. The lower extremities are more involved than the upper extremities. Initially, the most common complaint is difficulty in walking or weakness of the hands. Inability to release the hand grasp is another early symptom. As the weakness progresses, myotonia tends to disappear. The earlier the disease begins, the more severe the involvement of the bulbar musculature. Symptom-free preadolescents with bilateral temporal muscular atrophy, or teenagers with frontal baldness and gonadal atrophy, can be expected to follow the classic course of weakness and myotonia. Mental retardation or dementia is part of the syndrome, making the patient an unreliable historian who may deny the illness, length of illness, or the involvement of other family members.

Physical examination reveals an expressionless facies with a fish-mouth which is difficult to close (Fig. 3-3). Weakness of the orbicularis oculi leads to ptosis. Frontal baldness may be evident. Marked wasting of the

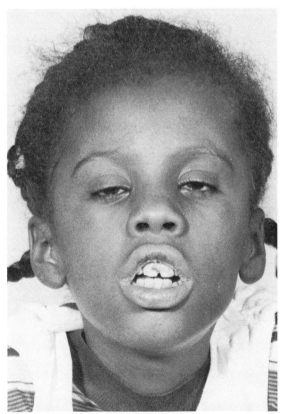

FIG. 3-3. A 5-year-old daughter of an involved woman shows lack of forehead wrinkling, ptosis, and a fish-mouth appearance.

neck muscles, especially the flexors, creates a slender neck. An early diagnostic clue is extreme weakness of the sternocleidomastoid muscle.[10] Wasting also occurs in the temporal and masseter muscles and results in hollowing of the muscles around the temple and jaw. Bulbar paralysis causes speech disturbances and difficulty in swallowing.

Myotonia is most pronounced in the hand grasp but may also be detected by percussion of the tongue and thenar eminence. Because myotonia tends to disappear as weakness progresses, a patient with severe wasting and weakness of the hands and forearms should be examined for myotonia of the elbow or shoulder. Deep-tendon reflexes are diminished or absent. Footdrop may be apparent. Examination of the back may demonstrate a structural scoliosis in the adolescent (Fig. 3-4).

An ophthalmologic slit-lamp examination done in children demonstrates no abnormalities. In adolescents, polychromatic spots are found under the anterior and posterior capsules of the eyes. Cataracts, which are found in the same area, are rare before adolescence. However, in the later stages of the disease, they often develop and are either radiating or stellate in formation.

Aural characteristics of an electromyogram resemble the mooing of a cow or the sound of a dive bomber. These myotonic discharges may occur in the young patient before clinical myotonia can be elicited and thus can be used to identify asymptomatic relatives.[52] Patients with the Schwartz–Jampel syndrome can be differentiated because their electromyogram, which lacks the waxing and waning of myotonia, has a repetitive activity of high frequency that can be eliminated by curare.

The biceps brachii is the best muscle to use for biopsy.[14] Histologically, multiple internal nuclei are present with an increased number of ring fibers that are superimposed on a myopathic-appearing biopsy. Atrophy of Type-1 fibers and hypertrophy of Type-2 fibers have been noted. Enzyme studies are nonspecific.

An electrocardiogram (ECG) shows changes characteristic of conduction defects, even though clinical symptoms of heart disease are not present. Adult patients may develop the Stokes–Adams type of cardio-

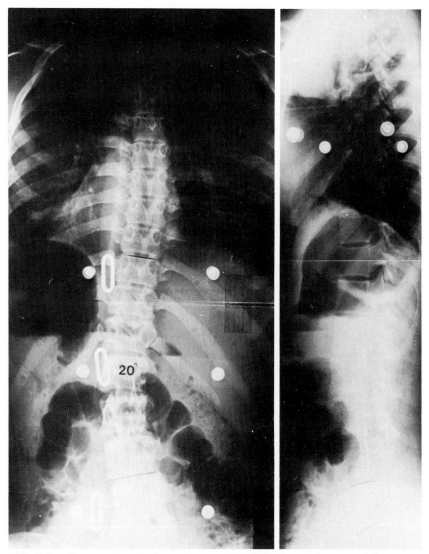

FIG. 3-4. Structural scoliosis rarely exceeds 30° in the adolescent. A few patients require orthotic control. The straight spine seen in the lateral roentgenogram is commonly found in myotonic dystrophy.

myopathy. Stroke has been associated with mitral valve prolapse.[15]

Clinically, the patient's condition deteriorates steadily with most patients losing the ability to ambulate within 15 to 20 years from onset. Postural drainage may be required because of severe pulmonary insufficiency caused by diaphragm and intercostal involvement. Death usually occurs in the fifth and sixth decades of life from chest infection or cardiac failure. The patient is at risk during surgery, especially when respiratory depressants such as thiopentone, barbiturates, and morphine are used. Obstetrical complications are common and include premature onset of labor and postpartum hemorrhage because of the inability of the uterus to contract after delivery. Hydramnios, an ominous sign, generally is associated with perinatal death.

Orthopaedic management may be required during the chronic phase. Weakness of the neck muscles may cause a painful subluxation of the cervical spine making it difficult for the patient to raise the head from a supine position. A soft cervical collar affords relief of this symptom. Ankle–foot orthoses afford control of drop-foot deformity.[70] Eventually, diffuse muscle weakness and increasing difficulty in maintaining balance will force the patient to accept a wheelchair level of activity. Scoliosis may be noted in adolescence (Fig. 3-5) but does not progress to the point where spinal fusion is required.

Myotonia Dystrophica in Infancy

Myotonic dystrophy is not common in infancy and childhood.[51,71] The newborn presents with hypotonia, facial diplegia, and diminished sucking and swallowing. Tube feedings may be necessary.[5,36,37,46,75] The expressionless facies has a triangular fish-shape mouth with the upper lip in the form of an inverted "V" (Fig. 3-6). The eyes cannot be closed completely. Approximately one half of these infants have rigid talipes equinovarus that has been associated with hydramnios and decreased fetal movement. Congenital dislocated hips have also been noted. Although fatal respiratory problems may occur in the newborn, prolonged survival is the rule after infancy. Swallowing improves after age 8 months. Cleft lip or palate, micrognathia, and a high-arched palate, as well as congenital heart disease, may be present. Later findings include a delay in motor development and hypotonia, which persists for many years. Delayed motor milestones may result in an awkward gait in the second year of life. Myotonia is not present clinically or demonstrated by an electromyogram until the latter half of the first decade of life. In later childhood, myotonia plus classic wasting of the sternocleidomastoid and temporal muscles are

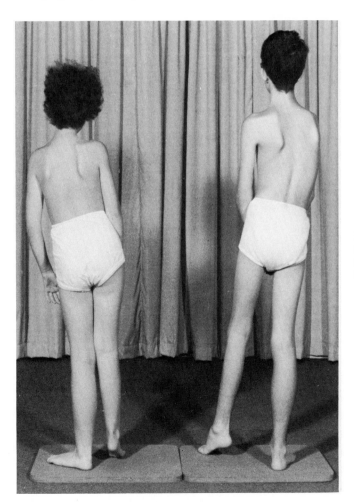

FIG. 3-5. Brother and sister of an affected mother demonstrate lordoscoliosis and pes cavus deformities. (Courtesy of Newington Children's Hospital)

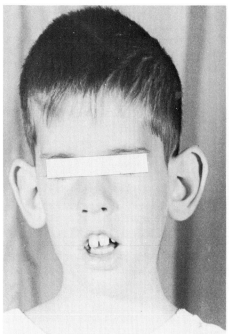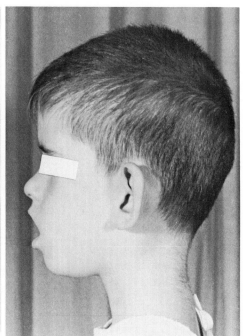

FIG. 3-6. A bland facies with a fish-mouth appearance is the hallmark of infantile myotonic dystrophy.

noted. Most patients show a steady improvement in motor function during the first decade of life, but subsequently weakness and wasting gradually increase.

These infants are almost always the offspring of an affected mother who often has forme fruste of the disease. Careful examination may demonstrate maternal subclinical or overt myotonia dystrophica. Even when she is symptom-free, mild facial weakness and fist myotonia can be demonstrated. Occasionally this form does not become apparent until 5 to 15 years of age when ptosis, facial diplegia, and myotonia are found. A combination of facial weakness and glossopharyngeal myotonia causes dyslalia and dysarthria. There is a high frequency of nonprogressive, borderline, or frank mental retardation.[12] Characteristic lenticular opacities do not occur until after age 14. The disease can be differentiated clinically from other forms of hypotonia by its multi-system pattern. An electromyogram may be required to rule out spinal muscular atrophy. Muscle biopsy will differentiate the disease from spinal muscular atrophy and congenital myopathies.

Talipes equinovarus or limited dorsiflex-

ion may be noted in infancy. Correction can be obtained by applying serial plaster casts and is maintained by bracing. The deformities will recur if immobilization is discontinued prematurely. Surgical correction may be required if the contracture is severe.

These patients are also prone to develop forefoot equinus which requires intrinsic release and long-term use of an ankle–foot orthosis (Fig. 3-7). A child with peroneal muscle weakness who develops talipes equinovarus will benefit from a Dwyer calcaneal osteotomy combined with a split anterior tibial transfer (Fig. 3-8). Persistent forefoot adduction can be managed by metatarsal osteotomies. These patients tend to develop contractures of other major joints in the lower extremities. Also they are very sensitive to anesthetics, particularly respiratory depressants, which may cause sudden death. Patients remain ambulatory until early adult life.

Myotonia Congenita (Thomsen's Disease)

Severity of myotonia congenita varies considerably. Usually it is present at birth, but it may not manifest itself until after age 10. My-

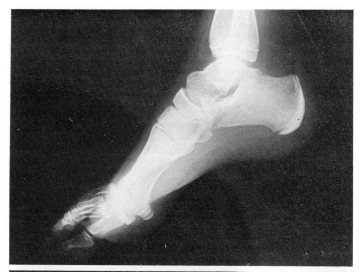

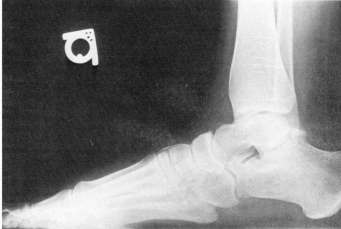

FIG. 3-7. An intrinsic release followed by corrective serial casts and long-term use of an ankle-foot orthosis is required to keep the feet plantigrade.

otonia is widespread and more marked in the lower extremities.[67,74] It is most evident with an initial movement; repetitive movement decreases the myotonia and facilitates later movements. Some patients appear herculean because of generalized muscle hypertrophy (Fig. 3-9). Patients with myotonia congenita have no associated weakness and none of the other endocrine or systemic abnormalities noted with myotonia dystrophica. This disease is compatible with a normal life span. The patient's disability is not great when the limits of the disease have been accepted. Procainamide and diphenylhydantoin (Dilantin) have both been used successfully in decreasing the myotonia, but they should be used only in severe cases.[30]

Paramyotonia Congenita (Eulenburg's Disease)

Paramyotonia congenita, which manifests itself in childhood, is characterized by episodes of paradoxical myotonia and flaccid paresis and is precipitated by exposure to cold.[69] Dystrophic features are absent, and the disease does not improve. Exposing the hand to cold demonstrates the myotonia, which develops initially in the ring and little fingers, and then spreads to the rest of the hand. This disease is associated with an elevated or lowered serum potassium. Generalized muscular hypertrophy and permanent weakness may occur in long-standing cases. Generally, the myotonia is relieved by the use of quinine sulfate or utilization of ion exchange resins in cases of hyperkalemia.

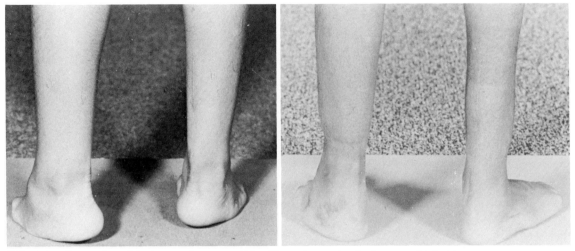

FIG. 3-8. Correction of foot varus is accomplished by calcaneal osteotomy and lateral plantar release. Muscle balance is achieved by placing the split anterior tibial transfer into the cuboid.

CONGENITAL MYOPATHIES

At birth, congenital myopathies present in the form of a "floppy baby." In early infancy or later in childhood, they present with features associated with muscle weakness.[20] The hypotonia is predominantly in the pelvic and shoulder girdles (Fig. 3-10). Some patients show generalized weakness or involvement of muscles innervated by cranial nerves. In most patients, involvement is mild, and generally the myopathies are nonprogressive. Inheritance usually follows an autosomal dominant pattern, but sporadic cases also occur. Serum enzymes are normal or slightly elevated. Electromyography demonstrates myopathic findings.

Differentiation of congenital myopathies is through histochemical and electron-microscopic evaluation of the structural changes within muscle.[23] The types include: 1) central core disease, 2) nemaline myopathy (rod body), 3) myotubular myopathy (centronuclear), and 4) congenital fiber-type disproportion.

Central Core Disease

Central core disease presents in infancy with hypotonia or delayed motor milestones.[61] Independent ambulation may not be achieved until 4 years of age. These children have an awkward form of running and are unable to jump. Distribution of muscle weakness may simulate Duchenne dystrophy, the lower extremities being more involved than the upper.[53] Other patients may demonstrate a more generalized weakness that spares only the facial and extraocular motor muscles. No deterioration in strength occurs, and the deep-tendon reflexes are retained. Muscle wasting is not marked. Congenital dislocated hip, flatfeet, pes cavus, lordoscoliosis, and dislocating patellae have occurred with this disease.[3]

Histochemical staining reveals that the center of the muscle fibers has been replaced with an amorphous substance devoid of oxidative and glycolytic enzymes. On electron microscopy, mitochondria and sarcoplasmic reticulum are absent in the core area. The disease appears to affect Type-1 fibers selectively.

Eng reports that these patients, particularly those with an elevated creatine phosphokinase (CPK) are more susceptible to malignant hyperthermia.[24] It is believed that there is an underlying defect in the sarcoplasmic reticulum that leads to an acute rise in the calcium within the aqueous sarcoplasm of the muscle fiber. Children and young adults, particularly males, are more commonly affected. In a susceptible person the attack may be induced by administering a skeletal muscle relaxant, especially a depolarizing agent such as succinylcholine chloride with or without the use of an inhalation

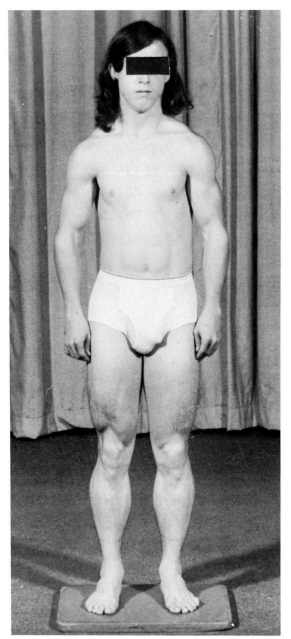

FIG. 3-9. Myotonia congenita, demonstrating generalized muscle hypertrophy. (Courtesy of Newington Children's Hospital)

rigid masseter muscle which makes intubation difficult. When succinylcholine chloride is used, there also may be excessive muscle fasciculations. The patient develops generalized and continuous rigor and the body temperature increases, often at an alarming rate. Profuse diapedesis, tachycardia, and tachypnea lead to metabolic acidosis with high blood lactate levels, hyperkalemia, and elevated serum CPK. Treatment must be prompt, since patients whose temperature exceeds 39° centigrade are unlikely to survive. Surgery and all anesthetic inhalation agents must be terminated.[40] The body temperature may be lowered with cooling blankets, ice packs, iced intravenous injections, or gastric or wound gavage. Careful monitoring of arterial gases permits early treatment of metabolic acidosis with sodium bicarbonate at an intravenous dose of 4 ml per kg of body weight. Hyperkalemia can be managed with insulin and glucose. Hyperventilation with 100% oxygen is also recommended. Dantrolene sodium is the drug of choice and is administered in the dose of 1 mg/kg/min up to 10 mg/kg for the total initial dose. The medication must be continued until all symptoms have been under control for at least 6 hours. Complications include a consumptive coagulopathy, renal shutdown from myoglobulinuria, and cardiac arrhythmia that leads to cardiac arrest. To prevent malignant hyperthermia, the physician should be suspicious when there is a history of anesthetic complications in the patient or his family, even when there is no history of neuromuscular disease. He must recognize that there is an increased risk of malignant hyperthermia in central core disease that requires close monitoring of patients who are given general anesthetics. Procaine is used as a local anesthetic, and nitrous oxide with barbituates, narcotics, or a neuroleptic drug are recommended as general anesthetics. Oral dantrolene sodium may be given the day before surgery in the dose of 1.5 mg/kg four times daily.

Nemaline Myopathy

Nemaline myopathy is more common in females. Most patients present in infancy or early childhood with a mild, nonprogressive myopathy.[60] An elongated facies with high-arched palate and a nasal, high-pitched voice are noted

anesthetic, especially halothane. Some patients experience episodes of malignant hyperthermia the first time such drugs are administered to them, but others are not affected until a second or later administration of the drug. The first sign of an attack is a

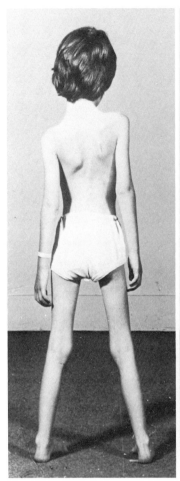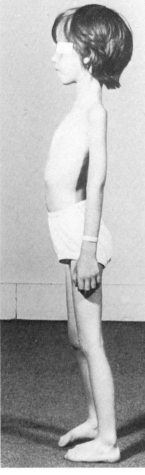

FIG. 3-10. A 6-year-old girl with progressive lordoscoliosis and femoral anteversion. A total-contact orthosis controls her spinal deformity, but the combination of reduced lordosis and pelvic-girdle weakness necessitates the use of a walker.

frequently. Skeletal changes may resemble those in arachnodactyly. There is generalized hypotonia, muscle wasting, and small muscle masses. Scoliosis (Fig. 3-11), pectus carinatum, and pes cavus have been reported. Facial weakness may be accompanied by a webbed neck or sternocleidomastoid weakness. Deep-tendon reflexes are decreased or absent. The autosomal dominant form is mild and nonprogressive. One third of the cases of nemaline myopathy are sporadic. The course may be fatal because of the severe involvement of pharyngeal and repsiratory muscles.[43] Patients with an early onset of this disease have a high incidence of respiratory infection.

LABORATORY DATA

The rods are easily overlooked on routine staining and do not show up on any of the histochemical enzyme reactions. When a Gomori trichrome stain is used, rod bodies become red, whereas muscle fibers appear blue-green. On electron microscopy the rods seem to be dense structures, usually rectangular in shape, and are in continuity with Z-bands. This may represent an abnormal deposition of Z-band material of a protein nature, possibly tropomyosin.

Myotubular Myopathy

Myotubular myopathy derives its name from the striking resemblance between the striated muscle in the biopsy and the myotubules of the fetus.[47,65] The patient presents with varying degrees of weakness generally noted in infancy, but occasionally the weakness may not become apparent until later in childhood (Fig. 3-12). There is generalized weakness of the

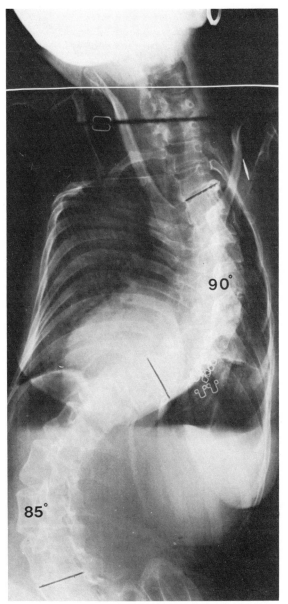

FIG. 3-11. Severe structural scoliosis in a 33-year old social worker with nemaline myopathy. The right shoulder is elevated to help maintain head balance. This grotesque deformity could have been prevented with current methods of correcting spinal deformity.

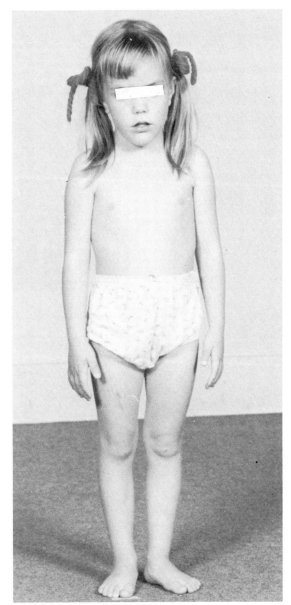

FIG. 3-12. Involvement of the extraocular and facial muscles causes the sad expression in a patient with myotubular myopathy.

axial musculature and neck flexors. Involvement of the extraocular and facial muscles may lead to a ptosis, squint, and a doleful expression. In early childhood these patients are subject both to asphyxia and recurrent, life-threatening, upper-respiratory infections.

The disease is nonprogressive and has been found in whites and blacks.

Histochemical studies reveal normal oxidative enzyme activity and unaffected fibers. Affected fibers have a central zone devoid of activity with adenosinetriphosphatase (ATPase) reaction and show an increased oxidative enzyme reaction. The majority of muscle fibers may demonstrate 1 to 4 centrally placed nuclei surrounded by an area devoid of myofibrils.

Congenital Fiber-Type Disproportion

Generalized hypotonia is noted at or shortly after birth. The degree of weakness may vary, and in some cases, it may progress during the first year of life. No progression has been noted after 2 years of age (Fig. 3-13). The majority of these patients eventually become ambulatory if life-threatening, recurrent respiratory infections are controlled during the first year of life. These patients are of short stature and have a high-arched palate. Contractures of the hands or feet and congenital dislocated hips were noted at birth in more than one half of the patients in Brooke's initial series.[11] Tor-

ticollis also has been reported. To prevent postural contractures from developing, the lower extremities should be splinted until the patient learns to walk. A minority of these patients will eventually achieve normal muscle strength. Neuromuscular scoliosis may be noted in the young child and can be successfully managed with a spinal orthosis until eventually a spinal arthrodesis is performed.

Some of these patients have been diagnosed as having spinal muscular atrophy Group I, which has a poor prognosis. The consistent clinical improvement of these patients after the first 2 years of life emphasizes the importance of establishing the correct diagnosis by muscle biopsy. On a normal biopsy Type-1 and Type-2 fibers are the same size. However, in this condition, the mean diameter of Type-

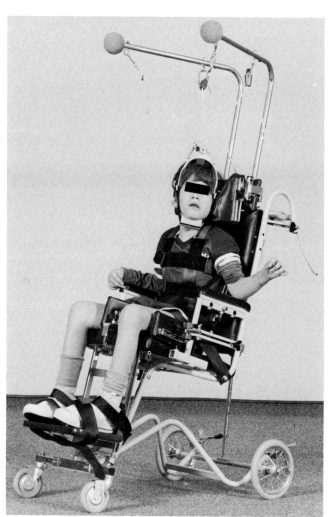

FIG. 3-13. Patients with congenital fiber-type disproportion may not gain independent head control. The Rancho-type of head suspension may provide valuable support.

1 fibers is smaller by a margin of at least 12%. There is frequently a Type 1-fiber predominance. Other laboratory studies are within normal limits.

Mitochondrial Myopathies

Mitochondrial myopathy represents a broad spectrum of metabolic abnormalities. Ragged-red fibers may be noted on the Gomori trichrome stain and the abnormal mitochondria, identified by electron microscopy, have giant bizarre forms. Weakness of the neck flexors and extraocular motor muscles occurs (Fig. 3-14), but facial weakness is absent. There is a consistent respiratory deficit, particularly on the forced expiratory volume (FEV) of pulmonary-function studies.

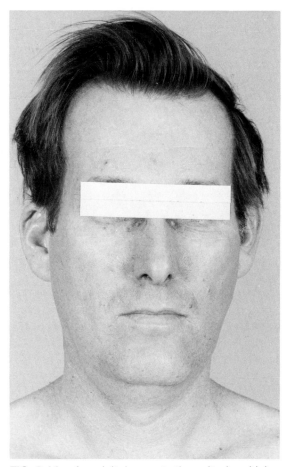

FIG. 3-14. An adult demonstrating mitochondrial facies with weakness of the neck flexors and extraocular motor muscles.

POMPE'S DISEASE (GLYCOGEN STORAGE DISEASE IIA)

A deficiency of α-1,4-glucosidase (acid maltase enzyme), which is required for glycogen metabolism, leads to the accumulation of glycogen in the lysozymes. The most severe form of glycogenosis (Pompe's disease) may clinically resemble spinal muscular atrophy, Group I. The infant appears normal for a few weeks but then develops severe hypotonia and an enlarged heart, liver, and tongue. The disease is progressive, and the child will die from cardiac and respiratory failure during the first year. This condition is distinguished from spinal muscular atrophy by the presence of myotonia on an electromyography and by a muscle biopsy.

Patients with milder forms of this disease may survive for several years. The age at onset of the disease and the pattern of the disease can mimic Duchenne muscular dystrophy. Like Duchenne patients, these patients demonstrate proximal weakness and their calf muscles develop a rubbery consistency. They develop heel-cord tightness and may or may not develop organomegaly. Affected adults develop girdle weakness, particularly in the pelvic area. Respiratory muscles become involved. The diagnosis is confirmed by a positive serum enzyme test, and a muscle biopsy distinguishes this type from limb-girdle dystrophy or polymyositis. Muscle biopsies demonstrate a vacuolar myopathy with excess glycogen apparent on the periodic acid-Schiff (PAS) stain.

THE INFLAMMATORY MYOPATHIES

Polymyositis and Dermatomyositis

Polymyositis is a protean disease with muscle weakness being the principal feature.[56] Polymyositis may present as an isolated disorder with clinical findings limited to muscle; if associated with skin manifestations, it is termed "dermatomyositis."[4,13,25] The disease is rare between the ages of 15 and 25. In childhood the disorder is always idiopathic and is not associated with malignancy. Dermatomyositis is more common in children than is polymyositis. The Brooke rule of thumb states "misery + muscle weakness = dermatomyositis," until proven otherwise.[23]

A febrile illness, immunization, or the

ingestion of drugs such as penicillin or sulfa may precipitate the onset of symptoms. The onset may be acute, insidious, or rapidly progressive leading to severe weakness, or the condition may remain mild. The child may present with systemic symptoms of a low-grade

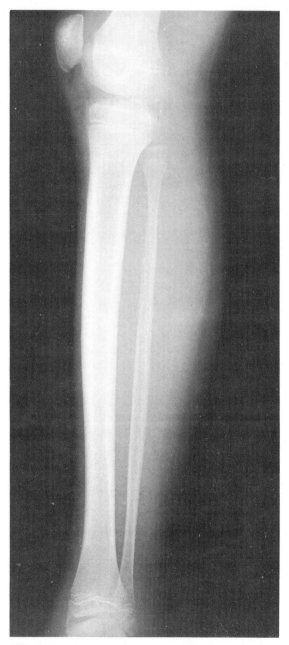

FIG. 3-15. In acute dermatomyositis, loss of soft-tissue shadows can be noted when there is soft-tissue swelling.

fever, malaise, listlessness, aching pain, and varying degrees of weakness in the shoulder and pelvic girdles (Fig. 3-15). An initial complaint may be difficulty in rising from the floor or climbing stairs. The appearance of Gowers' sign may cause confusion with Duchenne muscular dystrophy.

Dermatomyositis, more common in females, is rare before 2 years of age. Orbital edema, particularly of the upper eyelids, may be noted. Photosensitivity, common in dermatomyositis, may precipitate typical eruptions on the face and over the extensor surfaces of large and small joints. Erythema is noted over the extensor surfaces of the elbow and knee joints. The rash may appear before or after the onset of weakness. Characteristic skin lesions include a heliotropic or violaceous rash, particularly over the eyes and malar regions, in a classic butterfly distribution. This rash also may be noted on the upper chest and neck. Scaly erythematous lesions may develop over the metacarpal, phalangeal, and proximal interphalangeal joints (Gottrom's sign). The skin becomes discolored and thickened. Nodules may develop which will become necrotic and extrude calcified material.[48] This calcification is found only in severe cases and only when the disease is inactive (Fig. 3-16). In severe cases the skin changes are generalized, and the entire skin becomes tight, shiny, and red (Fig. 3-17).

In both polymyositis and dermatomyositis the muscles may become tender, brawny, and indurated as the disease progresses.[45] Approximately one third of the patients with polymyositis do not have pain accompanying the weakness. With polymyositis the discomfort is usually a deep ache or soreness made worse by continuing activity. The weakness in both disorders is symmetrical and begins proximally in the region of the pelvic girdle. Chronic dysphagia may develop with involvement of the oropharyngeal muscles. The remaining facial muscles are not involved. Weakness in the neck flexors is noted in contradistinction to myasthenia gravis where the posterior neck muscles are involved initially. The extremity weakness begins proximally and spreads distally as the disease progresses. Death may result from involvement of the respiratory musculature.[66]

The course is extremely variable, with spontaneous recovery to rapid fulminating

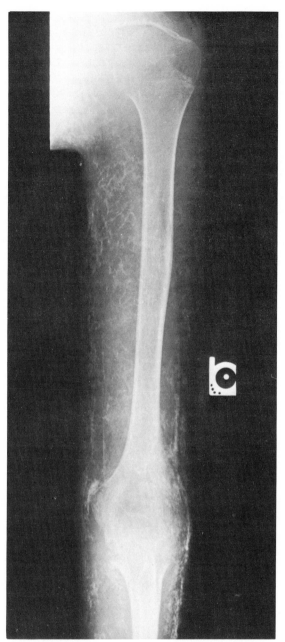

FIG. 3-16. The subcutaneous tissue may calcify when the dermatomyositis is inactive.

The diagnosis is made based on five major criteria[7,8]: (1) symmetrical weakness of the limb-girdle muscles and anterior neck flexors progressing over weeks to months with or without dysphagia or respiratory msucle involvement; (2) muscle biopsy necrosis of Types-1 and 2 fibers, phagocytosis, atrophy, and perifascicular distribution plus inflammatory exudate which is frequently perivascular; (3) an increase in skeletal muscle enzymes, particularly CPK, and, often, elevated adolase serum gluramic-oxaloacetic transaminase (SGOT) and serum glutamic-pyruvic transaminase (SGPT) levels; (4) an electromyographic record of short polyphasic motor units, fibrillation, and bizarre, high-frequency, repetitive discharges; and (5) dermatologic changes of lilac discoloration of the eyelids with periorbital edema and rash on the knees, elbows, malleoli, face, and upper torso. The diagnosis is established for dermatomyositis if the rash is accompanied by three or four of these criteria, probable if two criteria accompany the rash, and possible if one is found with the dermatologic condition. The diagnosis of polymyositis is established if four criteria are present, probable with three, and possible with two. The diagnosis is excluded if there is (1) evidence of central or peripheral neurologic disease, for example, fasciculation of long-tract signs, sensory change, decreased nerve conduction time or fiber-type atrophy and grouping on the muscle biopsy; and (2) muscle weakness that is slowly progressive and concurrent with a positive family history of Duchenne muscular dystrophy or calf enlargement. An infection such as trichinosis or toxoplasmosis also may indicate that this diagnosis is unlikely.

LABORATORY DATA

The CPK level and sedimentation rates frequently are elevated. Serial determinations in these studies may indicate activity of the myositis. The enzymes usually decrease 3 to 4 weeks before clinical improvement is noted in muscle strength and rise 5 to 6 weeks before clinical relapse. The sedimentation rate has been found to be of little practical use because it may return to normal levels when the acutely inflamed muscle responds to corticosteroid therapy.

Occasionally, children with classic clini-

death representing the extremes of the spectrum. Relapse must be guarded against. Bitnum reported that prior to the introduction of steroids, one third of the patients died of the disease, one third recovered with a minimal residual, and one third were left with moderate to severe physical restrictions.[6]

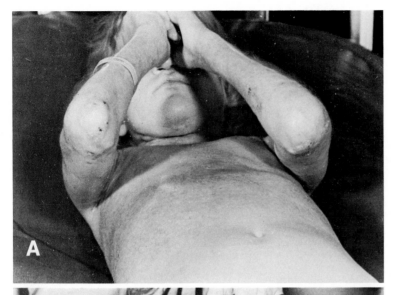

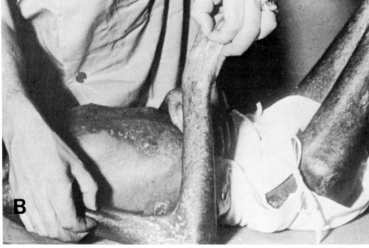

FIG. 3-17. **(A)** When ulcers persist, the thickened calcified tissue must be excised. **(B)** Chronic soft-tissue atrophy, subcutaneous calcifications, and contractures may develop. (Courtesy of Newington Children's Hospital)

cal dermatomyositis do not demonstrate elevations of CPK or erythrocyte sedimentation rates. Diagnosis is supported electromyographically by a record of polyphasic small, short motor unit potentials combined with fibrillation and bizarre, high-frequency, repetitive discharges. A baseline electromyogram is important because one of the most reliable early signs of effective treatment is the disappearance of fibrillation potentials; relapse is usually heralded by their reappearance. Muscle biopsy in children may show only minimal changes or the florid atrophy of all fiber types, particularly in a perifascicular distribution seen in adults. When a tumor is present in adults

with myositis, histopathologic examination shows no inflammation and phagocytosis despite massive necrosis of muscle.

MANAGEMENT OF THE ACUTE STAGE

Symptomatic management, including rest and moist heat, is necessary during the acute stage. Miller reports decreased mortality and morbidity rates in patients treated in this stage with adrenocorticosteroids.[45] The initial high dosage is reduced slowly until an effective level is reached. Dubowitz prefers a moderate dosage for short-term treatment.[21,22] He uses 1 mg per kg of body weight per day and recommends a gradual tapering of the drugs when progressive clinical remission is noted. He feels that long-term use causes a super-added steroid myopathy, which is a major complication of steroid treatment. Clinical response is a more reliable guide to prognosis than serum enzyme levels. The steroids are reduced every fourth day once clinical improvement is noted.

Orthopaedic management during the acute phase is designed to prevent the development of unnecessary, fixed deformities. The use of traction and splints is most appropriate.

MANAGEMENT OF THE CHRONIC STAGE

Active and passive exercises to preserve a normal range of motion, and the use of well-padded splints, may be important in preventing contractures in long-term dermatomyositis. The longer the symptoms persist after 6 months, the less the chance for remission. Most children have varying degrees of residual deficit which interfere with function. The discolored skin may break down over pressure areas where subcutaneous calcification has occurred. This condition is not found in adults. Excision of the thickened, calcified tissue may be required when contracture and calcification have taken place, since these plaques may break down and form suppurative ulcers. Oral aluminum hydroxide and disodium ethidronate (Algedrat) have also been used to reduce the intestinal absorption of phosphate and reverse the ectopic calcification. These drugs may be effective in treating widespread, subcutaneous calcification. The bedridden patient with generalized weakness and severe extremity contractures may die because of inanition, intercurrent infection, or respiratory failure. Intercurrent infection may be a complication, particularly if the patient is on long-term steroid treatment. Also, because the patients have vasculitis, they are vulnerable to widespread gastrointestinal ulceration. This can cause a perforated viscus which leads to mediastinitis and peritonitis and subsequently, death. Plasmapheresis has recently been used as an alternate method of treatment in chronic cases.*

---

*Zottoli EM. Unpublished observation.

Systemic Lupus Erythematosus

Systemic lupus erythematosus characteristically involves several organ systems. It is variably progressive and, if untreated, terminates in death. However, spontaneous remission for years is possible. The disease generally is more acute and severe in children than in adults.

Onset or exacerbation of the disease may be triggered by intercurrent infection, emotional factors, or exposure to drugs, such as anticonvulsants or sulfonamides. Systemic lupus erythematosus in children has a predilection for females, and usually the onset is after 8 years of age.

The onset of the disease may be acute or insidious. Frequently, early symptoms include malaise, fever, arthralgias, or a rash. Cutaneous manifestations, especially the classic "butterfly" rash, occur at some time in most affected children. Avascular necrosis of the femoral head may occur.[2] Spontaneous rupture of the patellar tendon has been reported following long-term corticosteorid therapy.[54,72] Raynaud's phenomenon may be present. Clinical renal involvement usually develops.

ETIOLOGY

The etiology is unknown, though generally it is considered to be a disease of altered immune reactivity. The inflammation is thought to be due to the formation of antideoxyribonucleic acid (anti-DNA) and anti-DNA complexes, and to a complement fixation. The last, initiates an inflammatory response, resulting in tissue injury.

LABORATORY DATA

Antinuclear antibodies, demonstrable in all patients with active systemic lupus erythematosus, provide the best screening test for the disease. DNA antibodies are disease-specific and provide a useful index of activity and severity. Lupus erythematosus cells generally are found in the synovial aspirate. Anemia is common.

MANAGEMENT

The majority of patients require long-term treatment but can lead useful lives.[28] Treatment with prednisone, the drug of choice because of its anti-inflammatory quality, usually results in the disappearance of the anti-DNA complexes. The dosage is tapered when signs of continuing disease activity have been eradicated. The aim is ultimate maintenance of the patient on the lowest level of prednisone compatible with the absence of clinical symptoms. Antimalarial drugs, proven effective in long-term suppression of systemic lupus erythematosus, may cause irreversible retinopathy and, therefore, are reserved for the occasional patient who requires an increased daily dose of prednisone. Incapacitating joint symptoms are managed with aspirin compounds. Physical therapy is instituted for range-of-motion and muscle-strengthening exercises. Sun-screening lotions are important in controlling the cutaneous manifestations. Those patients with systemic lupus erythematosus who are on long-term steroid therapy and who develop arthritis should be suspected of having an occult septic process. Diagnosis is established by arthrocentesis.

Discoid lupus erythematosus, the chronic cutaneous form of the disease, is uncommon in children. Infrequently it may convert to the systemic form. The cutaneous lesions, including persistent erythematosus, dry scales, and telangiectases in sun-exposed areas, may progress to scarring and disfigurement. Management is conservative, protecting the patient from excessive sun exposure and using local corticosteorid creams or ointments.

Scleroderma

Scleroderma in childhood is a rare and frustrating disease.[31] Both the localized cutaneous and systemic forms are recognized. Onset of the disease typically is at about age 5. It occurs in both sexes.

The localized cutaneous variety occurs either as morphea or linear scleroderma. The former is the more benign, with an insidious onset. The initial multiple purplish areas of skin generally resolve within 3 to 5 years. Systemic manifestations are rare. Linear scleroderma usually involves the head or an extremity and often is associated with atrophy of the underlying structure. Leg-length inequality, which may develop, is best managed by a shoe lift.

Systemic scleroderma is rare and less severe in children. The earliest clinical sign may be Raynaud's phenomenon or Sjögren's syndrome. The patient presents with muscle wasting, with the overlying skin atrophied and adherent to the subcutaneous tissue. Knees, ankles, and the small hand and foot joints may be involved. Frank polyarthritis is common early in the disease. The atrophy and tightening of the skin leads to a facial appearance of a pinched nose and pursed lips. In the chronic form, hands are shiny, with tapered finger tips, and motion is restricted.[59]

LABORATORY STUDIES

Diagnosis, established by a skin biopsy, reveals generalized atrophy of the dermis, with irregularity of the collagen bundles. A concomitant muscle biopsy may be necessary to differentiate scleroderma from dermatomyositis. The prognosis is poor in the presence of antinuclear-factor lupus erythematosus cells and an increased erythrocyte sedimentation rate.

MANAGEMENT

Management is primarily supportive.[28] Physical therapy, whirlpool treatments, and serial casts all may be used to prevent contractures. Rest and avoiding vasospasm-producing factors such as cold and tension are recommended. Polyarthritis is managed with aspirin compounds, and common gastrointestinal disturbances with a bland diet and antacids.

Myositis Ossificans

Myositis ossificans can be divided into two types, traumatic myositis ossificans and fibrodysplasia ossificans progressiva.

TRAUMATIC MYOSITIS OSSIFICANS

Traumatic myositis ossificans usually follow a crushing injury to muscle, causing hemorrhage.[68] Proliferation and metaplasia of muscle and connective tissue fibroblasts and, subsequently, osteoid formation occur. Eventually, the osteoid calcifies, leading to the formation of heterotopic bone.[1,35] Several weeks following trauma, a tender, firm mass gradually appears. This mass hardens as bone formation occurs. Roentgenograms, at this time, reveal feathery calcification distinctly separate from the normal-appearing cortex. Management, primarily, is to avoid further trauma to the injured tissue. This process is self-limited.

FIBRODYSPLASIA OSSIFICANS PROGRESSIVA (MYOSITIS OSSIFICANS PROGRESSIVA)

Fibrodysplasia ossificans progressiva is a rare, autosomal dominant disease first described by Patin in 1692.[49] It is characterized by progressive edema, calcification, and ossification of the fasciae, aponeuroses, ligaments, tendons, and interstitial tissue of muscle.[18,26,27,32,55,63] The basic defect is in the connective tissues; skeletal muscle remains fundamentally normal.

CLINICAL FEATURES. Both a hypoplastic thumb and hallux (Fig. 3-18) are present at birth.[44] Webbing, polydactyly, or deformed ears also may be noted in the newborn. Deafness occurs later because of ossification of the inner ear. The disease occurs more commonly in males and always appears in the first decade of life, usually before age 2.

Commonly, the neck muscles are involved first. Later the condition spreads to the paraspinal muscles and then to the face, shoulders, and arms. Initially, small, painful, hot areas of swelling appear in the dorsal neck and trunk over a 2- to 3-day period. These erythematous and warm lesions are attached to the deep fascia. The overlying skin is loose. The pain gradually subsides, and the lesions regress for several weeks, leaving an indurated lump in which calcification and ossification develop. The fasciae erector spinae and neck muscles are commonly involved and are responsible for the development of torticollis. As the masseter muscles become involved, the mandibular joint motion diminishes. The eyes, larynx, diaphragm, tongue, and heart are not involved. Eventually shoulder and pelvic girdles and proximal extremities are affected and the limbs may be locked into immobility causing a loss of function of both the arms and legs. Involvement distal to the knees and elbows is rare. Only the musculoskeletal system is involved. Death in adult life results from respiratory embarrassment.

LABORATORY STUDIES. No biochemical abnormalities have been demonstrated. Muscle biopsy is contraindicated because the trauma may lead to ossification. Muscle biopsies obtained during the acute stage demonstrate swelling and proliferation of connective tissue with interstitial edema. Classic inflammatory changes are absent. The centers of ossification occur between muscle fascicles or in association with tendons and aponeuroses. Muscle fibers undergo secondary atrophy and degenerative changes.[29] Dystrophic calcification and ossification develop gradually and are visible on roentgenograms within 48 months after onset (Fig. 3-18).[62] Ossification may occur in columns following the course of muscles, tendons, or ligaments, or may be irregular if fasciae or aponeuroses are involved. Angiographic studies are important in ruling out possible malignancy.[39,50]

MANAGEMENT. Since the course is one of steady progression with periods of remission and acute exacerbation, eventually the patient becomes totally disabled. No treatment has been proved universally effective.[42] Russel reports some success with the use of disodium ethane-1 hydroxy-1, 1-diphosphonate (EHDP), a compound which inhibits the crystal growth of hydroxyapatite.[57] Most patients are stabilized or are progressively improved with use of this low-toxicity drug. EHDP remains an experimental drug, and patients with this disease should be referred to health centers that use this medication. Surgery has proved disappointing, since attempted excision has resulted in aggravation of the disease process, with more extensive bone being formed.[64]

Fibrodysplasia ossificans progressiva should be distinguished from calcinosis universalis and dermatomyositis. Calcinosis universalis is a condition characterized by progressive accumulation of amorphous calcium phosphate and crystalline hydroxyapatite in subcutaneous lesions. The etiology of this rare condition is unknown. The lesions are more common in the extremities, beginning in the subcutaneous tissue and extending into the connective tissue of the ligaments and tendons. Cram recommends the use of EHDP for this condition. Surgical excision of the lesions followed by split-thickness skin grafts may be required.[16]

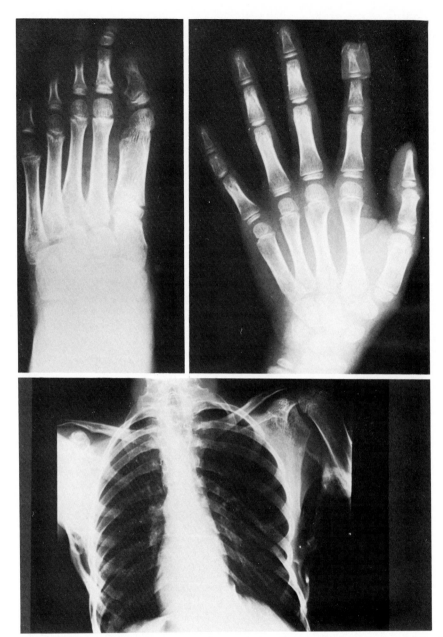

FIG. 3-18. These roentgenograms demonstrate columniation in plaques of ectopic bone in fibrodysplasia ossificans progressiva. The shortened hallux and pollex are universally found.

ARTHROCHALASIS MULTIPLEX CONGENITA

Arthrochalasis multiplex congenita is a rare clinical entity characterized by persistent generalized joint laxity.[19] The disease is transmitted as an autosomal dominant and occurs as an independent articular disorder lacking the cutaneous and systemic manifestations of Ehlers–Danlos syndrome. Criteria for establishing the diagnosis of arthrochalasis include apposition of the thumb to the flexor aspect of the forearm, passive hyper-

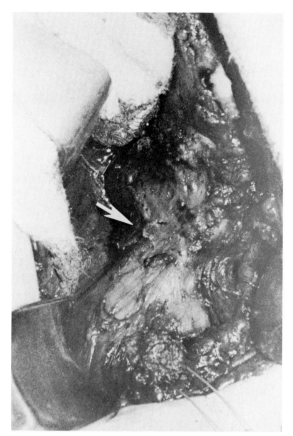

extension of the fingers so that they lie parallel to the extensor aspect of the forearm, hyperextension of the elbow of greater than 10°, hyperextension of the knee of greater than 10°, and increased ankle dorsiflexion and eversion of the foot. No neurological deficit can be demonstrated. Orthopaedic complications include congenital dislocated hips (Fig. 3-19) and dislocations of the patellae, elbows, and shoulders, as well as scoliosis. The persistence of the capsular laxity into adult life complicates the long-term management of these problems and in particular their hip dislocations. Older patients may require major hip reconstructive procedures in order to maintain independent ambulation. Histological and electron-microscopic evaluation has failed to demonstrate any underlying collagen deficiency.

PROGRESSIVE CONTRACTURE OF THE QUADRICEPS MUSCLE

Hněvkovský first described the gradual development of knee extension contracture due to progressive fibrosis of the quadriceps muscle in children.[34,38] Later, a causal relationship was established between quadriceps contracture and multiple intramuscular injections.[33,41,58]

Williams classifies the infantile presentation into three categories[73]: (1) a stiff, extended knee, (2) congenital recurvatum (Fig. 3-20), and (3) congenital dislocation. Young

FIG. 3-19. Congenital dislocated hips result from excessive capsular redundancy and laxity. The arrow indicates the hourglass narrowing caused by gentle traction on this markedly redundant capsule. No collagen abnormalities have been identified by electron microscopy or fibroblast culture.

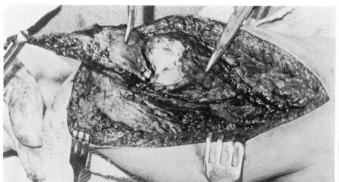
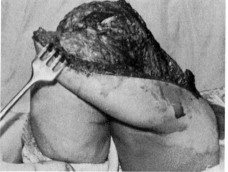

FIG. 3-20. Formal quadriceps, lengthening should permit full flexion at the time of correction of the congenital recurvatum. The surgical instruments point to the undersurface of the patella and its abnormal bed, both of which were covered with fibrous tissue.

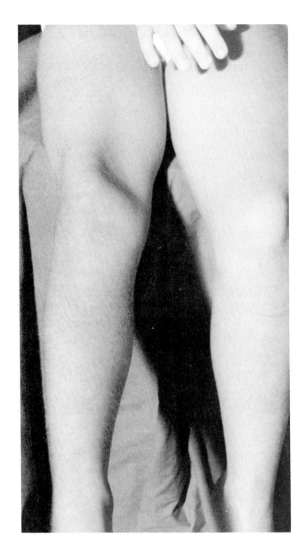

FIG. 3-21. Progressive loss of knee flexion in this 5-year-old girl limits range of motion.

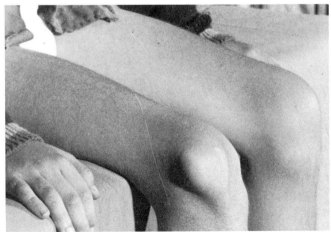

FIG. 3-22. Dislocation occurs every time this 9-year-old boy flexes his knees more than 45°.

children may develop progressive loss of knee motion during the first few years of life. In later childhood, the patient may present with a habitual patellar dislocation.

Stiff Knees

Children with a progressively more limited range of knee flexion usually present at about 3 years of age (Fig. 3-21). The contracture is distributed equally among all components of the quadriceps, except the vastus medialis. Bose and Williams recommend quadriceps-

plasty to lengthen these shortened muscles.[9,73]

Habitual Dislocation of the Patella

The average age of presentation is 6 years. Lateral patellar dislocation occurs every time the knee is flexed (Fig. 3-22). Physical findings are demonstrated by holding the patella in the midline and finding it impossible to flex the knee more than 30°. Further flexion is possible only if the patella is allowed to dislocate; then a full range of motion is readily obtained. Anatomic findings and surgical management are similar to those in patients with stiff knees.

REFERENCES

1. Ackerman LV: Extra-osseous localized non-neoplastic bone and cartilage formation (so-called myositis ossificans). Clinical and pathological confusion with malignant neoplasms. J Bone Joint Surg 40A:279, 1958
2. Aptekar RG, Decker JL: Orthopaedic aspects of systemic lupus erythematosus. In Proceedings of American Academy of Orthopaedic Surgeons, J Bone Joint Surg 57A:1027, 1975
3. Armstrong RM, Koenigsberger R, Mellinger J, Lovelace RE: Central core disease with congenital hip dislocation: study of two families. Neurology 21:369, 1971
4. Banker BQ, Victor J: Dermatomyositis (systemic angiopathy) of childhood. Medicine 45:261, 1966
5. Bell DB, Smith DW: Myotonic dystrophy in the neonate. J Pediatr 81:83, 1972
6. Bitnum S, Daeschner CW, Travis LB, Dodge WF, Hopps HC: Dermatomyositis. J Pediatr 64:101, 1964
7. Bohan A, Peter JB: Polymyositis and dermatomyositis (First of two parts). N Engl Med J 292:344, 1975
8. Bohan A, Peter JB: Polymyositis and dermatomyositis (Second of two parts). N Engl Med J 292:403, 1975
9. Bose K, Chong KC: The clinical manifestations and pathomechanics of contracture of the extensor mechanism of the knee. J Bone Joint Surg 58B:478, 1976
10. Brooke MH: A clinician's view of neuromuscular diseases. Baltimore, The Williams & Wilkins Company, 1977
11. Brooke MH: A neuromuscular disease characterized by fibre types disproportion. In Kakulas BA (ed): Proceedings of the Second International Congress on Muscle Diseases, Perth, Australia, November, 1971. Amsterdam, Excerpta Medica, 1973
12. Calderon R: Myotonic dystrophy. A neglected cause of mental retardation. J Pediatr 68:423, 1966
13. Carlisle JW, Good RA: Dermatomyositis in childhood: Report of studies on seven cases and a review of the literature. Lancet 79:266, 1959
14. Carroll JE, Brooke MH, Kaiser K: Diagnosis of infantile myotonic dystrophy. Lancet 2:608, 1975
15. Cook AW, Bird TD, Spence AM, Pagon RA, Wallace JF: Myotonic dystrophy, mitral-valve prolapse, and stroke. Lancet 1:335, 1978
16. Cram RL, Barmada R, Geho WB, Ray RD: Diphosphonate treatment of calcinosis universalis. N Engl J Med 285:1012, 1971
17. Denny-Brown D, Nevin S: The phenomenon of myotonia. Brain 64:1, 1941
18. Dixon TF, Mulligan L, Nassim R, Stevenson FH: Myositis ossificans progressiva. J Bone Joint Surg 36B:445, 1954
19. Drennan JC: Hip dislocation in arthrochalasis multiplex congenita. Orthopaedic Transactions 2:47, 1978
20. Dubowitz V: Diagnostic advances in neuromuscular disease. Arch Dis Child 47:149, 1972
21. Dubowitz V: Muscle Disorders in Childhood. Philadelphia, WB Saunders, 1978
22. Dubowitz V: Treatment of dermatomyositis in childhood. Arch Dis Child 51:494, 1976
23. Dubowitz V, Brooke MH: Muscle Biopsy: A Modern Approach. London, WB Saunders, 1973
24. Eng GD, Epstein BS, Engel WK, McKay DW, McKay R: Malignant hyperthermia and central core disease in a child with congenital dislocating hips. Arch Neurol 35(4):189, 1978
25. Everett MM, Curtis AC: Dermatomyositis: A review of 19 cases in adolescents and children. Arch Intern Med 100:70, 1957
26. Fairbank HAT: Myositis ossificans progressiva. J Bone Joint Surg 32B:108, 1950
27. Frejka B: Heterotopic ossification and myositis ossificans progressiva. J Bone Joint Surg 11:157, 1929
28. Gellis SS, Kagan BM: Current Pediatric Therapy, ed. 7. Philadelphia, WB Saunders, 1976
29. Deschiekter CF, Maseritz IH: Myositis ossificans. J Bone Joint Surg 20:661, 1938
30. Geschwind N, Simpson JA: Procaine amide in the treatment of myotonia. Brain 78:81, 1955

31. Goel KM, Shanks RA: Scleroderma in childhood: Report of 5 cases. Arch Dis Child 49:861, 1974
32. Griffith G: Progressive myositis ossificans. Arch Dis Child 24:71, 1949
33. Gunn DR: Contracture of the quadriceps muscle. J Bone Joint Surg 46B:492, 1964
34. Hagen R: Contracture of the quadriceps muscle in children. Acta Orthop Scand 39:565, 1968
35. Hardy AG, Dickson JW: Pathological ossification in traumatic paraplegia. J Bone Joint Surg 45B:76, 1963
36. Harper PS: Congenital myotonic dystrophy in Britain. I. Clinical aspects. Arch Dis Child 50:505, 1975
37. Harper PS: Myotonic Dystrophy, ed. 12. Philadelphia, WB Saunders, 1979
38. Hněvkovský, O: Progressive fibrosis of the vastus intermedius muscle in children. A cause of limited knee flexion and elevation of the patella. J Bone Joint Surg 43B:318, 1961
39. Hutcheson J, Klatte EC, Kremp R: The angiographic appearance of myositis ossificans circumscripta. A case report. Radiology 102:57, 1972
40. Kolb M, Horn ML, Martz R: Dantrolene in human malignant hyperthermia—multi-center review. Anesthesiology 56:254, 1982
41. Lloyd-Roberts GC, Thomas TG: The etiology of quadriceps contracture in children. J Bone Joint Surg 46B:498, 1964
42. Lutwak L: Myositis ossificans progressiva: Mineral, metabolic, and radioactive calcium studies of the effects of hormones. Am J Med 37:269, 1964
43. McComb RD, Markesbery WR, O'Connor WN: Fatal neonatal nemaline myopathy with multiple congenital anomalies. J Pediatr 94:47, 1979
44. McKusick FA: Fibrodysplasia ossificans progressiva. In Heritable Disorders of Connective Tissue, ed. 4, p 687. St Louis, CV Mosby, 1966
45. Miller JJ: Later progression in dermatomyositis in children. J Pediatr 83:543, 1973
46. Moosa A: The feeding difficulty in infantile myotonic dystrophy. Dev Med Child Neurol 16:824, 1974
47. Munsat TL, Thompson LR, Coleman RF: Centronuclear ("myotubular") myopathy. Arch Neurol 20:120, 1969
48. Ozonoff MB, Flynn FJ, Jr: Roentgenologic features of dermatomyositis of childhood. American Journal of Roentgenology: Radium Therapy and Nuclear Medicine 118:206, 1973
49. Patin G: Lettres choisies de Feu Mr. Guy Patin. Cologne, Vol. 1:28, 1692
50. Peck GT, Braund RR: The development of sarcoma in myositis ossificans. JAMA 119:776, 1942
51. Pinsky L, DiGeorge AM: Congenital familial sensory neuropathy with anhidrosis. J Pediatr 68:1, 1966
52. Polgar JG, Bradley WG, Upton ARM, Anderson J, Howat JML, Petito F, Roberts DF, Scopa J: The early detection of dystrophia myotonica. Brain 95:761, 1972
53. Ramsey PL, Hensinger RN: Congenital dislocation of the hip associated with central core disease. J Bone Joint Surg 57A:648, 1975
54. Rascher JJ, Marcolin L, James P: Bilateral, sequential rupture of the patellar tendon in systemic lupus erythematosus. J Bone Joint Surg 56A:821, 1974
55. Riley HD, Christie A: Myositis ossificans progressiva. Pediatrics, 8:753, 1951
56. Rosenkranz E: Ueber kongenitalie kontraktruren der oberen extremitäten: im anschluss an die mitteilung eines einschlägigen falles. Z Orthop 14:905, 1905
57. Russell RGG, Smith R: Diphosphonates: Experimental and clinical aspects. J Bone Joint Surg 55B:66, 1973
58. Sacristan HD, Sanchez-Barba A, Lopez-Duran Stern L, Mendez Martin J, Linan C, Fernandez L: Fibrosis of the gluteal muscles. Report of 3 cases. J Bone Joint Surg 56A:1510, 1974
59. Schlenker JD, Clark DD, Wecksser EC: Calcinosis circumscripta of the hand in scleroderma. J Bone Joint Surg 55A:1051, 1973
60. Shy GM, Engel WK, Somers JE, Wanko T: Nemaline myopathy. A new congenital myopathy. Brain 86:793, 1963
61. Shy GM, Magee KR: A new congenital nonprogressive myopathy. Brain 79:610, 1956
62. Singleton EB, Holt JF: Myositis ossificans progressiva. Radiology 62:47, 1954
63. Smith DM, Zeman W, Johnson CC, Jr, Deiss WP Jr: Myositis ossificans progressiva. Metabolism 15:521, 1966
64. Smith R, Russell RGG, Woods CG: Myositis ossificans progressiva: Clinical features of eight patients and their response to treatment. J Bone Joint Surg 58B:48, 1976
65. Spiro AJ, Shy GM, Gonatas NK: Myotubular myopathy. Persistence of fetal muscle in an adolescent boy. Arch Neurol 14:1, 1966
66. Sullivan DB, Cassidy JT, Petty RE: Prognosis in childhood dermatomyositis. J Pediatr 80:555, 1972
67. Thomsen J: Tonisch krampfe in willkurlich beweglichen muskeln in folge von erebter psychischer disposition. Arch Psychiatr Nerven 6:706, 1876
68. Thorndike A: Myositis ossificans traumatic. J Bone Joint Surg 22:315, 1940
69. Thrush DC, Morris CJ, Salmon MV: Paramyotonia congenita: A clinical, histochemical and pathological study. Brain 95:537, 1972
70. Tuck WH: The Stanmore cosmetic caliper. J Bone Joint Surg 56B:115, 1974
71. Vanier TM: Dystrophia myotonia in childhood. Br Med J 2(5208):1284, 1960
72. Wener JA, Schein AJ: Simultaneous bilateral rupture of the patellar tendon and quadriceps expansions in systemic lupus erythematosus. A case report. J Bone Joint Surg 56A:823, 1974
73. Williams PH: Quadriceps contracture. J Bone Joint Surg 50B:278, 1968
74. Winters JL, McLaughlin LA: Myotonia congenita. J Bone Joint Surg 52A:1345, 1970
75. Zellweger H, Ionasescu V: Early onset of myotonic dystrophy in infants. Am J Dis Child 125:601, 1973

Chapter 4

Acquired Paralytic Conditions

Poliomyelitis

Anterior poliomyelitis is an acute viral infection with special localization in the anterior-horn cells of the spinal cord in certain brain stem motor nuclei. Generally, it is caused by one of three types of poliomyelitis virus, although other members of the enteroviral group, for example Coxsackie and the ECHO viruses, can also clinically and pathologically produce a disease indistinguishable from polio.

Humans are the sole natural reservoir, transmitting poliomyelitis by the oropharyngofecal route. Initial invasion occurs through the gastrointestinal and respiratory tracts, and spreads to the central nervous system through the blood. Each type of polio virus has strains of varying virulence. The types do not offer cross-immunity, and reinfection in an individual is possible. Although the disease has been known for centuries, it was not until the latter half of the 19th century that epidemics were recorded. Those epidemics occurred most commonly in summer and autumn and in temperate-zone countries that had made recent improvements in levels of sanitation. This rise in health standards lead to a lowering of the "pool of immune resistance" to the disease. Recent development of prophylactic vaccines has greatly reduced the incidence of polio.[160,162] From 1950 to 1954, 190,000 cases of poliomyelitis were reported in the United States.

EPIDEMIOLOGY

The control of poliomyelitis through immunization involves not only the direct protection of individuals, but uses the concept of herd immunity.[91] Therefore, immunization of a sufficient proportion of the population acts as a barrier to the introduction and spread of the virus, thus indirectly protecting susceptible individuals.

In the prevaccine era, attack rates were higher in the more favored socioeconomic groups, with the peak incidence in the 5- to 14-year-olds. In the past decade, paralytic poliomyelitis has occurred chiefly in unimmunized infants and preschool children and often in inner-city or other poverty-stricken areas. In 1970, 32 cases were reported, 29 of which occurred in patients under the age of 5 years who had received inadequate or no immunization, with Type 1 polio virus accounting for the majority.

Not all patients who receive oral poliomyelitis vaccine develop adequate levels of antibodies. Those who do may have an appreciable decrease in the titer over a 2- to 5-year period. The protective role of persisting serum antibodies is not clear. Ogra and Karzon have shown that local intestinal secretory antibodies afford protection against reinfection with polio in the absence of detectable serum antibodies.[142] The American Academy of Pediatrics recommends booster doses to maintain a protective level of antibodies in those who have been immunized by an initial series of oral vaccine. Since 1970, fewer than 100 cases per year have been reported. These sporadic cases can occur even among those who have received oral vaccination.

PATHOLOGY

The poliomyelitis virus invades the body through the oropharyngeal route and multiplies in the alimentary-tract lymph nodes before spreading by the hematogenous route. The incubation period varies from 6 to 20 days. It is estimated that 1% to 2% of those infected suffer neural disease. The histologic diagnosis of poliomyelitis is made by studying the distribution of the lesions. The anterior-horn ganglion cells of the spinal cord are acutely attacked, especially in the lumbar and cervical enlargements. The medulla, cerebellum, and midbrain also are involved. Except for the motor area, the white matter of the spinal cord and the entire cerebral cortex are spared.

Damage to the anterior-horn motor cells may be due directly to viral multiplication or toxic by-products of the virus, or may be due indirectly to the results of ischemia, edema, and hemorrhage in the glial tissues surrounding the anterior-horn cells. The ganglion cells in the involved area swell within 48 hours and undergo chromatolysis of the Nissl substance in the cytoplasm. In addition, an acute inflammatory cellular reaction and edema with perivascular mononuclear cuffing take place. Destruction of the spinal cord occurs focally, with wallerian degeneration evident throughout the length of the individual nerve fiber after 3 days. Peripheral trauma, such as an intramuscular injection or surgery within the fortnight preceding onset of the disease, can affect localization of the paralysis in anatomically related segments of the cord.

A tonsillectomy performed during an epidemic may lead to the development of bulbar poliomyelitis within 7 to 14 days following surgery. It is postulated that excessive physical exercise, such as strenuous contact sports, late in the incubation period of polio poses a high risk for extensive and severe paralysis.

The inflammatory response gradually subsides, and the necrotic ganglion cells are surrounded and partially dissolved by macrophages and neutrophils.[5] A histologic cross-section through a focal area may reveal complete absence of ganglion cells from the anterior horn. After 4 months, the spinal cord is left with residual areas of gliosis, with lymphocytic cell collections occupying the area of the destroyed motor cells. There is focal proliferation of the reparative neuroglial cells. The remaining ganglion cells show no evidence of progressive histologic abnormality. The involved motor unit skeletal muscle demonstrates gross atrophy, and replacement by fat and connective tissue appears histologically.

Extreme variation can be found in the number and severity of individual muscles involved in the resultant flaccid paralysis. The percentage of motor units destroyed in an individual muscle varies markedly, and the resultant clinical weakness is proportional to the number of lost motor units. All muscle fibers in an individual motor unit supplied by an anterior-horn cell are affected by its destruction. Sharrard states that clinically detectable weakness is present only when more than 60% of the motor nerve cells supplying a muscle have been destroyed.[176] The muscles involved can vary from one or two to those of all four extremities, the trunk, and the bulbar musculature.

Muscles innervated by the cervical and lumbar enlargements are most commonly affected. Paralysis occurs twice as frequently in lower extremity muscles than in those in the upper extremity. Sharrard, by combined clinical and histologic studies, demonstrated that muscles with short motor nerve cell columns often are severely paralyzed, while those with long motor cell columns more frequently are left paretic.[173,174] The quadriceps, glutei, tibialis anterior, medial hamstrings, and hip flexors are the lumbar-innervated muscles most commonly involved. The deltoid, triceps, and pectoralis major are those most frequently affected in the upper extremity. The sacral nerve roots are spared, resulting in characteristic sparing of the intrinsic muscles of the foot.

PROGNOSIS FOR MUSCLE RECOVERY

Recovery of muscle function is dependent upon the return to function of those anterior-horn cells damaged, but not destroyed. The major clinical recovery occurs during the first month following acute illness, and is nearly complete by the sixth month. Limited potential for recovery persists through the second year. The rate of recovery is slightly better in the upper extremities, and it is particularly rapid in young children. Total paralysis of the muscle persisting beyond the second month is an ominous sign of severe motor-cell destruction. Sharrard states that the average final grade of a muscle is two grades above its assessment at 1 month and one grade above at 6 months.[173] A muscle paralyzed at 6 months remains paralyzed. Green feels that muscle assessment can be carried out 2 weeks after the onset of poliomyelitis, at which time a muscle demonstrating a flicker of activity would result in a fair rating at 18 months.[60] A muscle rated poor at 2 weeks would rate fair to good, and

a muscle rating fair on early examination eventually would rate as good when assessed at 18 months. A muscle with a particular grade is less likely to show significant recovery when surrounded by severely paretic muscles.

ACUTE STAGE

Acute poliomyelitis infection may cause symptoms ranging from mild malaise to generalized encephalomyelitis with widespread paralysis. Diagnosis is based on clinical findings, because no laboratory tests performed during this period are diagnostic for poliomyelitis.

The clinical course in younger children may be biphasic. Systemic symptoms, including listlessness, sore throat, and a slightly elevated temperature, may be followed by several days of well-being. Symptoms that recur and culminate in paralysis include hyperesthesia or paresthesia in the extremities, severe headache, sore throat, vomiting, nuchal rigidity, back pain, and limitation of straight-leg raising, due to pain caused by meningismus. Characteristically, the paralysis is asymmetric, and in younger children the lower extremity is involved more commonly than the upper extremity. The patient's temperature rarely exceeds 103° F. Although a high infant mortality is noted, the disease tends to be milder in children than in older patients.

In older children and adults, poliomyelitis frequently occurs without a previous minor illness or fever. The preparalytic patient may have a low-grade temperature, may appear markedly flushed, and may be very apprehensive. The onset may be gradual, over 1 week, with little increase in temperature. In contrast to younger children, muscular pain is a prominent symptom.

The acute phase of poliomyelitis generally lasts 7 to 10 days. Asymmetrical paralysis is noted on the third or fourth day, and may increase in severity over several days. This may be associated with a decrease in temperature. The return to normal temperature for 48 hours and the absence of progressive muscular involvement signals the end of the acute phase.

The orthopaedist should be familiar with the clinical signs of acute poliomyelitis. Meningismus is reflected in the characteristic flexor posturing of the upper and lower extremities.

Muscles are tender, even to gentle palpation. The patient's discomfort may limit the examination to assessment of those muscles most commonly involved, and may necessitate serial examinations.

The superficial reflexes are usually the first to be abolished. The initially normal deep-tendon reflexes may become increased or decreased 12 to 24 hours later, indicating impending paresis of the extremity. The deep-tendon reflexes are absent when that muscle group is paralyzed. No objective sensory changes are noted in poliomyelitis.

Additional clinical signs can be elicited during the acute stage. The patient may assume a characteristic tripod position when asked to sit up unassisted. The patient with flexed knees and hands positioned behind him for support is exhibiting spinal rigidity. Nuchal rigidity also may be detected by asking the sitting patient to flex his chin toward his knees.

Passive assessment includes the Kernig and Brudzinski tests for nuchal irritation. In addition, the patient may be placed supine with head and neck drawn over the edge of a bed. Support is given under the patient's shoulders while he attempts to raise his trunk. Normally, the head follows the plane of the trunk, but in poliomyelitis it frequently falls back limply.

Cervical-innervated muscle paresis usually is asymmetrical, and is most commonly found in the muscles of the shoulder girdle, arms, neck, the intercostals, and the diaphragm. Patients with upper-extremity involvement, especially of the shoulder girdle, must be watched carefully for intercostal and diaphragmatic weakness, which may lead to severe respiratory embarrassment. The diaphragm and deltoid have common innervation, and involvement of the deltoid muscle warrants fluoroscopic examination to determine diaphragmatic function. Weakness of the anterior neck muscles may be associated with a nasal quality of speech and may indicate difficulty in swallowing. These patients require intensive care, possibly including assisted ventilation or tracheotomy.

Lumbar-innervated muscle involvement is reflected in paralysis of abdominal, back and leg muscles. The presence of the Beevor's sign indicates asymmetrical involvement of the abdominal muscles, with a shift of the umbilicus toward the stronger side. Temporary loss of bladder function also may be noted.

Differential diagnosis includes Guillain–Barré syndrome and other forms of encephalomyelitis. Cerebrospinal fluid analysis performed at the onset of the acute stage of poliomyelitis demonstrates 20 to 300 white blood cells, which are initially polymorphonucleocytes, but which rapidly shift to become 90% lymphocytes. The protein level is unremarkable.

Paralysis in Guillain–Barré syndrome is symmetrical, and cerebrospinal fluid analysis during the acute phase demonstrates an elevated protein level with little or no increase in the cell count. The protein elevation peaks at 2 to 4 weeks and then slowly declines to normal.

Management

Acute-stage management requires the combined efforts of the pediatrician and the orthopaedist. It is necessary to minimize the patient's activity, generally by bedrest. Analgesics are most effective when combined with the application of hot packs for 15 to 30 minutes every 2 to 4 hours. Sedatives may be necessary for anxiety, and good general nursing care is required. Constipation and fecal impaction are common complications in this phase.

Flexion patterns of the upper and lower extremities during the acute stage lead to the prompt development of fixed contractures. The fascia contracts, and muscular aponeurosis and secondary shortening of partially involved muscles occur later in the disease. The involved muscles are sensitive to palpation, and efforts to stretch the irritated muscles increase the reflex muscle spasm.

Correct anatomic positioning of the limbs on a firm mattress is necessary to avoid development of flexion posturing (Fig. 4-1).[60] Irritated muscles, combined with the effects of gravity, cause the extremity to assume a deformed position, while the antagonistic muscles are too weak to oppose those that are irritated. The spastic triceps surae cause rapid development of a fixed equinus, preventing recovery of the overstretched dorsiflexors. This can be avoided by the use of a padded footboard. Sufficient space should be allowed at the lower end of the mattress so that the foot

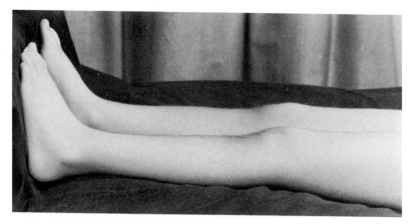

FIG. 4-1. Proper positioning during the acute and convalescent stages of poliomyelitis prevents fascial contractures. (Courtesy of Newington Children's Hospital)

can rest in neutral position when the patient is placed in the alternate prone position. Spasticity in the hip flexors, abductors, and external rotators may create a frog-leg position, which becomes permanent as the tissues shorten. Irwin considers the iliotibial band to be the greatest deforming force in the lower trunk and lower extremities during this phase.[100] Sandbags around the thighs hold the hips in neutral position and may prevent excessive external rotation. In order to relax the hamstrings, the knees should be held in slight flexion by placing a padded roll beneath them. The upper extremities can be controlled with judicious use of slings. Patients with marked spasm may require other temporary devices during the acute stage. Pillows may be required for extreme lordosis, and the pillow height may be decreased gradually as the amount of back spasm decreases. The extreme sensitivity of the limbs to movement precludes the use of braces.

Gentle, passive range-of-motion exercises should be carried out on all joints, within the limits of the patient's tolerance, several times a day.[167] These are most effective when preceded by the application of moist heat. An active exercise program should be discouraged until the muscles are no longer sensitive to touch.

CONVALESCENT STAGE

The convalescent phase begins 2 days after the temperature returns to normal and progression of the paralytic disease ceases. The phase continues for 2 years, with spontaneous improvement in muscle power occurring during this period. Muscle strength increases rapidly through the fourth month and much more gradually thereafter. The important exceptions to this pattern include the deltoid, with a marked diminution of improvement at 4 months, and the triceps surae, in which the end result is achieved by 18 months.

The orthopaedist's goals during the patient's convalescent phase are to obtain maximum recovery of the individual muscles, to maintain or restore the normal range of joint motion, and to prevent or correct deformities that do occur.

The first few weeks of the convalescent stage are characterized by acute inflammation in the fasciae and muscle aponeuroses which cause rapid development of fibrous flexion contractures. A fixed deformed position in an extremity favors the subsequent secondary shortening of the partially involved muscles and places those muscles antagonistic to the flexors at a mechanical disadvantage.

Muscles in the early convalescent phase remain hypersensitive to palpation and attempted therapy. Orthopaedic goals and management vary little from the acute stage. Proper positioning in bed, intermittent hot packs, and limited passive range-of-motion exercises four to six times daily continue to be important in keeping the extremities free from deformity.

Limited muscle examinations can be performed during this period and can approximate the degree and distribution of weakness. The muscles must lose their sensitivity before a thorough assessment and grading of individual muscles can be accomplished.

The rate of recovery noted on serial examinations is the best guide to potential recovery. Muscle assessment should be carried out monthly for 6 months and then every 3 months. Formal examination of the young child may be unrewarding. Much information can be obtained by observing the child in the performance of daily activities or at play. Lower-extremity function can be demonstrated by observing the child during ambulation and at play on a mat; upper-extremity function can be assessed by watching the child grasp and play with toys. Palpation of the limbs during activity also aids in the orthopaedist's appreciation of the muscle strength.

Johnson stated that an individual muscle demonstrating less than 30% of its normal strength at 3 months should be considered permanently paralyzed.[101] Muscles that have recovered more than 80% of their strength will recover spontaneously, requiring no specific therapy. He emphasized that muscles that fall between these two parameters retain the potential for useful function, and therapy should be directed toward creating hypertrophy of the remaining fibers.

The physical therapy program should be directed toward making individual muscles assume maximum capability. The muscles must be made to work in their normal pattern of motor activity. Paretic muscles should be exercised to their maximum level of function in a carefully designed program that does not allow already normally functioning muscles to become hypertrophic.

Overactivity in the early convalescent phase of disease may lead to eventual loss of some of the recovery potential of individual muscles. These muscles fatigue quickly, for example, after two or three contractures, and must not be exercised beyond their capability, since the recovery of function will be inhibited. Muscles that rate less than good (Grade 3 on the Medical Research Council rating) should be put through an active range-of-motion in a plane that eliminates gravity. General exercises such as crawling, sitting up, and walking can be added by the fourth month. Alignment of the extremities is maintained in bivalved casts or plastic orthoses to prevent overfatigue and deformity at times when physical therapy is not being carried out.

Contractures in an antagonistic muscle must be stretched before an active exercise program is initiated for a paretic muscle. Both vigorous passive stretching exercises and wedging casts are helpful in the management of mild and moderate degrees of contracture. The surgical release of tight fascia and muscle aponeurosis, as well as the lengthening of short tendons, may be necessary if the contracture persists longer than 6 months. This is particularly true in the lower extremity, although occasionally a shortened pectoral fascia and the tendons about the elbow may require lengthening.

Hydrotherapy can be used in patients with extensive paralysis. Weak muscles may require reinforcement slings or support in warm water, but as the strength increases, the workload also may be increased. This policy should be followed from the sixth week to the sixth month. The initial goal in the severely paralyzed patient is to achieve standing balance and, later, ambulation in the pool until adequate control of the trunk and lower limbs is gained. Then, to develop a four-point gait, the patient should advance to standing at the parallel bars before crutches are used.

Orthoses should be withheld as long as further recovery is anticipated. Their use in the convalescent phase is limited to avoiding development of an abnormal gait. The particular combination of motor weakness determines when the patient should be allowed to walk and what minimal orthoses are required to assist ambulation. Early walking may be beneficial in mild paralysis, but in more severe forms this activity level may be a frustrating and sometimes harmful experience for the patient. Dynamic assist-type bracing is preferred. An ambulatory brace may also be used as a night splint to prevent deformity.

Weakness in the foot dorsiflexors and inverters requires a short leg brace with a T-strap, drop-foot stop, and dorsiflexion spring-assist. Quadriceps strength of less-than-good quality may require use of a long leg brace with a knee-locking mechanism. Severe hip involvement may require a pelvic band or corset with hip hinges. The strength of the upper extremity must be considered when anticipating the possibility of walking, because marked paralysis may preclude the use of crutches. Spring-loaded splints to control flail wrist or fingers are sometimes used. A spinal orthosis may be required for paralytic scoliosis.

Amyotrophic Lateral Sclerosis

Mulder has reported a group of patients with progressive muscle weakness which occurred many years after an episode of acute poliomyelitis.[133] The average age of the patient at the time of illness was 5 years and the initial severe paralysis was followed by significant improvement. All patients reached adult life and were able to work but noted a progressive weakness developing in middle life. The onset was asymmetrical and insidious. Although fasciculations and progressive decrease in muscle bulk were noted, they were not accompanied by sensory or bulbar dysfunction or extrapyramidal symptoms. Therefore, there appeared to be the suggestion that this syndrome represented a forme fruste of amyotrophic lateral sclerosis but that it lacked the increased deep-tendon reflexes and abnormal plantar responses of this disease.

CHRONIC STAGE

The chronic stage, beginning after 24 months, is that in which the orthopaedist must manage the long-term consequences resulting from muscle imbalance. The greatest degree of muscle recovery occurs within the first year; no improvement can be expected during the chronic stage.

The goal of the orthopaedist is the achievement of maximum functional activity. Securing muscle balance, preventing or correcting soft-tissue deformity or subsequent osseous complications, and directing allied personnel, such as the physical therapist and the orthotist, are integral parts of the orthopaedic design of treatment.

Flaccid paralysis, muscle imbalance, and growth all contribute to fixed deformity in the chronic stage.[61] Soft-tissue contractures permit an increased mechanical advantage for the stronger muscles and continued attenuation of their weaker antagonists. The greater the disparity in muscle balance, the sooner the deformity becomes apparent. Even a slight difference in muscle power produces deformity over a long period of time.

Purely static (negative) joint instability does not result in fixed deformity, except in cases in which it is allowed to occur over a period of years in a growing child.[148,149] Static instability can be controlled readily and indefinitely by orthoses. Dynamic (active) joint instability readily produces a fixed deformity, and orthotic control is difficult. Deformities initially are confined to soft tissue, but later bone growth and joint alignment are affected. Deformity continues to worsen until growth of bone and soft tissue ceases.

The age of onset of poliomyelitis is important. The osseous growth potential of young children makes them more vulnerable to bony deformity than adults, who rarely develop severe early joint changes.[155] The worst deformities occur with early age and severe muscle imbalance.[18] Soft-tissue surgery, especially tendon transfers, performed in the young child prior to the development of structural changes is particularly important. Bony procedures must be postponed until skeletal growth is adequate (e.g., triple arthrodesis or spinal fusion may be performed on 12-year-old patients).

Physical therapy stresses the achievement of maximum functional activity through a variety of techniques. The therapist employs active hypertrophy exercises to change muscles with marginal function to a level of functional activity. The patient is instructed to recognize his motor deficits and to use all available muscles to successfully perform and complete a task. The substitution of functional muscles and the development of trick movements to compensate for individual motor weaknesses are encouraged. A passive stretching regimen is continued to prevent or correct soft-tissue contractures.

Orthotic use in the chronic phase may enable the patient to increase his functional activity, for example, walking or augmenting the action of weak muscles and protecting paretic muscles from overstretching.[196] The use of orthoses before the development of a fixed deformity is important in control of the lower extremity. Dynamic rather than static splinting, including the use of spring-assisted devices, is more effective (Fig. 4-2). External tibial torsion commonly is associated with a paralytic equinus deformity and the short leg orthosis must have not only a dorsiflexion spring-assist attachment, but also must be designed to accommodate torsion or secondary increase in forefoot inversion and heel varus will occur.

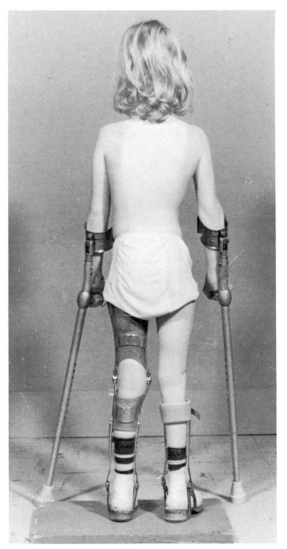

FIG. 4-2. Asymmetrical paralysis requires careful orthotic prescription. (Courtesy of Newington Children's Hospital)

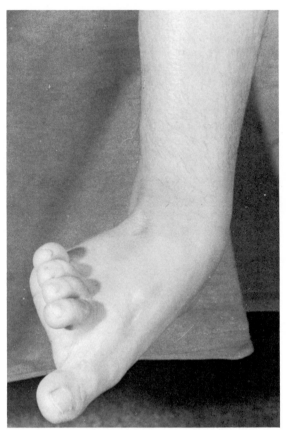

FIG. 4-3. The prescence of unopposed peronei and extensor digitorum longus muscles will result in fixed valgus deformities. (Courtesy of Newington Children's Hospital)

The achievement of muscle balance in the patient with dynamic instability effectively halts the progression of paralytic deformity (Fig. 4-3).[165] A tendon transfer is performed when dynamic muscle imbalance is sufficient to produce deformity and brace protection is required. The transfer should be delayed until the paralyzed muscle has been given adequate postural treatment, to ensure that is has regained maximum strength and that the proposed tendon transfer is required. Timing of

the tendon transfer should be considered in relation to the total rehabilitation program.

The objectives of a tendon transfer are to: (1) provide active motor power to replace the function of a paralyzed muscle or muscles; (2) eliminate the deforming effect of a muscle when its antagonist is paralyzed; (3) produce stability through better muscle balance.

The principles of tendon transfer are well established[81,124,125,126,129,132,137]: (1) The muscle to be transferred should rate good or normal before transfer and must have adequate motor strength to actively carry out the desired function. Muscles of subnormal strength can be transferred if they are a factor in dynamic instability or when they can be combined with another subnormal muscle, thus upgrading the total grade of the transfer. On the average, one grade of motor power is lost after muscle transfer. The patient with extensive paralysis benefits least from this procedure. (2) The strength and range-of-motion of the transferred muscle and that of the muscle being replaced must be similar. Phasic muscle transfers are more effective than those of antagonistic muscles. Antagonistic muscles transferred in the lower extremity, (e.g., the posterior transfer of the tibialis anterior to the os calcis) can be trained to become active. Mixing phasic and nonphasic transfers uniformly dooms the latter to failure of conversion unless it is done as a separate second procedure. (3) The loss of original function resulting from tendon transfers must be balanced against potential gains (Fig. 4-4). The removal of a muscle without consideration of the strength of its antagonist leads to the development of a secondary iatrogenic deformity. Consideration of muscle balance of the ankle and foot illustrates this. The transfer of the peroneus longus in the presence of a strong anterior tibial muscle results in a dorsal bunion as the forefoot supinates. It must be combined with a lateral transfer of the tibialis anterior to the base of the second metatarsal bone. (4) Free passive range-of-motion is essential in the absence of deformity at the joint to be moved by the tendon. (5) A transplant is an adjunct to bony stabilization and cannot be expected to overcome a fixed bony deformity.[107] Prior to tendon transfer, osseous deformity must be corrected by serial casting, soft-tissue surgery, or corrective bony procedures. (6) A smooth-gliding channel for the tendon transfer is essential. Preferably, the tendon is passed through the subcutaneous tissue, since tendons passed under deep fascia retinaculum frequently become adherent and function only as a passive tenodesis. A window resected through an interosseous membrane to allow a tendon to be transferred must be large enough to permit the tendon to glide without binding and to allow muscle fibers, rather than tendon, to be in contact with the osseous membrane. (7) Atraumatic handling of muscle tissue ensures an intact neurovascular supply in the transferred muscle and prevents adhesions. (8) The tendon should be routed in a straightline direction between its origin and its new insertion. (9) Attachment of the tendon transfer should be under suffi-

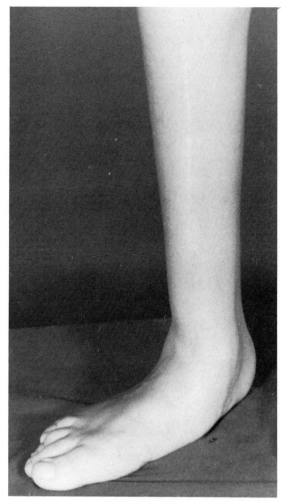

FIG. 4-4. An injudicious tibialis anterior transfer in a patient with functioning peroneal muscles results in iatrogenic pes planovalgus. (Courtesy of Newington Children's Hospital)

cient tension to correspond to normal physiologic conditions and should allow the transferred muscle to achieve a maximum range of contracture. A transfer that is too loose permits the muscle belly to shorten, with accompanying loss of power. A transfer that is attached too tightly results in muscle degeneration. Lower-extremity tendon transfers should be attached to bone, to allow firm incorporation.

Careful postoperative management of a tendon transfer enhances its functional result. The transfer is immobilized for a minimum of 4 weeks, with the joint held in a slightly overcorrected position, and it is followed by 3 weeks of carefully guarded motion before protective functional activity is begun. The limb is supported by a bivalved overcorrected plaster or brace, except during exercise periods, until the transfer achieves fair strength and there is no tendency toward recurrence of deformity. The cast or brace is then discontinued gradually during the day. However, prolonged use of a bivalved night cast or brace is required to prevent contracture. Resistive exercises are initiated when the transfer attains normal range-of-motion and fair strength. The final stage of training is incorporation of the transfer into a functional pattern, such as gait. A brace should be used until the transfer has achieved adequate muscle power to assume its intended function.

Stability of the foot depends on the outline and conformation of bones and joints, the integrity of the soft tissues, including joint capsules and ligaments, and the coordinated activity of the extrinsic and intrinsic muscles.

The movement of the ankle complements the movement of the hindfoot and creates the equivalent of a universal joint. Motion in one of these joints directly influences the others. For example, equinus of the hindfoot leads to inversion of the subtalar joint and forefoot. The axis of movement of the ankle joint passes from the anteromedial to the posterolateral direction, and the subtalar joint is always inverted when the talus is plantar flexed. The subtalar joint, a determining factor in the foot, influences performance of the more distal articulations. The superior articular surface of the talus is longer on the lateral side than on the medial side, thus further inverting the subtalar joint. The talus also serves as the fulcrum between the short hindfoot lever, with its powerful plantar flexor antigravity muscles, and the long forefoot lever, with its small dorsiflexor muscle mass.

Movement is achieved by coordinated muscle activity. The plantar flexor muscles are the triceps surae, tibialis posterior, flexor hallucis longus, flexor digitorum longus, peroneus longus, and peroneus brevis. Muscles that produce dorsiflexion are the tibialis anterior, extensor hallucis longus, extensor digitorum longus, and peroneus tertius. Inversion is produced by the tibialis posterior, tibialis anterior, and flexor hallucis longus, while eversion is effected by the peroneus brevis, extensor digitorum longus, and peroneus tertius.

The Foot and Ankle

Satisfactory long-term ambulation requires a stable plantigrade foot, with weight evenly distributed at the heel and forefoot during standing and walking. No significant fixed deformity is acceptable. Muscle transfer is performed to prevent development of contracture, to achieve balance between dorsiflexion and plantar flexion, as well as inversion and eversion, and to re-establish a walking pattern as normal as possible. Bony procedures are generally delayed until the patient reaches approximately 12 years, when foot growth is adequate, and they are performed to correct or prevent deformity or to achieve stability.

SOFT-TISSUE SURGERY

PARALYSIS OF DORSIFLEXORS. This allows a foot in the nonweight-bearing position to fall into plantar flexion, due to the pull of gravity and the weight and length of the forefoot. The anterior soft-tissue structures, including the ankle joint capsule and ligaments, gradually stretch. In poliomyelitis, the majority of tendon transfers are performed for dropfoot deformity.[62] Substitution of muscle power sufficient to allow the toes to clear the ground precludes the need for foot and ankle orthoses.

PARALYSIS OF THE ANTERIOR TIBIAL MUSCLE. This type of paralysis results in the loss of dorsiflexor and invertor power and results in the development of equinovalgus deformity. This is observed initially in the swing phase of gait as a moderate equinovalgus with forefoot eversion. Later, evidence of dorsiflexor and invertor insufficiency is found in both phases of gait. The long toe extensors, which normally function as auxiliary dorsiflexors, become overactive during the swing phase, in an attempt to replace the paralyzed tibialis anterior. Hyperextension of the proximal phalanges and depression of the metatarsal heads result (Fig. 4-5). An equinus contracture of the ankle gradually develops as the functioning triceps surae contracts. Occasionally, the un-

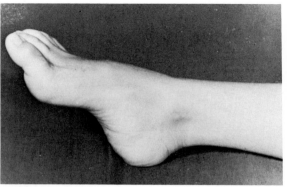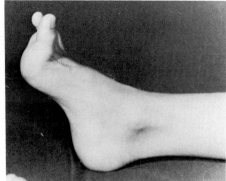

FIG. 4-5. Tibialis anterior paralysis caused toe extensor overactivity during attempts at ankle dorsiflexion. Eventually cock-up toe deformities develop. (Courtesy of Newington Children's Hospital)

opposed activity of the peroneus longus, which depresses the first metatarsal, combines with an active tibialis posterior to cause the formation of a cavovarus deformity.

Orthopaedic management of paralysis of the tibialis anterior begins with passive stretching exercises and serial casts to correct the equinus. The triceps surae is not lengthened, since stretching might weaken this powerful muscle.[58] Occasionally, a posterior ankle capsulotomy is required. These procedures are combined with an anterior transfer of the peroneus longus to the base of the second metatarsal.[81,97] The peroneus brevis is sutured to the distal stump of the peroneus longus to preserve the activity of the peroneus longus on the first metatarsal and to prevent formation of a dorsal bunion. Alternatively, the extensor digitorum longus may be recessed to the dorsum of the midfoot to supply active dorsiflexor power.[54] Claw-toe deformity is managed by transferring the long toe extensors into the metatarsal necks.

A fixed cavovarus deformity may require a plantar fasciotomy and an intrinsic muscle release prior to tendon surgery. The peroneus longus then is transferred to the base of the second metatarsal and the extensor hallucis longus to the neck of the first metatarsal.[105] The extensor hallucis longus has a strong tendency to reattach itself, leading to recurrence of the original claw-toe deformity.[190] This is controlled by suturing its distal stump to the extensor hallucis brevis. This also prevents the development of flexion deformity of the interphalangeal joint.

PARALYSIS OF BOTH THE TIBIALIS ANTERIOR AND THE TIBIALIS POSTERIOR MUSCLES. This results in more rapid development of hindfoot and forefoot equinovalgus (Fig. 4-6). Initially, this is evident only during weight-bearing, but it becomes fixed as secondary shortening of the heel cord and peroneal muscles occurs. On a lateral weight-bearing roentgenogram, this mimics cogenital convex pes valgus. The apparent "vertical talus" is not confirmed when a lateral roentgenographic view is obtained with the foot in a dependent position.

The tight heel cord is stretched with serial casts in inversion to avoid surgical weakening of the triceps surae. Paralysis of both tibial muscles in the presence of normal peronei requires transfer of one of the peronei. The peroneus longus, selected because of its greater excursion, is transferred to the base of the second metatarsal to replace the tibialis anterior, and one of the long toe flexors is substituted for the paretic tibialis posterior. The peroneus brevis is sutured to the stump of the peroneus longus.

ISOLATED PARALYSIS OF THE TIBIALIS POSTERIOR. This is uncommon and results in hindfoot and forefoot eversion.[54] Both the flexor hallucis longus and flexor digitorum longus have been used successfully in tendon transfers. Through a posterior medial incision, the plantar intrinsic muscles are sharply dissected from their calcaneal origin, and exposure and division of one of the long toe flexors is accomplished. The flexor digitorum

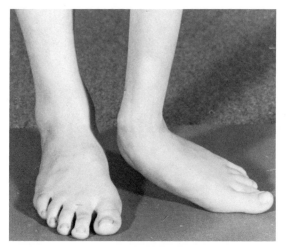

FIG. 4-6. An equinovalgus deformity develops when the tibialis anterior and tibialis posterior muscles are paralyzed. (Courtesy of Newington Children's Hospital)

longus, used commonly, is then dissected from its retromalleolar tendon sheath and is rerouted through the tibialis posterior tunnel and attached to the navicular bone. Posterior transfer of the extensor hallucis longus through the interosseous membrane, and thence through the tibialis posterior tunnel to the navicular bone, has also been used.

Axer recommends a different approach to paralytic valgus feet in children between the ages of 3 and 6 years.[4] Moderate paralytic valgus is managed by bringing the conjoined extensor digitorum longus and the peroneus tertius tendons through a transverse tunnel in the talar neck and suturing the tendon back onto itself (Fig. 4-7). A preliminary heel cord lengthening may be required for fixed equinus. More severe valgus is controlled by transferring the peroneus longus onto the medial aspect and the peroneus brevis onto the lateral

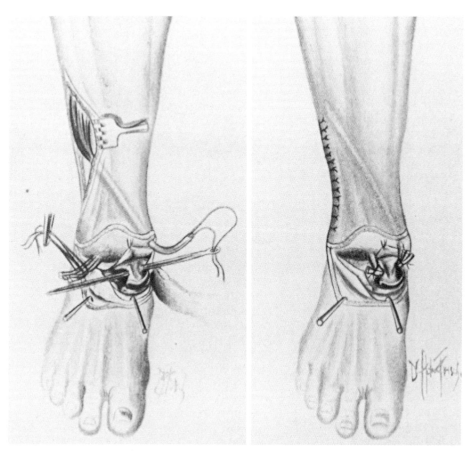

FIG. 4-7. Inserting the conjoined tendon through the medial talar neck creates an active midline dorsiflexor. (Axer A: Into-talus transposition of tendons for correction of paralytic valgus foot after poliomyelitis in children. J Bone Joint Surg 42A:1119, 1960)

aspect of the talar neck. Isolated transfer of the peroneus brevis is contraindicated, because eventually it leads to forefoot inversion deformity, particularly if muscle power remains in the tibialis posterior. A cast is applied for 6 weeks, and a short leg orthosis is used for 6 months.

PARALYSIS OF TIBIALIS ANTERIOR, TOE EXTENSORS AND PERONEI

The unopposed activity of the tibialis posterior and triceps surae leads to progressive severe equinovarus deformity.[69] The tibialis posterior increases forefoot equinus and cavus by depressing the metatarsal heads and shortening the medial arch of the foot. The contracted triceps surae causes equinus and secondary varus and acts as a fixed point towards which the plantar intrinsic muscles pull, leading to increased forefoot adduction. The plantar fascia is shortened and the cavus fixed.

Passive stretching in corrective serial casts is attempted with equinus, but a heel cord lengthening may be required. Preliminary soft-tissue release of the cavus also may be necessary. Anterior transfer of the tibialis posterior to the base of the third metatarsal is effective and may be supplemented by a similar anterior transfer of the long toe flexors.[191] Tendon transplantation without stabilization usually is sufficient, and the deformity can be controlled through physical therapy and bracing.[24] The most favorable results obtained by Watkins with anterior transfer of the tibialis posterior occurred in varus feet in which an overactive tibialis posterior combined with good calf muscles and a power deficit in the dorsiflexors.[199] My preferred method is to create a bony tunnel through either the base of the third metatarsal or the third cuneiform and, in preference to using a pull-out wire, to suture the transfer to a button over a felt pad placed on the nonweight-bearing aspect of the plantar surface of the foot. The suture can be tied over the plantar fascia, should the viabiliy of the plantar skin be questionable.

ISOLATED PARALYSIS OF THE PERONEI.
This is rare in poliomyelitis. It results in severe hindfoot varus, due to the unopposed tibialis posterior activity. The os calcis is inverted, the forefoot adducted, and the varus deformity increased by the dynamic action of the invertor muscles in gait (Fig. 4-8). The increased mechanical advantage of the tibialis anterior increases the forefoot varus. The unopposed activity of the tibialis anterior also allows the first metatarsal to become dorsiflexed, and a dorsal bunion may result. Balance is restored by lateral transfer of the tibialis anterior to the base of the second metatarsal bone.[113] This transfer rarely decreases the motor power by more than one half grade. The foot retains lateral stability, and a good result can be expected. Isolated tibialis anterior transfer may leave the extensor hallucis longus in a position of overactivity and may lead to hyperextension of the great toe and development of a painful callus under the first metatarsal head. In children over the age of 5 years, transfer of the extensor hallucis longus to the first metatarsal head should be performed before the bony deformity becomes fixed.[105]

PARALYSIS OF PERONEAL AND LONG-TOE EXTENSORS.
A less severe equinovarus deformity that develops when these muscles are paralyzed is managed by transferring the tibialis anterior to the base of the third metatarsal bone. Hemitransplantation of the tendocalcaneus has proven unsatisfactory.[22]

PARALYSIS OF TRICEPS SURAE MUSCLE.
Ankle plantar flexion is functionally more important than dorsiflexion. The triceps surae is the strongest muscle group in the body and must be able to lift the entire body weight with each step. Paralysis of the triceps surae, while active functional power remains in the dorsiflexor group, leads to a rapidly progressive calcaneal deformity of the foot. The deformity increases as a result of unopposed dorsiflexor function, combined with attenuation of the triceps surae. The patient is unable to stabilize his calcaneus or to transfer his body weight distally to the metatarsal heads and thus loses push-off power in walking.

The earliest clinical signs that suggest talipes calcaneus are an increase in the range of ankle dorsiflexion as the talus is displaced upward and as the os calcis rotates under and into a more vertical position.[63] The posterior lever arm is decreased as the tuber calcanei shortens and the insertion of the triceps surae migrates upward on the tuber. The stimulus to normal longitudinal growth of the tuber is diminished, and a shortened os calcis results.

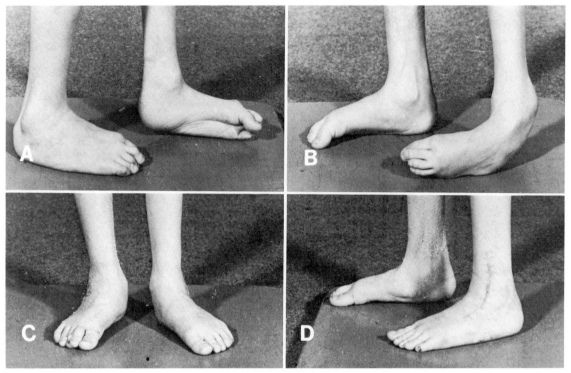

FIG. 4-8. **(A,B)** Unopposed tibialis anterior activity produces severe pes varus and dorsal bunion deformity. **(C,D)** Correction is achieved by triple arthrodesis and a staged lateral transfer of the tibialis anterior. (Courtesy of Newington Children's Hospital)

The foot shortens as the os calcis rotates into an increasingly more vertical position. The remaining muscles force the forefoot into equinus, thereby creating a cavus deformity (Fig. 4-9).

Adequate tension on the tendo Achillis is important in the normal function of the long toe flexors and extensors, as well as the intrinsic foot muscles. When the triceps surae is weak, the tibialis posterior, peronei, and long toe flexors are ineffective hindfoot plantar flexors. However, they can depress the metatarsal heads, thus causing forefoot equinus. The vertical position of the os calcis allows the intrinsics and plantar fascia to shorten and act as a bowstring, drawing together the metatarsal heads and the os calcis. The long axis of the tibia and the os calcis coincide, and any residual triceps surae power is abolished.

Management. Overstretching of the paretic triceps surae during the acute phase of poliomyelitis is managed by keeping the foot in a position of slight equinus.[63] This position is maintained during the convalescent phase, during which the exercise program is increased gradually. In the presence of a weak triceps surae, early walking is discouraged. The patient should learn to walk with the involved extremity and the crutches striking the ground simultaneously. The rapid development of this deformity necessitates the taking of serial standing roentgenograms, especially in children under the age of 5 years.

Surgical correction is performed to prevent the development of calcaneal deformity and to restore functional hindfoot plantar flexion. This prevents retrograde displacement of the tibia, provides a more stable base for stance and gait, and creates a counter-thrust against which the remaining intact muscles can function. There will be a recurrence if the deforming tendons are not transferred and muscle balance and lateral stability are not achieved.

In acute poliomyelitis, development of a progressive calcaneal deformity is the only absolute indication for tendon transfers in children under the age of 5 years.[57,82]

The degree of residual triceps surae strength and the pattern of remaining muscle function determine the amount and combination of muscles requiring posterior transfer. When the motor strength of the triceps surae rates fair, the posterior transfer of two or three muscles may lead to a normal gait. Complete triceps surae paralysis is managed by posterior transfer of as many muscles as are available, saving the tibialis anterior for a possible secondary procedure or, if necessary, a move to the dorsum of the midfoot. A fixed cavus deformity requires a plantar fasciotomy and an intrinsic muscle release before tendon transfer can be performed.

Tendon Transfers for Calcaneal Deformity. The tibialis anterior, the strongest muscle in comparison with the triceps surae, may be transferred posteriorly as early as 18 months after the acute stage of poliomyelitis, or as soon as no further return of triceps strength is obvious.[82] The posterior transfer can be performed as an isolated procedure if the lateral stabilizers are balanced and the strong toe extensors can be utilized for dorsiflexion. Later, the toe extensors may require transfer to the metatarsal heads, together with interphalangeal fusions, to prevent development of claw toes.

Care must be taken to achieve maximum length of the tibialis anterior tendon, which may have shortened secondary to the calcaneal deformity. Its muscle belly is bluntly freed in the anterior compartment and is then transferred through the interosseous membrane. The insertion of the tendo Achillis is split longitudinally, and osteoperiosteal flaps are developed on the tuber. The foot is placed in a position of maximum plantar flexion to ensure that the transfer is attached under appropriate tension. To achieve adequate plantar flexion, occasionally it is necessary to release other dorsal soft-tissue structures (including the ankle joint capsule), or to lengthen long toe extensors. The attenuated tendo Achillis may also require shortening, accomplished by a Z-plasty, with resection of redundant tendon from the proximal part. The transferred tibialis anterior is attached to the tuber and the distal stump of the tendo Achillis, which has retained its normal attachment

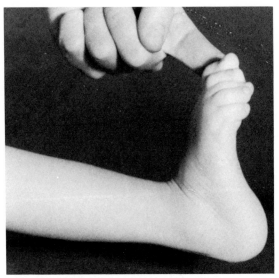

FIG. 4-9. Calcaneal deformity resulting from triceps surae paralysis. (Courtesy of Newington Children's Hospital)

to the tuber calcanei. Plantar flexion position is maintained by long leg casts for 5 weeks and a brace for an additional 4 months.

Pure calcaneocavus develops when the invertors and evertors are balanced. Posterior transfer of only one set of these muscles leads to instability and secondary deformity. Transfer of the peroneus brevis and the tibialis posterior to the heel controls the calcaneus and provides sufficient power to augment the strength of a "fair" triceps surae and to allow the patient to regain a normal gait pattern. Cavus with lateral imbalance requires transposition of the acting invertor or evertor to the heel. Calcaneocavovalgus is managed by transferring both peronei to the heel (Fig. 4-10), whereas the tibialis posterior and flexor hallucis longus are the preferred muscle transfers for cavovarus deformity.[81]

Makin recommends translocation of the peroneus longus, in the presence of a mobile calcaneal deformity.[121] The tendon is translocated into a groove cut in the posterior calcaneus, with no interference to the origin or insertion of the peroneus longus.[11] The tendon is freed proximal to the lateral malleolus and at the cuboid groove. The foot is placed into maximal plantar flexion, allowing the peroneus longus to displace posteriorly into the calcaneal groove, where it eventually unites

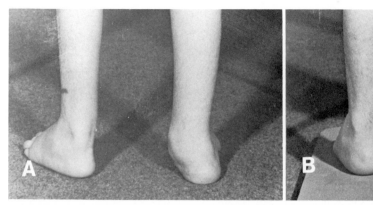

FIG. 4-10. (**A**) Retained peroneal and long-toe extensor function produces a calcaneo-cavovalgus deformity. (**B**) Correction is achieved by a triple arthrodesis and transfer of the peroneii into the heel and the extensor digitorum longus muscles to the midfoot. Indications for this procedure must be carefully followed. (Courtesy of Newington Children's Hospital)

with the bone. Postoperatively, an equinus cast is applied for 6 weeks in growing children. An extra-articular subtalar arthrodesis may be necessary as a second procedure.

In cases where no invertors or evertors are present for transfer, hamstrings have been used to replace the triceps surae.[49] The requirements include complete paralysis of the triceps surae, strong medial hamstrings or biceps femoris muscles, and strong ankle dorsiflexors and quadriceps muscles. The insertions of the semitendinosus and gracilis and, occasionally, semimembranosus are mobilized, are passed subcutaneously, and are attached to the sagittally cut tendo Achillis (Fig. 4-11). A mattress suture at the upper end of the tendo Achillis prevents this cut from extending proximally. The tendons are sutured with the knee flexed to 25° and the foot in plantar flexion.

FLAIL FOOT. Paralysis of all muscles distal to the knee results in equinus deformity, due to passive plantar flexion (Fig. 4-12). The intrinsic muscles generally retain function, as sacral sparing is common in poliomyelitis. This may lead to forefoot equinus or cavoequinus deformity, which can be controlled by Steindler stripping, sometimes combined with a plantar neurectomy. A second-stage midfoot wedge resection for forefoot equinus may be required in the older patient who will require a polypropylene ankle–foot orthosis.

ARTHRODESIS OF THE FOOT AND ANKLE

Structural bony deformity must be corrected before a tendon transfer can be performed. The type of correction is determined by the age of the patient and the rate of progression of the deformity. Because the cartilage of the small bones of the foot is responsible for growth as well as articulation, arthrodesis must be delayed until the patient is over 10 years of age to avoid producing an excessively short foot. Bony deformity in younger children is corrected by procedures not involving cartilage.[117]

Stabilizing procedures for the foot and ankle may be classified as follows: (1) extra-articular subtalar arthrodesis, (2) triple arthrodesis, (3) anterior or posterior bone blocks to limit motion at the ankle joint, and (4) ankle arthrodesis. These can be performed singly or in combination.

EXTRA-ARTICULAR SUBTALAR ARTHRODESIS. Paralytic equinovalgus results from paralysis of the tibialis anterior and posterior, together with unopposed action of the peronei and triceps surae. The os calcis is everted and is displaced laterally and posteriorly. The sustentaculum tali can no longer function as the calcaneal buttress for the talar head, which shifts medially and into equinus. Hindfoot and forefoot equinovalgus rapidly develops and with growth the deformity becomes fixed.

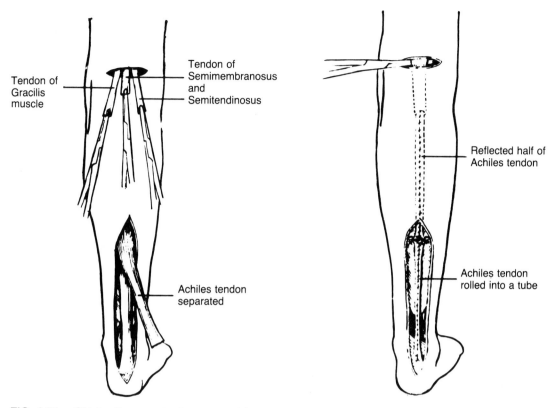

FIG. 4-11. Strict adherence to the prerequisites are required for control of calcaneo-cavus deformity. (Emmel HE, LeCocq JF: Hamstring transplant for the prevention of cal-caneocavus foot in poliomyelitis. J Bone Joint Surg 40A:911, 1958)

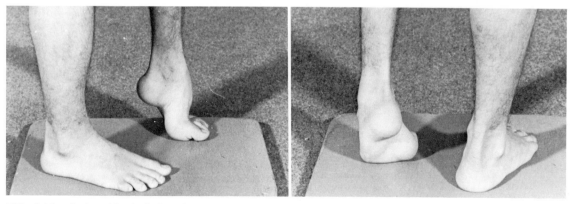

FIG. 4-12. Isolated intrinsic function causes talipes equinocavus. (Courtesy of Newington Children's Hospital)

Initial management of this deformity by a short leg brace with a varus-producing T-strap is not always successful, and surgical correction may be indicated. Grice developed an extra-articular subtalar fusion for patients between the ages of 3 and 8 years, with resultant restoration of the height of the medial longitudinal arch (Fig. 4-13).[64,65] In the ideal situation, the valgus is localized to the subtalar joint and a calcaneus that can be ma-

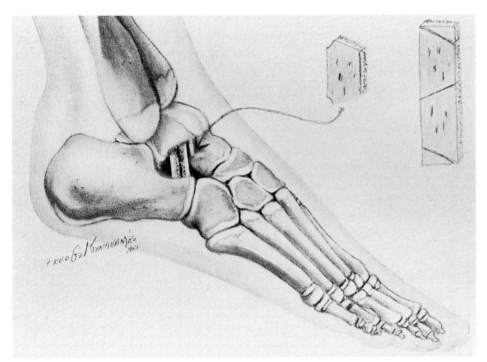

FIG. 4-13. Subtalar joint instability can be corrected by extra-articular subtalar fusion. Iliac bone graft is recommended. (Grice, DS: An extra-articular arthrodesis of the subastragalar joint for correction of paralytic flat feet in children. J Bone Joint Surg 34A:927, 1952)

nipulated into its normal position beneath the talus. Prerequisites for the procedure include careful clinical assessment and weight-bearing roentgenograms of the foot and ankle to determine whether the valgus is primarily located in the subtalar or the ankle joint. The procedure is contraindicated, unless the forefoot is sufficiently mobile to be made plantigrade when the hindfoot is corrected. Failure to heed this precaution results in the development of a painful callosity over the fifth metatarsal head. A second-stage tendon transfer may be necessary to achieve dynamic hindfoot balance and to prevent recurrence of the equinovalgus, which may develop in spite of a successful extra-articular subtalar arthrodesis.[95]

Technique. An Ollier approach centered over the sinus tarsi is used. No skin flaps are developed and the incision is carried down to bone. The origin of the extensor digitorum brevis is sharply freed from the calcaneus and retained as a distal pedicle. Any remaining soft tissue is curetted from the sinus tarsi because it would interfere both with the seating and the stability of the graft procedure. Reduction of the os calcis beneath the talus is attempted by manipulating the foot into equinus and inversion. The capsules of the subtalar joints generally are not violated. Occasionally it is necessary to perform a capsulotomy of the anterior and part of the posterior subtalar joint in order to obtain satisfactory reduction. The anterior calcaneofibular collateral ligament must be separated during this capsulotomy from the underlying subtalar capsule to prevent injury to the ligament that might result in anterior talar subluxation.[153]

The os calcis is reduced and broad, straight osteotomes of varying widths (¾ in to 1¼ in) are inserted into the sinus tarsi to block the subtalar joint and to determine the length and ideal position of the bone graft. The long axis of the graft is placed with the distal end of the strut slightly forward, in order to be at a right angle with the subtalar joint axis when the ankle is dorsiflexed to neutral. The hind-foot should be in slight valgus or neutral but never in varus. The flexibility of the forefoot again should be assessed.

With a straight osteotome, the optimum location for the recipient graft bed is outlined on both the talar neck and calcaneus. The width of the bed is determined by the width of the graft to be inserted. The depth of the recipient bed should be only to the hard sub-chondral bone since the tarsal bones may be osteoporotic and penetration of the graft into the soft cancellous bone would lead to sub-sequent loss of correction. The lateral cortical margin of the calcaneal graft bed is retained as an additional support for the bone block.

A bone graft of appropriate size is taken from the lateral iliac crest and fashioned into two trapezoidal bone grafts with the cancel-lous surfaces face to face. The corners of the graft base are removed and serve to lock over the preserved lateral cortical margin, thus preventing lateral displacement postopera-tively. The foot is inverted and the bone graft inserted into the prepared bed, then tamped into a countersunk position. Initial position-ing of the graft should be accurate since re-positioning may lead to either fracture of the graft or destruction of the created graft bed. The graft is locked firmly into place when calcaneal eversion is allowed. I have found it unnecessary in the management of paralytic equinovalgus to transfix the graft with Kirschner wires. The distal soft-tissue pedicle of muscle and fibrous tissue is then sutured to the talus and calcaneus. A single layer of interrupted sutures is used to close the sub-cutaneous tissue and skin.

Reduction of the valgus may accentuate an equinus contracture. A formal heel-cord lengthening can be accomplished through a separate incision performed simultaneously with the subtalar fusion. If the stability of the graft is questionable, the heel-cord lengthen-ing can be deferred for six weeks. A long leg cast is applied with the knee flexed 45° and the foot in a neutral position. The patient is maintained in a nonweight-bearing program

FIG. 4-14. The Dennyson modification of the subtalar arthrodesis affords more rigid fixation than the original Grice procedure.

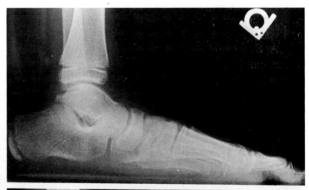
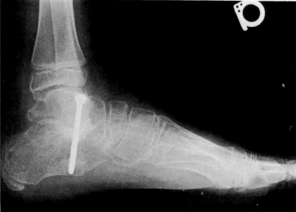
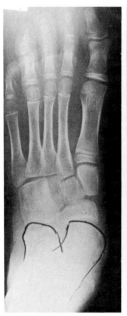
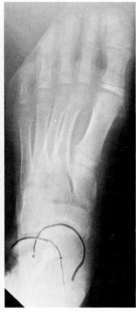

for eight weeks. An additional month in a long leg walking cast with the knee in extension is recommended. Plaster immobilization should be maintained until there is radiographic evidence of trabecular union on both sides of the graft. Generally this is best appreciated from an oblique view of the hindfoot. I prefer the Dennyson modification of the subtalar arthrodesis which uses cancellous grafts and metallic internal fixation (Fig. 4-14).[41] The technique is described in Chapter 10.

Smith found that the majority of Grice procedures performed for poliomyelitis gave a satisfactory long-term result and did not require further bone surgery.[177] However, additional tendon procedures were frequently required. The unsatisfactory results that occurred in a minority of cases were identified early in the postoperative course. Overcorrection resulting in varus deformity (Fig. 4-15) and increased ankle joint valgus, the two most common complications, were found most frequently in calcaneovalgus feet.[143] Pseudarthrosis, graft resorption and degenerative arthritis of the metatarsal joints also occurred. Bone infection was managed by sequestrectomy, and, eventually, by triple arthrodesis.

A Grice procedure resulting in hindfoot varus can be corrected by realigning the original graft or by inserting a new graft.[152] The majority of these secondary procedures are successful.

Seymour obtained extra-articular fusion of the subtalar joint by inserting a fibular graft through the talar neck into the calcaneus.[171] This procedure is limited to mobile equinovalgus feet in which the deformity can be corrected passively, without requiring exposure of the sinus tarsi.[93] A longitudinal excision is made over the neck of the talus and its periosteum divided. A series of Paton burrs are passed posteriorly and distally through the talar neck into the manually-corrected calcaneus to reach its plantar posterior cortex. A fibular graft, generally 4 cm to 6 cm in length, is obtained through a second incision; it is shaped to a point, tamped to the bottom of the tract, and trimmed flush with the talar neck. This procedure is not recommended, due to the high risk of fatigue fracture and resorption of the fibular graft. In addition, proximal migration of the distal fibula from nonunion at the fibular donor site may result in an unacceptable ankle valgus.

Makin noted fibular underdevelopment leading to ankle valgus, particularly in patients who contracted poliomyelitis before reaching the age of 2 years.[120] The distal tibial growth plate remains intact and horizontal, but the epiphysis becomes deformed. The distal fibular epiphysis is delayed in ossification, while the tibia ossifies on schedule. By the time the distal fibula is visualized by roentgenogram, the main fibular shortening has already occurred. The proximal tibia may also undergo underdevelopment, leading to genu

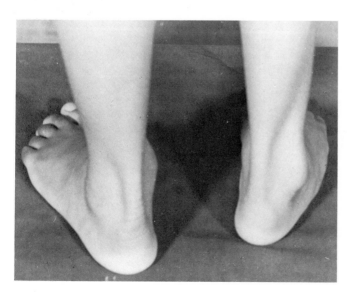

FIG. 4-15. Overcorrection with the Grice arthrodesis produces heel varus. A painful callus develops over the weight-bearing, right, fifth metatarsal head. (Courtesy of Newington Children's Hospital)

valgum, as the fibular collateral ligament tethers the knee. The knee also may develop a secondary external tibial torsion.[146] Initial management is attempted with a short leg brace with a wide varus-producing T-strap. An epiphysiodesis of the medial distal-tibial growth plate can be performed in patients over the age of 8 years.[151] Eventual correction of a marked valgus deformity in the ankle may be accomplished by a supramalleolar osteotomy. This procedure should be reserved for final correction, when the patient is nearing skeletal maturation.

Calcaneal Osteotomy. A hindfoot varus or valgus deformity in growing children can be corrected by calcaneal osteotomy (Fig. 4-16).[47] This procedure can be combined with release of the intrinsic muscles and the plantar fascia in the management of cavovarus deformity.[40] The procedure is used most commonly in management of heel varus. A closing wedge resection, based laterally, is used when the heel is of adequate height and size. Exposure of the lateral os calcis is gained through an oblique incision ½ inch below the palpable tendon of the peroneus longus. The width of the graft to be removed, generally not exceeding ¼ inch, is determined by the amount of heel varus to be corrected. Two parallel osteotomes outline the lateral aspect of the graft and are directed to meet on the medial aspect of the os calcis. An effort is made to retain an intact medial cortex to act as a hinge. An awl placed in the tuber assists in the satisfactory closure of the osteotomy site. Occasionally, the closure cannot be accomplished until the medial hinge is osteotomized. Stability can be achieved by use of a Kirschner wire, which is maintained in place for six weeks.

Mitchell recently described a posterior displacement osteotomy of the os calcis.[131] This improves the mechanical advantage of the tendon transfers that are done to increase plantar flexion. He combines an extensive plantar release with an oblique transverse osteotomy that permits upward and backward displacement of the weight-bearing part of the os calcis.

Evans obtains correction of a calcaneal valgus deformity by lengthening the os calcis.[50] The osteotomy is performed proximal to the calcaneal cuboid joint and in a plane parallel to that joint. A special spreader is used to allow insertion of a tibial cortical graft.

TRIPLE ARTHRODESIS. This is the most effective stabilizing procedure in the foot, results in a fusion of the subtalar, calcaneocuboid, and talonavicular joints. In 1923, Ryerson recognized the need to consider the three joints as a physiologic unit that is critical to the development of hindfoot lateral stability.[159] He observed that the talus is securely held in position by the malleoli. Arthrodesis is designed to fasten the remaining hindfoot bones to the talus, thereby controlling lateral stability (Fig. 4-17A). Triple arthrodesis reduces motion of the foot and ankle to plantar flexion and dorsiflexion. It is indi-

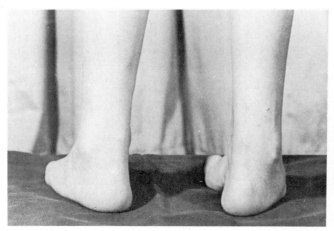
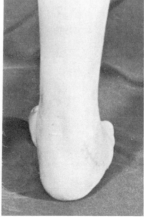

FIG. 4-16. Correction of a cavovarus deformity with a Dwyer osteotomy and plantar fascial release. (Courtesy of Newington Children's Hospital)

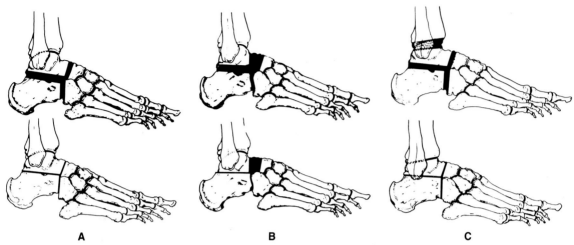

Fig. 4-17. Triple arthrodeses. The shaded areas indicate the amount of bone removed. The position of bones after surgery is shown. (**A**) Ryerson triple arthrodesis, (**B**) Hoke triple arthrodesis, (**C**) pantalar arthrodesis. (Patterson RL, Parrish, FF, Hathaway EN: Stabilizing operations on the foot. J Bone Joint Surg 32A:1, 1950)

cated when most of the weakness and deformity occurs at the subtalar and midtarsal joints.

The goals of triple arthrodesis include: (1) a stable and static realignment of the foot; (2) removal of deforming forces; (3) arrest of the progression of deformity; (4) elimination of pain and decrease of limp; (5) elimination of a short leg brace with a corrective shoe, or sufficient foot correction to allow fitting of a long leg brace, and (6) a normal-appearing foot.

Stability of the talus in the ankle mortise is essential for a successful result. Failure to recognize ankle instability may result in instability of the foot on weight-bearing and, possibly, a recurrence of the deformity. Preoperative roentgenographic evaluation is a necessary complement to clinical assessment. A paper tracing should be made of the lateral roentgenographic image of the ankle. It should be divided into its tibiotalar and calcaneal components, as well as a component comprising all of the bones of the foot distal to the midtarsal joint. They are reassembled with the foot in the corrected position, allowing accurate measurement of the size and shape of the wedges to be removed.

Age is another important preoperative consideration. Forty-seven percent of triple arthrodeses in one series failed when done on children under the age of 9 years, whereas the rate of failure was only 9% when done on children over the age of 10 years.[145] This rate of failure was due primarily to undercorrection. No major growth disturbances were noted in the older group.

Ryerson's triple arthrodesis may be used in poliomyelitis when dorsiflexion and plantar flexion of the ankle are sufficiently strong. The procedure does not allow the posterior displacement of the foot sometimes necessitated by muscle imbalance, especially weakness of the triceps surae. Posterior displacement effectively lengthens the posterior lever arm of the foot, as the ankle fulcrum is transferred to a position closer to the center of the foot. Dunn accomplished this displacement by excising the navicular bone and a portion of the talar neck and head.[46] The Hoke method achieves less displacement and combines subtalar arthrodesis with resection, reshaping, and reinsertion of the talar head and neck (Fig. 4-17B).[89] This last technique can be adapted successfully to the correction of any of the combinations of foot deformities. Williams and Menelaus have described a triple arthrodesis with a tibial inlay graft for the undeformed or valgus foot.[205]

The operative technique varies with the type of deformity.[15] In talipes equinovalgus, the medial longitudinal arch is depressed, the talar head enlarged and plantarflexed, and the forefoot abducted. The arch may be restored by raising the talar head and shifting the sustentaculum tali medially beneath the talar neck and head. This is accomplished by resecting a portion of the talar neck and head by a subtalar joint wedge based medially (Fig. 4-18 *Top*). The tendency to forefoot supination with correction of the hindfoot valgus must be controlled at the time of the triple arthrodesis by a midtarsal joint resection, with the wedge based medially. In talipes equinovarus (Fig. 4-18 *Bottom*), the enlarged talar head blocks dorsiflexion and lies lateral to the midline axis of the foot. This must be reduced to a position slightly medial to the midline axis of the foot, and it is accomplished by a subtalar wedge based laterally, combined with a midtarsal joint resection with a wedge based laterally.

At the time of surgery the foot must be aligned with the ankle mortise, not with the knee. Any associated rotational or angular deformity in the remainder of the extremity should be corrected by a separate procedure.

Operative Technique. Exposure is gained through a modified Ollier approach. The incision extends from the extensor digitorum longus tendon in the midtarsal region laterally toward the calcaneocuboid joint and then curves posteriorly to terminate 1 cm below and posteriorly to the lateral malleolus. No skin flaps are developed and the dissection is carried directly to bone. The contents of the sinus tarsi are sharply freed from the talus and calcaneus and elevated in a single soft-tissue pedicle based distally. The capsules of all three joints are thoroughly incised to mobilize the bones of the hindfoot for repositioning, in order to decrease the amount of bone resection necessary for adequate correction. Periosteal stripping of a short segment of the cuboid allows for adequate soft-tissue retraction to expose the plantar surface of the calcaneocuboid joint. The cartilaginous surfaces of this joint are cleanly removed with an osteotome followed by excision of the talonavicular joint. Maximum bony contact in feet not requiring correction of valgus or varus is insured by minimal decortication of the talar head and navicula. The previously described midtarsal wedge would be required to correct either varus or valgus of the midfoot. A severe valgus deformity may require an accessory incision

for adequate talonavicular exposure. The hook of the navicula must be resected flush with the navicular body in cases where severe varus is noted or will act to prevent lateral displacement of the forefoot.

The articular surfaces of the anterior subtalar joint, including the sustentaculum tali, are next excised with an osteotome. The posterior subtalar joint capsule is incised anteriorly and laterally along the calcaneal dome. Care must be taken to separate the capsule from the anterior fibulocalcaneal ligament. Division of this ligament may result in postoperative anterior subluxation of the talus.[153] Improved exposure of this joint is gained by removal of the anterior lip of the posterior talar facet level with and parallel to the dome of the calcaneus. A wide osteotome is used to allow for removal of the calcaneal wedge in one block. Concern about the higher rate of avascular necrosis in the talus limits the amount of the wedge removed from the posterior talar facet. Apposition of the bony surfaces is carefully scrutinized and any defects packed with chips of the removed bone until maximum bony contact is obtained. Staple fixation of an individual joint occasionally is indicated. The distal soft-tissue pedicle is rotated into the sinus tarsi and reattached to the talus and os calcis. The subcutaneous tissue and skin are reapproximated with a single layer of interrupted suture, and a well-molded long leg cast is applied with knee flexed to 45°. The plaster and sterile cast padding are divided down to the skin along the medial aspect of both the foot and the leg to accommodate postoperative swelling. This opening must be packed with cast padding to avoid the development of window edema.

The patient is maintained in a cast suspended by slings from an overhead frame until all swelling has subsided. Two weeks later the cast is changed under general anesthesia and the patient is allowed to ambulate on crutches. A short leg walking cast, applied after an additional 6 weeks, is worn until solid bony union is demonstrated by clinical and radiographic examination, usually 10 to 12 weeks later.

Complications. Pseudarthrosis is the most frequent complication, especially in the talonavicular joint.[145,206] Loss of mobility of the hindfoot places additional stress on the ankle

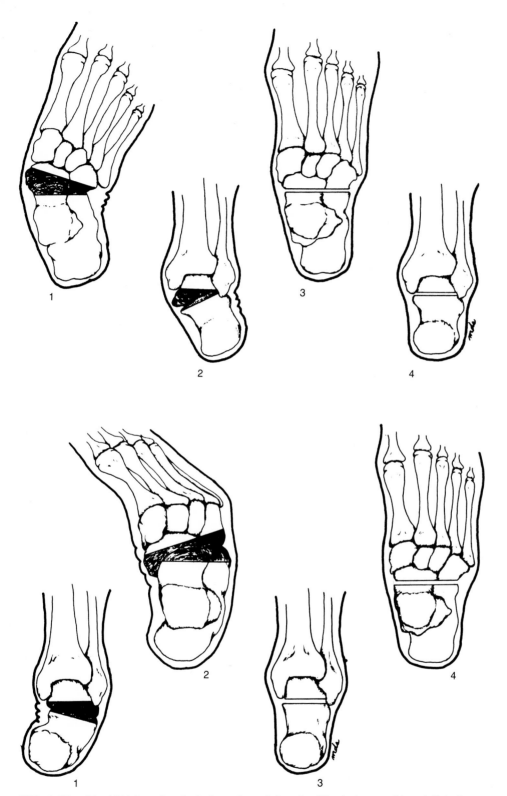

FIG. 4-18. (*Top*) Triple arthrodesis for valgus deformity. Shaded areas (*1* and *2*) indicate wedge resections necessary to correct forefoot abduction and heel valgus. The position of the bones after surgery (*3* and *4*). (*Bottom*) Triple arthrodesis for varus deformity. Forefoot inversion and hindfoot varus are corrected by wedge resections (*1* and *2*). The position of the bones after surgery (*3* and *4*).

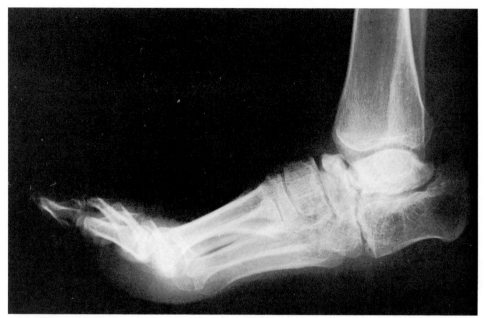

FIG. 4-19. Excessive talar resection produces avascular necrosis and nonunion in the foot of the adolescent who undergoes triple arthrodesis.

joint and may lead to the development of degenerative arthritis. Development of ankle joint ligamentous laxity following triple arthrodesis may require ankle fusion.[52,153] Excessive resection of the talus may result in avascular necrosis (Fig. 4-19). This is particularly true in the adolescent and is demonstrated by roentgenograms obtained 3 to 4 weeks following triple arthrodesis.[122] It should be treated with nonweight-bearing until vascular healing is evident. Failure to appreciate muscle imbalance following hindfoot stabilization leads to a significant incidence of secondary forefoot deformity.[39] Unopposed tibialis anterior or peronei function is the most common cause of secondary deformity.

Fixed equinus deformity can be corrected at the subtalar joint by a Lambrinudi drop-foot arthrodesis (Fig. 4-20).[108] The drop foot results from retained activity in the triceps surae, combined with inactive dorsiflexors and peronei.[51,77] The posterior talus abuts the undersurface of the tibia, and the posterior ankle joint capsule contracts, creating a physiologic bone block. The procedure uses the fixed plantar-flexed position of the talus, against which the rest of the foot can be brought up to the desired degree of dorsiflexion. Bernau recommends that the plane of the talar osteo-

tomy be made parallel to the transverse axis of the ankle joint in plantar flexion.[10] Surgical correction should permit a line drawn through the longitudinal axis of the talus to pass through the shaft of the first metatarsus. Patients with less than an extreme degree of equinus gradually stretch the dorsal capsule and tendons, and a recurrence of the deformity can be expected. The Lambrinudi drop-foot arthrodesis should not be performed on patients under 9 years of age. Residual active muscle power requires either a tendon resection or transfer to prevent development of varus or valgus deformity.[145]

The procedure is not recommended for a flail foot.[118] It is less successful when done for pain, hindfoot instability, or as an attempt to free the patient from a caliper. It is not indicated if paralysis in the remainder of the limb will still require a caliper because of hip or knee instability. The success of the operation depends upon the strength of the dorsal ligaments of the ankle joint.[52] Anterior talar subluxation noted on a weight-bearing lateral roentgenogram indicates the need for a two-stage pantalar arthrodesis.

Technique. Using a Kocher incision, a subtalar joint excision is performed by removing an anteriorly based wedge which includes the

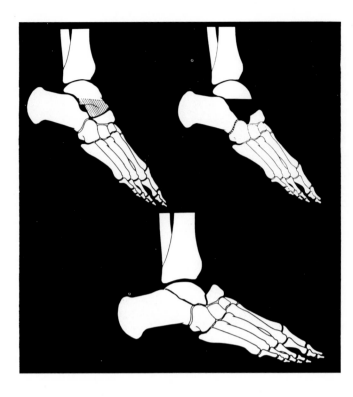

FIG. 4-20. Lambrinudi triple arthrodesis for paralytic drop-foot. The talar beak is wedged into the prepared navicular trough, and the remaining osseous surfaces are apposed. (Hart VL: Lambrinudi operation for drop-foot. J Bone Joint Surg 22:937, 1940)

talar head and neck. The remaining portion of the talus forms an angle of 100° with the tibial shaft. This angle is important since it allows the patient to wear normal heels and to achieve a toe-off at the end of the stance phase of gait. The foot is dorsiflexed against the talus. The talar beak is inserted into a horizontal notch fashioned in the posteroinferior navicular. The calcaneocuboid joint is decorticated prior to fitting the talar beak into the navicular notch. A long leg cast is applied and weight-bearing allowed 3 weeks later. The cast is left on until radiographic evidence of fusion is demonstrated, generally in 8 to 10 weeks.

One complication of this arthrodesis is pseudarthrosis at the talonavicular joint, particularly in patients over 20 years of age. This is due to inadequate contact of the talar beak and the navicular bone. Other complications are ankle instability and residual varus or valgus deformities secondary to muscle imbalance.

Talipes Calcaneus. This rapidly progressive deformity results from triceps insufficiency combined with unopposed dorsiflexor activity. The powerful triceps surae is responsible for toe-off at the end of the stance phase of gait, and its paralysis results in a fatiguing calcaneal gait. The tension of the tendo Achillis is also critical for stabilizing the os calcis and for normal function of the dorsiflexors and plantar flexors, as well as the intrinsic foot muscles.

Peabody emphasizes that progressive calcaneus can be prevented by redistribution of muscle power in the early postparalytic stages (2 to 3 years after onset).[149] Triceps surae paralysis and the subsequent development of progressive calcaneal deformity are the only absolute indications for tendon transfer in children under the age of 5 years with poliomyelitis.

An astragalectomy performed for calcaneus or calcaneovalgus deformity provides stability and posterior displacement of the foot, and is recommended for children between the ages of 5 and 12 when an arthrodesis cannot be performed (Fig. 4-21).[111,195] A talectomy limits motion between the leg and foot, especially in dorsiflexion, and creates a physiologic tibiotarsal bone block or ankylosis.[116] The procedure produces even weight distribution and good lateral stability and places the lower tibia over the center of the weight-

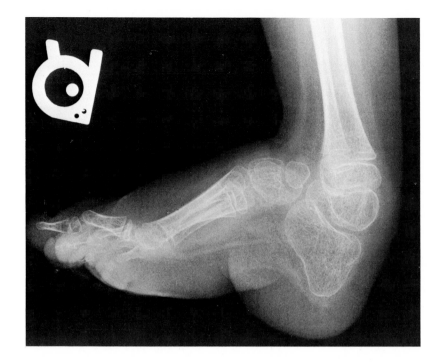

FIG. 4-21. The pistol-grip deformity of severe paralytic calcaneocavus. (Courtesy of Newington Children's Hospital)

bearing area by displacing the foot posteriorly. The result is a painless foot with a satisfactory cosmetic appearance not requiring special shoes or external support.

Technique. An astragalectomy is performed through a Kocher incision. The lateral collateral ligaments are divided and the foot turned medially, permitting adequate exposure of the talus. The talus is excised *in toto,* because any remaining fragments would lead to further ankle joint deformity. The ligaments are stripped from both malleoli and the lower one-half inch of the tibia, and the foot is displaced posteriorly.

The malleolar articular cartilage must be tailored to the contour of the calcaneus. Posterior displacement of the foot places the medial malleolus over the talonavicular joint and the lateral malleolus over the calcaneocuboid joint. Additional stability is achieved by suturing the anterior soft-tissue flap to the lateral malleolus. The foot must be rotated externally beneath the leg, often 30° to 40°, to place the long axis of the foot at a right angle to the ankle joint rather than to the patella. Whitman recommends posterior transfer of the peronei when a valgus component is present.[203]

Initially a long leg cast with the knee in flexion is applied with the foot held backward in marked equinus and valgus. Three weeks later, a short leg cast with the foot again in equinus, slight valgus, and external rotation, is used, and a few weeks later a walking heel in equinus is included. Plaster immobilization is maintained for twelve weeks following surgery. A shoe with a one-inch heel elevation to maintain equinus is worn for an indefinite period. The patient is not allowed to walk barefoot for at least one year following surgery. The average shortening following talectomy is one-half inch and can be compensated for by wearing an inner heel lift, thus allowing for the wearing of a normal shoe.

Thompson finds that muscle imbalance is the most common cause of failure of astragalectomy.[195] The presence of a strong tibialis anterior or tibialis posterior is the most frequent cause of secondary deformity.[90] Forefoot equinus also can develop from intrinsic muscle activity, causing a secondary contracture of the plantar fascia. Surgery performed on youngsters under 5 years leads to the recurrence of the deformity. In those over 15 years, pain frequently results.

A tibiocalcaneal arthrodesis is the only alternative following an unsuccessful talectomy. Carmack employs an anterior approach, leaving the foot in slight equinus.[25] This arthrodesis is most commonly performed for residual pain at an average of 7 years after astragalectomy. Staples recommends a posterior arthrodesis, in which an iliac graft is slotted into the os calcis and is fixed to the tibia by a screw.[184]

Calcaneal deformity in patients over 10 years of age is most effectively managed by the Elmslie double tarsal wedge osteotomy (Fig. 4-22).[32,48] Other types of triple arthrodesis require substantial resection of bone from both the os calcis and the talus.[164] The first stage of the Elmslie procedure is the release of the plantar soft tissue through a lateral incision, combined with a dorsal wedge excision arthrodesis of the talonavicular and calcaneocuboid joints. Complete correction of the cavus component of the deformity results. A cast is applied in a position of marked dorsiflexion. Sufficient soft padding between the leg and foot is necessary to prevent maceration. The second-stage procedure, performed 6 weeks later, is done through a vertical incision along the medial border of the tendo Achillis. The long toe flexors are divided distally, and a posterior wedge excision arthrodesis of the subtalar joint is performed. This wedge should extend distally to the point of the previous osteotomy. The foot is then plantar flexed, bringing the bony surfaces together. The now redundant tendo Achillis is surgically shortened. The posterior surface of the tibia is exposed, and a strip of the distal tendo Achillis is anchored to the tibia, with the foot in moderate plantar flexion. The long toe flexors also are inserted into the tendo Achillis.

ANKLE FUSION AND PANTALAR ARTHRODESIS. *Ankle fusion* has been performed primarily for dangle or flail foot.[198] It also may be indicated when deformity recurs following triple arthrodesis.[184] The Charnley compression arthrodesis has been widely accepted in poliomyelitis.[28,29] The ankle joint is exposed through an anterior incision. Division of all the dorsal soft-tissue structures is carried out. Both malleoli and the distal tibia are divided in a horizontal plane. The foot is placed in the desired position and appropriate correction is obtained through a talar wedge resection. A Steinmann pin is placed into the talus anterior to its axis to increase compression and to counterbalance the activity of the tendo Achillis. A second Steinmann pin is located in the distal tibia at a point determined after the compression clamps have been applied, confirming that the pins will be parallel. The pins are maintained in place for 8 weeks. An additional 4 weeks immobilization in plaster is necessary.

Chuinard describes an ankle fusion for skeletally immature patients with flail feet.[33] The procedure is indicated in children, since it does not disturb the distal tibial growth plate.

Pantalar arthrodesis (Fig. 4-17C) is indicated for flail foot with paralyzed quadriceps, to eliminate the need for a long leg brace.[74,187] A strong gluteus maximus is required to initiate toe-off at the end of the stance phase in a normally aligned knee that has attained full extension, or a few degrees of hyperextension. The presence of hamstrings and the posterior joint capsule controls the knee and prevents genu recurvatum. The ankle should be fused in 10° of equinus to produce the backward thrust on the knee joint necessary for stable weight-bearing.[112] It is essential that lateral roentgenograms be obtained at surgery to accurately determine the plantar flexion, since excessive equinus in the ankle fusion will result in pain and increased pressure under the metatarsal heads. Waugh identified a compensatory increase in forefoot motion that as-

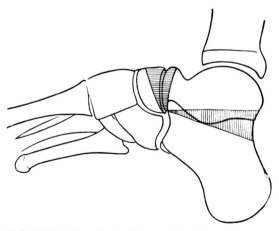

FIG. 4-22. Elmslie double tarsal-wedge osteotomy. The shaded areas indicate the two-stage wedge resections. (Cholmeley JA: Elmslie's operation for the calcaneus foot. J Bone Joint Surg 35B:46, 1953)

sists in the stance-gait pattern.[201] The younger the patient, the greater the compensatory motion achieved.

Complications of pantalar arthrodesis are pseudarthrosis, painful plantar callosities secondary to unequal weight distribution, and excessive heel equinus, leading to increased pressure on the forefoot.

Claw-toe deformity, characterized by hyperextension of the metatarsophalangeal joints and flexion of the interphalangeal joints, may develop when long toe extensors are needed during the swing phase to substitute for severely weakened ankle dorsiflexors. Generally, no toe deformity is noted during the stance phase. However, marked deformity occurs when the tendo Achillis is contracted. Management includes correction of any fixed ankle equinus and appropriate tendon transfers to restore active ankle dorsiflexion.

Clawing may also develop when the long toe flexors are used to substitute for a paretic triceps surae in the toe-off phase of stance gait. Suitable tendon transfer to restore active ankle plantar flexion generally eliminates the need for corrective toe surgery. Claw toes may also be associated with cavus deformity. Correction of the cavus by appropriate soft-tissue or osseous surgery usually results in spontaneous resolution of the toe deformity.

Clawing of the lateral toes caused by overactivity of the long toe flexors can be corrected by a Girdlestone–Taylor transfer of the long toe flexors into the dorsal hood of the extensor tendon (Fig. 4-23).[193] A dorsolateral incision is made extending from the neck of the metatarsus to the distal interphalangeal joint. Extraperiosteal dissection exposes the plantar structures. A blunt hook is used to isolate the long toe flexor which is then tenotomized and advanced to the expansion of the extensor tendon. Fixed soft-tissue contractures may require extensor tenotomy or plantar capsulotomy before the flexor tendon is attached.

Residual clawing of the great toe may result following corrective surgery for ankle dorsiflexor insufficiency. This can be corrected by a Jones transfer of the extensor hallucis longus tendon to the neck of the first metatarsal.[105] The great toe interphalangeal joint is arthrodesed and stabilized with an intramedullary wire, and the distal stump of the extensor hallucis longus tendon is sutured to the extensor hallucis brevis. Clawing of the great toe resulting from ankle plantar-flexion insufficiency can be managed by a Dickson–Diveley procedure (Fig. 4-24).[45] The extensor hallucis longus tendon is tenotomized, routed medially, and inserted into the flexor hallucis longus tendon at the plantar aspect of the first metatarsal head. Arthrodesis of the interphalangeal joint is required.

Pes cavus generally is a symptom of an underlying neuromuscular disease for which a diagnosis should be sought. In addition to the

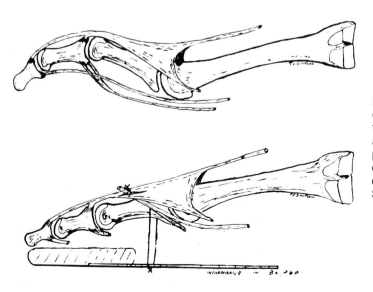

FIG. 4-23. Immediate and permanent correction of the deformity can be obtained by this transfer into the dorsal and lateral aspect of the extensor expansion. (Taylor RG: The treatment of claw toes by multiple transfers of flexors into extensor tendons. J Bone Joint Surg 33B:539, 1951)

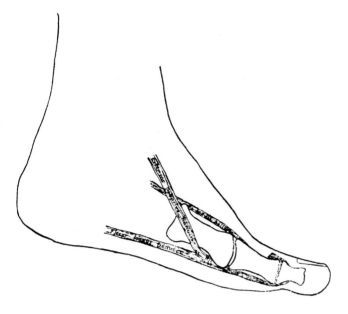

FIG. 4-24. This procedure is recommended when clawing of the great toe persists after appropriate foot stabilization and tendon transference to restore active ankle plantar flexion. (Dickson, FD, Diveley RL: Operation for correction of mild claw foot, the result of infantile paralysis. JAMA 87:1275, 1926 Copyright 1926, American Medical Association)

anterior-horn cell involvement with poliomyelitis, the pathologic lesion may be located in the spinal cord (myelomeningocele), spinal cerebellar tract (Friedreich's ataxia), peripheral nerves (Charcot–Marie–Tooth disease and Déjérine–Sottas disease), and skeletal muscle (myopathies). The majority of these deformities demonstrate a "forefoot drop" on a fixed hindfoot, with the triceps surae either of normal length or slightly contracted. In poliomyelitis, the development of cavus may follow this pattern or may represent a calcaneocavus deformity, due to weakness or overstretching of the triceps surae. The differential diagnosis can be determined by lateral roentgenograms, with the foot stressed in maximum dorsiflexion. Treatment of the calcaneocavus has been discussed earlier in this chapter.

The pathogenesis of pes cavus is obscure. The deformity can develop due to weakness or imbalance between both intrinsic and extrinsic muscle groups, which control foot dynamics. The factor identified by investigators has influenced their choice of management. According to Bentzon, cavus deformity results from plantar flexion of the first metatarsal, resulting from a strong peroneus longus and a paretic tibialis anterior.[8] He recommends division of the peroneus longus, with imbrication of the proximal stump into the tendon of the peroneus brevis. Hallgrimsson describes isolated peroneus brevis weakness,

with compensatory hypertrophy of the peroneus longus and resultant overpowering of tibialis anterior function.[72] Garceau and Brahms identify specific overactive intrinsic muscles.[55] They recommend selective denervation of the abductor hallucis, the flexor hallucis brevis, the flexor digitorum brevis, and the quadratus plantae; they report their best results in young children without a fixed deformity.

Soft-tissue procedures for fixed cavus deformity are indicated before adaptive bony changes have occurred. Although the Steindler stripping—lengthening the medial longitudinal arch—is the procedure of choice, it results in excessive tension on the traditional medial Steindler incision (Fig. 4-25).[185] I prefer an Elmslie lateral heel incision, which is carried forward from the os calcis to the calcaneocuboid joint. Following release, the foot is forced into the corrected position. A short leg cast is applied, with no molding on the plantar surface and with double-thickness felt under the forefoot. The cast is changed after 7 days when remanipulation is performed. A walking boot cast with a rubber platform placed beneath the forefoot, applied 3 weeks postoperatively, is worn for an additional 3 weeks. Long-term protection of the correction is afforded by a short leg brace. Dwyer combines the plantar release with a closing wedge calcaneal osteotomy

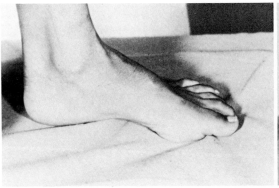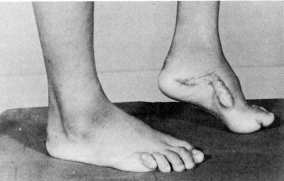

FIG. 4-25. Pes cavus correction through the traditional medial incision causes frequent complications because of increased skin tension resulting from lengthening of the medial longitudinal arch.

when heel varus accompanies the cavus deformity (Fig. 4-26).[47]

Bony procedures are indicated for severe cavus deformity, and generally are preceded by plantar release. Cole describes a dorsal tarsal wedge osteotomy for cavus without varus of the calcaneus or gross muscle imbalance.[35] The cavus is corrected without loss of motion in the subtalar joint. Severe cavovarus deformity requires a triple arthrodesis.

Technique. Cole exposes the midfoot through a dorsal longitudinal incision and a plane developed between the third and fourth extensor tendons. The periosteum is divided longitudinally. A vertical transverse osteotomy is made from the middle of the navicular and cuboid to their plantar surfaces (Fig. 4-27). An oblique second osteotomy begun distal to the first is connected at the plantar cortex. The width of the resected wedge is determined by the amount of residual cavus after plantar release. The wedge is removed and the forefoot elevated to close the defect. Staples may be used to maintain correction. This type of procedure usually corrects secondary toe deformity.

POSTERIOR BONE BLOCK. This negates the need for a drop-foot brace by eliminating ankle plantar flexion, while retaining a functional range of dorsiflexion.[197] It is particularly useful in patients with a completely flail foot and weak quadriceps muscles who may be made brace-free by a combination of triple arthrodesis and posterior bone block.[80] Best results are obtained in patients between the ages of 10 and 20 years in whom there is a discrepancy of less than two grades between plantar-flexion and dorsiflexion muscles, and in whom plantar flexion of at least a Grade 3 is retained.[98] The procedure is contraindicated in full-time brace wearers.

Campbell constructs a bone buttress on the posterior aspect of the talus and the superior surface of the calcaneus, which impinges on the posterior lip of the distal tibia and prevents ankle plantar flexion.[23] Inclan combined a Hoke triple arthrodesis with a second-stage posterior bone block, using the resected talar head.[96] An osteochondral flap was raised from the posterior superior talus and the graft wedged beneath this, thereby widening the posterior talus, while retaining a congruous cartilaginous joint surface.

Ingram and Hundley reviewed the long-term results in 90 patients treated with a Campbell posterior bone block.[98] Half of the patients developed degenerative arthritis of the ankle joint, and a quarter of them developed avascular necrosis of the talus. The procedure in the flail foot may lead to ankle joint ankylosis.

The Knee

FLEXION CONTRACTURE OF KNEE

Contracture of the iliotibial band may cause knee-flexion contracture, genu valgum, and external tibial rotation deformity. Retained

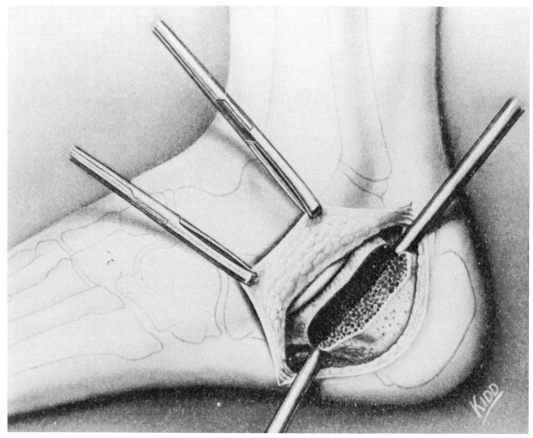

FIG. 4-26. The ideal time for the calcaneal osteotomy is about 3 or 4 years of age. The procedure is contraindicated when the heel is very small. (Dwyer FC: Osteotomy of the calcaneum for pes cavus. J Bone Joint Surg 41B:80, 1959)

function of the hamstrings, combined with paralysis of the quadriceps, may also lead to the development of knee-flexion contracture (Fig. 4-28). Flexion deformities of less than 30° may be corrected by serial casts, but posterior subluxation of the tibia due to short hamstrings must be carefully avoided.[37] Hughes recommends hinged casts, while Hart prefers open wedge casting, with relief of tension at night.[76,94]

More pronounced knee-flexion contractures require surgical correction.[207] A Yount fasciotomy may be combined with hamstring lengthening before instituting traction or a wedging cast.[36,209] The anterior cruciate ligament may undergo adaptive shortening with persistent flexion contracture, causing the tibia to be hinged at its anterior edge, instead of gliding around the femoral condyle. Somer-

ville recommends division of the isolated anterior cruciate through a meniscectomy incision to correct the contracture.[180]

Flexion contractures exceeding 70° are accompanied by adaptive flattening of the knee articular surfaces.[71] There is increased growth on the anterior surface of the tibia and femur, due to a decrease in pressure and a tendency toward posterior tibial subluxation and recurrence of contracture in the growing child. The quadriceps expansion becomes adherent over the femoral condyles, and the collateral ligaments lose their ability to glide. Severe knee-flexion contractures in the growing child can be managed by dividing the iliotibial band, and performing a patellar retinacular expansion and a posterior capsulotomy. Postoperative skeletal traction is achieved by placing a pin in the distal tibia, while a second pin placed

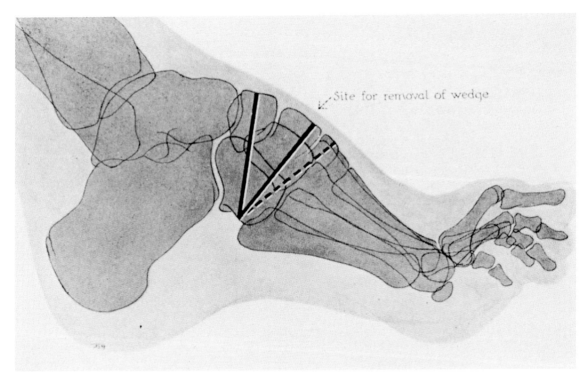

FIG. 4-27. This technique preserves the midtarsal joints in cavus deformity without calcaneal varus or gross muscle imbalance. Triple arthrodesis is preferred if heel varus is associated with pes cavus. (Cole WH: The treatment of claw-foot. J Bone Joint Surg 22:895, 1940)

in the proximal tibia pulls anteriorly to avoid posterior tibial subluxation. Harandi reported severe hypertension following a combination of surgical release of knee-flexion contractures and the use of wedging casts.[75] Management by release of the stretching force resulted in the prompt return to a normotensive state. The long-term use of the Hessing type of long leg brace may be necessary to allow the joint to remodel. A supracondylar osteotomy may

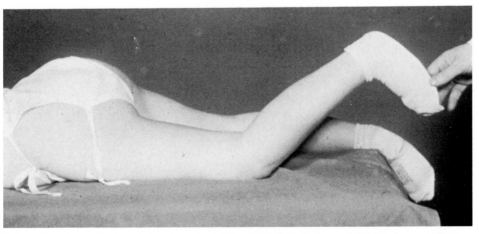

FIG. 4-28. Knee-flexion deformity caused by dynamic imbalance between the quadriceps and the hamstring muscles. (Courtesy of Newington Children's Hospital)

be indicated as a second-stage procedure in patients nearing skeletal maturity.[36]

PARALYSIS OF QUADRICEPS MUSCLE

Quadriceps paralysis is common in poliomyelitis and may result in knee instability. Patients who retain strong hip extensors and ankle plantar flexors are able to gain stability by locking the knee in hyperextension. The knee remains unsteady when it cannot be hyperextended passively during stressful activities, such as climbing stairs or walking on uneven ground. The presence of a knee-flexion contracture caused by active hamstrings also prevents the knee from achieving hyperextension.

MANAGEMENT. Tendon transfers about the knee generally are performed to reinforce weak or paralyzed quadriceps. Hamstring paralysis does not require transfer, because knee flexion is accomplished by gravity, as the hip is flexed in walking. Transfers are most effective when they supplement activity of the weak quadriceps.

Anterior transfer of the hamstrings is recommended for quadriceps insufficiency.[38] Sutherland demonstrated that the majority of these transfers function as extensors of both the hip and knee during the stance phase.[192] Surgical transfer is reserved for patients who have sufficient muscle power to warrant the expectation of becoming brace-free, the ideal patient retaining a fair or better-than-fair rating in the hip flexors, gluteus maximus, hamstrings, and triceps surae.[168] The hip extensors and flexors are essential for walking up and down stairs, and the triceps for active knee flexion, as well as control against genu recurvatum. Flexion deformity of the hip and knee must be corrected before transfer, as their later correction may compromise the transfer function.

Technique.[38,168] Anterior transfer of the biceps femoris and semitendinosis is the procedure of choice (Fig. 4-29). A longitudinal incision is made over the posterolateral thigh from the junction of the proximal and mid-thirds to the fibular head. The common peroneal nerve is identified and freed from its location posteromedial to the biceps tendon. The biceps femoris tendon is dissected from

the lateral collateral ligament and divided at its attachment to the fibular head. The muscle bellies of the short and long heads of the biceps are freed proximally to allow the transfer to achieve a vertical line of pull.

A second incision is made over the lower pole of the patella, and a subcutaneous tunnel is created to join the two incisions. A segment of the lateral intermuscular septum and the iliotibial band are resected to allow the muscle transfer to be directed obliquely toward the patella. The semitendinosis is detached from the upper tibia and the tendon mobilized through a third short incision along the posteromedial aspect of the thigh. The semitendinosis tendon is threaded through an oblique subcutaneous tunnel toward the patella. Both transfers are anchored under tension into the body of the patella. An I-shaped incision is made in the quadriceps tendon and two oblique longitudinal tunnels are drilled, starting superiorly and emerging on each side of the patellar tendon. Postoperatively, the knee is placed in extension in a long leg cast; functional training of the transfer is begun toward the end of the first week. After maintenance in recumbency for 3 weeks, the cast is bivalved, and an active physical therapy program is instituted. Short-time use of a long leg orthosis may be required until the transfer has achieved sufficient power to stabilize the knee in extension.

The most common complication of this procedure is lateral dislocation of the patella, which occurs when only the biceps femoris is transferred. Other factors leading to failure of transfer are presence of a paretic triceps surae, resulting in postoperative genu recurvatum, and the selection of muscles for transfer that lacked sufficient muscle power.

GENU RECURVATUM. This results from adaptive bone changes in the proximal tibia following a lack of quadriceps power, or following relaxation of soft tissues of the posterior knee. The first of these occurs when the triceps surae are normal and the quadriceps and hamstrings lack enough power to lock the knee in extension in walking. The proximal tibia is forced into hyperextension, and adaptive depression of the anterior tibial articular surface and overgrowth of the posterior tibial condyles occur.

Alignment of the extremity can be re-

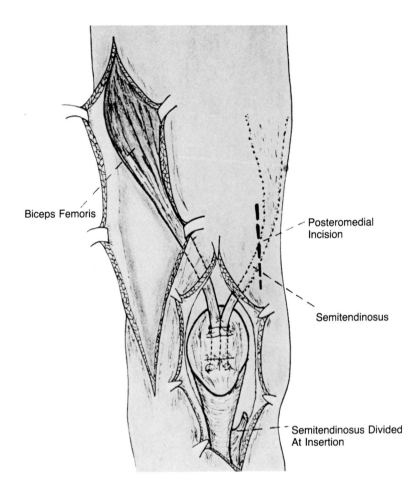

Biceps Femoris

Posteromedial
Incision

Semitendinosus

Semitendinosus Divided
At Insertion

FIG. 4-29. Transference of the hamstring tendons is contraindicated unless one other knee flexor, as well as the gastrocnemius muscle, is functioning. Transfer of a strong biceps reinforces a weak quadriceps while the medial hamstring transfer serves as a check rein on the patella to prevent lateral dislocation. (Schwartzmann JR, Crego, CH, Jr: Hamstring-tendon transplantation for the relief of quadriceps femoris paralysis in residual poliomyelitis. A follow-up study of 134 cases. J Bone Joint Surg 30A:541, 1948)

stored by either an opening or closing wedge osteotomy of the proximal tibia, in patients nearing skeletal maturity.[99] A second-stage anterior transfer of the hamstring corrects the muscle imbalance.

Genu recurvatum also occurs with weakness of the triceps surae and hamstring muscles (Fig. 4-30). Stretching of the muscles is followed by relaxation of the posterior knee-capsular ligaments. This type of recurvatum develops rapidly, with considerable functional disability, and it usually requires management with a long leg orthosis.

Heyman uses the peronei to construct posterior ligaments.[84,85] He recommends the procedure only when the quadriceps is strong enough to lock the knee and when walking without a brace is possible postoperatively. The procedure is most effective when performed prior to secondary bony changes, and

is indicated in patients under the age of 12 years.

Heyman developed a procedure that corrects lateral instability, as well as genu recurvatum.[85,86] The lateral collateral ligament is recreated by dividing the biceps femoris tendon proximal to the knee joint (Fig. 4-31). A flap of fascia lata is fashioned, and it is folded into a tube. The knee is flexed 70°, and the biceps femoris tendon is stapled to the posterior aspect of the lateral femoral condyle. The fascia lata band is advanced and is secured in a similar fashion to the fibular head. In a similar procedure, using the divided gracilis and semitendinosis, transfers can be fashioned to replace the medial collateral ligament. The combination of these transfers blocks hyperextension. Heyman reports favorable results in 5 out of 7 patients in a long-term follow-up study.[87] His outstanding re-

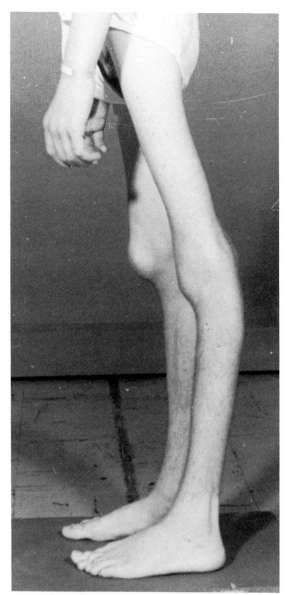

FIG. 4-30. Functional genu recurvatum becomes structural when adaptive joint changes occur in a patient with paralysis of the triceps surae and hamstrings. (Courtesy of Newington Children's Hospital)

sults are in contrast to those of most other authors who found that soft tissues eventually stretch again after repair, requiring a long leg orthosis to prevent recurrence of this deformity.

Perry recently reported a triple tenodesis of the knee for posterior soft tissue laxity which permitted greater than 30° of genu recurvatum.[150] This procedure includes advancing the posterior capsule proximally with the knee joint in 20° of flexion, passing semitendinosis and gracilis tendons through transverse tunnels in the tibia and femur, and creating two diagonal fascial strips from the biceps femoris tendon and iliotibial band. This combination blocks hyperextension and may result in the patient eventually becoming brace-free.

FLAIL KNEE

A flail knee is unstable and requires either a long leg orthosis with a knee-locking device, or arthrodesis. The latter is rarely indicated and should be deferred until skeletal maturity is achieved and the patient's needs clearly established. Arthrodesis may be required in an adult who performs heavy manual labor. It should be considered as a unilateral procedure in a patient with marked paralysis in both lower extremities. The technique of knee fusion should be determined after careful analysis of the various patterns of knee deformity and after primary correction of any associated severe knee deformity. The Charnley compression arthrodesis is recommended.[29]

ILIOTIBIAL BAND

The iliotibial band plays a unique role in the development of hip, knee, or lower trunk deformity. This thickened portion of the fascia lata arises posteriorly from the coccyx and sacrum, laterally from the iliac crest, and extends anteriorly to Poupart's ligament and the superior ramus of pubis.[100] It attaches to a lateral tibial tubercle (tubercle of Gurdy) and the patella. Its superficial layer covers the gluteus maximus and tensor fascia lata; its second layer is beneath these muscles. These two layers converge to form the iliotibial band, which, with the lateral intermuscular septum, adheres to the linea aspera, extending from the greater trochanter to the posterior lateral femoral condyle. The iliotibial band serves as a major insertion for the gluteus maximus and is the site of origin for the short head of the biceps femoris. Contracture of the iliotibial band leads to a flexion-abduction external rotation deformity of the hip, as well as valgus flexion and external rotation of the knee.[102]

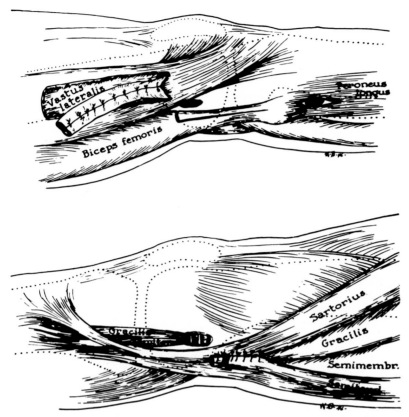

FIG. 4-31. This shows reconstruction of both collateral ligaments with the attachments secured by staples to the femoral condyle. (Heyman, CH: Operative treatment of paralytic genu recurvatum. J Bone Joint Surg 29:644, 1947)

Because of spasm in the hip flexors, hip abductors, hamstrings, and tensor fascia lata during the acute stage of poliomyelitis, the patient assumes a frog-leg position. This posture can be avoided through correct anatomic limb positioning on a firm mattress, with sandbags about the thighs. The irritated muscles make joint movement painful and lead to rapid contracture of the iliotibial band. The tensor fascia lata rarely is paralyzed in poliomyelitis.[53] Partially paralyzed muscles shorten due to contracture of replacement fibrosis; adaptive shortening of normal muscles occurs only late in the disease process.

An established contracture of the iliotibial band is the most common indication for surgical intervention (Fig. 4-32).[144] Passive stretching and plaster casting are unsuccessful because the pelvis cannot be controlled adequately, thus the force applied is transferred to the anterior and lateral abdominal walls.[100] Surgical correction should be limited to the release of the tight fascia, while avoiding injury to those muscles only secondarily contracted.

An Ober procedure releases the fascia that lies over the sartorius, the rectus femoris, the tensor fascia lata, and the anterior portion of the gluteus maximus.[138] Blunt dissection augments the release and may create a gap of 1 to 2 inches in the fascia. The Yount fasciotomy (resection of a 1-inch block of the iliotibial band and the lateral intermuscular septum from the distal lateral femur) should be done in conjunction with the proximal release, as recommended by Irwin.[100,209]

Severe hip flexion-abduction contractures warrant more radial surgical techniques, such as lengthening of the major hip flexors and, occasionally, division of the anterior hip cap-

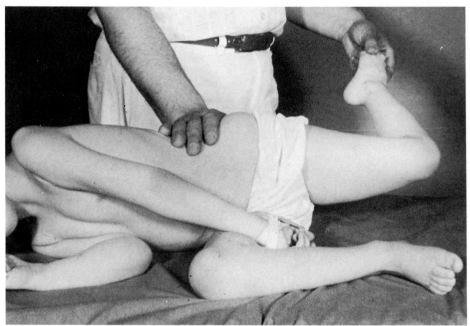

FIG. 4-32. The Ober test for iliotibial band contracture. The flexed contralateral limb locks the pelvis. The ipsilateral hip is flexed, then abducted and extended with the knee maintained in right-angle flexion. Normally the extremity drops well below a horizontal line parallel to the table. The angle that the thigh makes with the horizontal line represents the degree of abduction contracture. (Courtesy of Newington Children's Hospital)

sule.[181] The Barr transfer of the iliotibial band to the erector spinae muscle will be discussed in the section on gluteus maximus paralysis.[6] Soft-tissue procedures must be performed before a proximal femoral osteotomy is considered for final correction of residual deformity.

PELVIC OBLIQUITY

The development of a paralytic pelvic obliquity can result from contractures above or below the level of the pelvis, or both. A fixed hip abduction contracture requires the ipsilateral pelvis to be tilted down, allowing the contralateral side to rotate upward. The obliquity creates an apparent ipsilateral leg lengthening. A flexion abduction contracture caused by the iliotibial band can hold the pelvis in this oblique position.[100] The ipsilateral trunk muscles may lengthen, while those on the opposite side may undergo myostatic contracture to conform to the oblique pelvic position. Eventually, structural lumbar vertebral changes may occur. The uninvolved hip tends

to sublux. Conversely, an adduction contracture leads to apparent shortening, and the ipsilateral hip may sublux. These two deformities in combination create a windblown pelvis, with the adducted hip in jeopardy of dislocating.[141]

Mayer emphasizes the role of asymmetric weakness of the spinal and abdominal muscles in the development of the pelvic obliquity.[127] The strong trunk muscles and ligaments contract, while the weakened muscles stretch and allow the sides to tilt downward.[3,114,115] Thoracolumbar scoliosis and fixed pelvic obliquity may result from asymmetrical paralysis of the obliquus and quadratus lumborum. Asymmetrical paralysis of the abdominals and the obliquus, combined with a normal quadratus lumborum, causes thoracolumbar scoliosis that is convex to the side of paralysis, but a fixed pelvic obliquity does not occur because the downward pelvic tilt is prevented. The combination of weak anterior abdominal muscles and unopposed erector spinae muscles causes an increased lumbar lordosis.

The Hip

GLUTEUS MEDIUS PARALYSIS

Gluteal muscles are necessary for hip abduction, and they are responsible for maintaining the pelvic level during the stance phase of gait. The power of the gluteal muscles is demonstrated by the Trendelenburg test. Normally, an individual stands on one extremity while flexing the opposite hip; the pelvis is held in a horizontal plane, and the gluteal folds remain at the same level. In the presence of gluteal weakness, weight borne on the extremity causes the pelvis on the normal side

to drop lower than the affected side. To compensate for this, the patient leans toward the involved side, thereby transferring the body weight directly over the hip joint (Fig. 4-33). During ambulation, gluteus medius weakness forces the trunk to sway over the affected limb, while the pelvis sags on the opposite side. Weakness of the ipsilateral gluteus maximus is common and produces a marked lurching type of gait.[66]

TREATMENT.   Transfer of the iliopsoas to the greater trochanter is effective in restoring lateral hip stability. Careful assessment of its pretransfer strength is made by flexing the knee

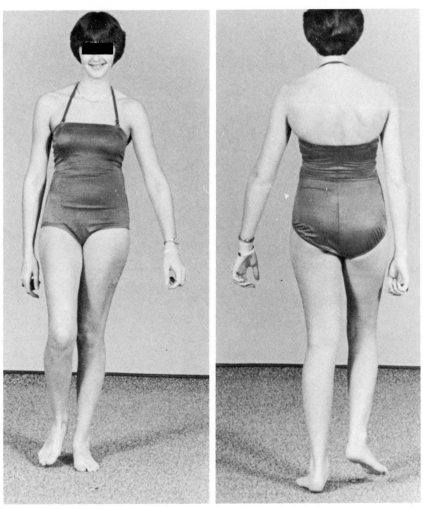

FIG. 4-33.   Paralysis of the gluteus medius muscle causes the trunk to sway toward the affected side and causes the opposite side of the pelvis to sag, resulting in an unsightly limp.

to the chest from a right angle, against resistance.[135] Good abdominal muscle strength is also a prerequisite for transfer. The normal sartorius becomes the primary hip flexor after iliopsoas transfer.

Mustard noted clinical improvement continuing for 1 to 2 years following transfer.[134,135] He achieved his best results in patients with a normal or good gluteus maximus function to assist with pelvic stability, but found that even when combined with poor gluteus maximus function, results of the transfer were satisfactory.

TECHNIQUE.[134,135] The incision extends anteriorly from the middle third of the iliac crest and passes below the anterosuperior iliac spine. It is carried distally along the medial border of the sartorius for an additional 6 cm to 10 cm. The lateral femoral cutaneous nerve is identified. A plane is developed between the tensor fascia lata and sartorius. The sartorius and the anterosuperior iliac spine are divided and the tensor fascia lata and residual gluteal muscles are stripped by subperiosteal dissection. The origins of the abdominal muscles and the iliacus are released from the iliac crest.

The femoral neurovascular structures are identified and retracted medially. Ligation of the medial circumflex vessels may be necessary to gain adequate exposure of the lesser trochanter. Flexion, external rotation, and abduction of the hip at this point, assist in exposure of the lesser trochanter. The psoas insertion is divided with a meniscotome under direct vision. Sharp dissection detaches remaining attachments of the psoas and iliacus to the femoral neck.

The femur is rotated medially to expose the greater trochanter. A trough is cut in the ilium beginning anteriorly between the two spines. The trough is rongeured posteriorly to accommodate the transferred muscle as posterior as possible to allow for more direct line of pull (Fig. 4-34). The remaining hip abductors are split longitudinally, allowing the psoas to be pulled through towards the trochanter. The thigh is abducted and internally rotated and the psoas attached to the greater trochanter. The vastus lateralis is sutured to the edge of the iliopsoas tendon and the fascia lata reattached to the anterior crest of the ilium. The patient is placed in a one-and-a-half hip spica in abduction and internal rotation for 5

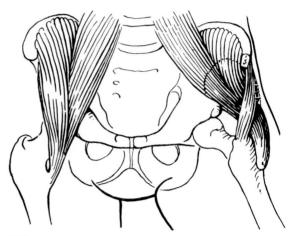

FIG. 4-34. Transferring the iliopsoas below the greater trochanter is most effective when there is good or normal gluteus maximus muscle strength to assist in stabilizing the pelvis and a normal sartorius to act as a hip flexor. (Mustard WT: Iliopsoas transfer for weakness of the hip abductors; preliminary report. J Bone Joint Surg 34A:647, 1952)

weeks. The hips should be protected with crutches until the transfer rates at least a fair plus and the Trendelenburg test is negative.

Sharrard transfers the psoas tendon and the entire iliac muscle posteriorly through a window cut through the iliac wing, immediately anterior to the sacroiliac joint (Fig. 4-35).[175] He creates a tunnel in the greater trochanter with Paton burrs, and advances the tendon through the tunnel to the anterolateral surface of the greater trochanter. The entire iliac muscle is taken down and mobilized, resulting in devascularization of the muscle. The Sharrard procedure is more extensive and technically more difficult than the others, and transfer of the psoas tendon alone by this method is recommended only when both the gluteus medius and maximus are paralyzed. The posterior iliopsoas transfer for the gluteus maximus can supplement the function of a weakened muscle, but the iliopsoas is not strong enough to act independently in hip extension.

The external oblique muscle has also been transferred to the greater trochanter for paralysis of the gluteus medius. This muscle has a spinal segment innervation different from that of the hip abductors and, therefore, it may remain functional when the glutei are paralyzed. A muscle with antigravity strength is

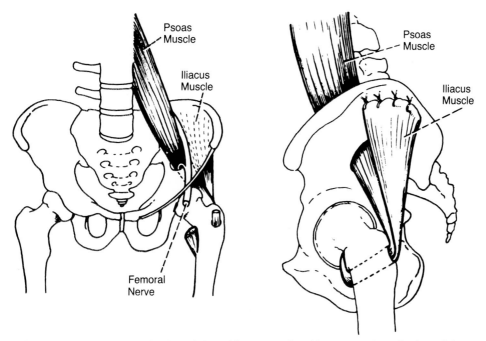

FIG. 4-35. An adequate division of the adductors and stable concentric reduction of the hip are required for a successful Sharrard transfer. (Sharrard, WJW: Posterior iliopsoas transplantation in the treatment of paralytic dislocation of the hip. J Bone Joint Surg 46B:426, 1964)

required for transfer, but sufficiently strong abdominal muscles should remain to maintain the integrity of the abdominal wall after its transfer. Thomas describes a procedure where the entire muscle belly is freed, leaving its origin on the rib cage, and its insertion is released from the ilium and Poupart's ligament to obtain sufficient length for transfer (Fig. 4-36).[194] I reserve this method as an alternative, to be used only when other transfers are not available. Legg's posterior transfer of the tensor fascia lata is reserved for patients with hip instability and gluteus medius weakness who have no other active muscles available for transfer.[43,110]

GLUTEUS MAXIMUS PARALYSIS

Isolated paralysis of the gluteus maximus causes the body to lurch backward when weight is borne on the involved hip. The paretic gluteus maximus can be further weakened by the development of an increasing flexion deformity caused by active hip flexor muscles.

Accurate assessment of the strength of the gluteus maximus can be made only after hip-flexion contractures have been corrected. The most reliable test is to place the patient in a prone position, with the lower extremities flexed at the hip over the end of the examining table. The knee also is flexed to eliminate the extensor action of the hamstrings on the hip. The patient then is required to extend the hip against gravity and against varying levels of manual resistance. A side-lying position is chosen to eliminate the force of gravity if the muscle is of less than fair strength.

MANAGEMENT. Transfers to restore hip extension in poliomyelitis generally function as does a tenodesis. They must be preceded by surgical correction of flexion and abduction contractures.

My experience with posterior iliopsoas transfer in poliomyelitis has been disappointing. Hogshead and Ponseti recommend transfer of the erector spinae and tensor fascia lata, combined with an anterior hip release (Fig. 4-37).[88] The fascia lata is divided at its tibial insertion and a strip of fascia, including the

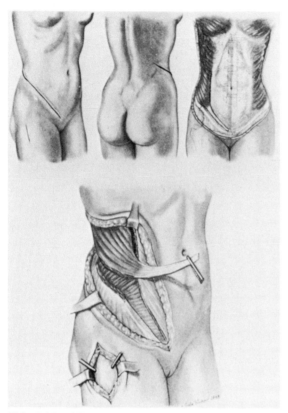
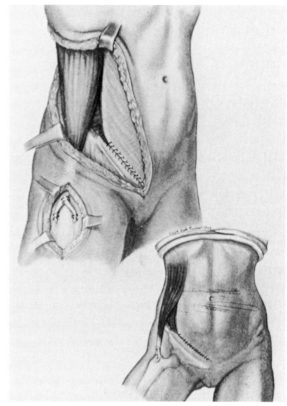

FIG. 4-36. Hip stability during weight-bearing and active abduction will be restored only if the external oblique muscle has nearly normal strength. (Thomas CI, Thompson, TC, Straub CR: Transplantation of the external oblique muscle for abduction paralysis. J Bone Joint Surg 32A:207, 1950)

iliotibial band, is dissected proximally. The attachment to the greater trochanter is preserved as an anchor, and the fascial strip is passed subcutaneously across the buttock to a mobilized flap of the erector spinae muscle. Their long-term results indicate that the removal of the deforming iliotibial band is effective for permanent relief of hip flexion and abduction deformities, and it assists in the control of lumbar lordosis.

PARALYTIC DISLOCATION OF THE HIP

Dislocation of the hip is rare in poliomyelitis. It may occur in children who contract polio before the age of 2 years (before weight-bearing has been established).[144] Generally, these youngsters have flexors and adductors that retain normal strength, while the gluteal muscles are paralyzed. Dislocation may also develop because of a fixed pelvic obliquity in which the contralateral hip is held in a position of marked abduction, usually by the iliotibial band or a structural scoliosis. Failure to correct a pelvic obliquity allows the vulnerable hip to dislocate gradually.[141]

Abductor muscle weakness causes growth retardation of the greater trochanter. The proximal femoral capital epiphysis continues to grow away from the stunted trochanter, thus increasing the valgus deformity of the femoral neck. An adaptive increase in femoral neck anteversion also may develop. The hip joint in both categories of dislocation becomes mechanically unstable and gradually subluxes. The capsule becomes stretched, and secondarily, the acetabulum increases in length, but it becomes more shallow as the femoral head presses against its superior rim.

MANAGEMENT. The treatment goals are reduction of the dislocation, restoration of mus-

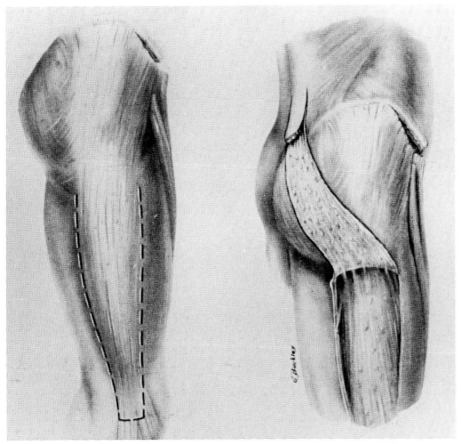

FIG. 4-37. The erector-spinae transfer must be combined with appropriate soft-tissue releases to correct severe flexion abduction deformities of the hip and secondary lumbar lordosis. (Hogshead, HP, Ponseti IV: Fascia lata transfer to the erector spinae for the treatment of flexion abduction contractures of the hip in patients with poliomyelitis and meningomyelocele. Evaluation of results. J Bone Joint Surg 46A:1389, 1964)

cle balance, and establishment of weight-bearing. Muscle balancing procedures must be deferred until bony deformity has been corrected and the critical amount of tension necessary for the transfer can be determined.

Reduction of the hip generally can be achieved by simple abduction, which sometimes is facilitated by an open adductor tenotomy.[179] Adaptive soft-tissue contractures may develop, requiring an adductor tenotomy combined with effective skin or skeletal traction. Traction must bring the femoral head opposite the acetabulum before closed reduction is attempted. Concentric reduction in the growing child takes advantage of the remaining useful depth and remodeling potential of the acetabulum. The reduced hip is maintained in an abduction spica, until the necessary muscle balancing procedures are accomplished.

A dislocation that cannot be reduced by traction requires an open reduction and an adductor tenotomy. The patient over age 3 whose femoral head cannot be brought opposite the acetabulum may need an open reduction, combined with a femoral shortening procedure, to avoid excessive pressure on the femoral head in its reduced position. Jones recommends a closing wedge varus osteotomy to both shorten the femur and correct excessive femoral neck valgus and anteversion.[103,104] Nail-plate fixation is used to maintain the neck shaft angle at 105° in the child under age 5, and at 125° in the older child.

Redislocation did not occur after weight-bearing had been established. Ashley accomplishes femoral shortening in the child over age 3 by allowing the osteotomized femoral shaft to overlap in the trochanteric area.[2] Stability is obtained with plate and screw fixation.

The shallow, elongated acetabulum associated with this type of dislocation relatively contraindicates a pelvic osteotomy. Salter's prerequisites for innominate osteotomy include a complete and concentric reduction of the femoral head into the true acetabulum.[163] This cannot be accomplished in an acetabulum that has gradually wandered superiorly and laterally. Weissman reports the results on a small series of patients in which a Colonna arthroplasty was used to salvage unstable painful hip dislocation in children between the ages of 3 and 6 years.[202] A second-stage supracondylar osteotomy was performed to correct anteversion.

Dislocation occurring because of a predisposing cause, such as pelvic obliquity or another contracture, is managed by eliminating the predisposing factor and restoring muscle balance around the hip. Mild acetabular dysplasia can be corrected by the creation of a bone shelf.[87] The combination of a shallow acetabulum, coxa valga, and extensive hip muscle paralysis may require hip arthrodesis. A Schanz pelvic support osteotomy with a Blount plate fixation stabilizes the hip and improves the gait but further shortens an already short extremity. The procedure is indicated in the skeletally mature patient with a fixed pelvic obliquity.

ARTHRODESIS. Hallock recommends hip arthrodesis for the skeletally mature patient with a painful dislocation or a severe limp secondary to extensive muscle paralysis.[73] Prerequisites include good quadriceps and knee ligament stability, as well as good foot and ankle stability, and good abdominal muscle, paravertebral muscle and ipsilateral quadratus lumborum strength. He prefers intra-articular fusion, with the hip placed in 35° of flexion and in a neutral lateral and rotatory position. An additional 15° of abduction can be used for a short limb. Sharp reported a high incidence of fracture of the ipsilateral limb when hip fusion was performed in the skeletally immature patient.[172] Its application is limited to the patient with one flail limb and one normal limb having sufficient contralateral gluteus medius strength to elevate the fused unit.

The Shoulder

Shoulder stability is essential for all upper extremity activities (Fig. 4-38).[44,186] Scapulothoracic rotation and stability affect humeral placement, which is necessary for effective use of the mobile hand.[42,109] A satisfactory level of function of the hand, forearm, and elbow is a prerequisite for any shoulder reconstructive surgery. Saha classifies muscles acting at the glenohumeral joint into three functional groups: prime movers, steering muscles, and

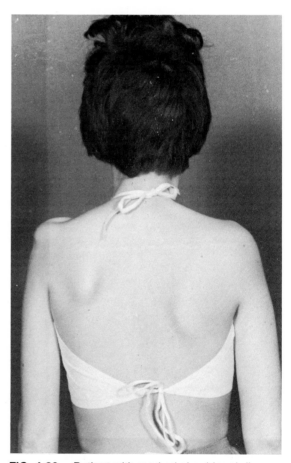

FIG. 4-38. Patient with marked shoulder girdle paralysis from poliomyelitis. Tendon transfers or arthrodesis may be required when the hand, the forearm, and the elbow remain serviceable. (Courtesy of Newington Children's Hospital)

depressors.[161] The prime movers are the deltoid and pectoralis major (clavicular head). Their insertion at the junction of the proximal and middle thirds of the humeral shaft afford them the mechanical advantage to exert considerable force in flexion, abduction, and extension. The steering group includes the rotator cuff muscles (subscapularis, supraspinatus, and infraspinatus). Their motor power is exerted at the junction of the axis of the humeral head and neck and the humeral shaft. They serve to stabilize the humeral head in the glenoid cavity in varying degrees of abduction. The vertical gliding of the humeral head is accomplished by muscle fibers acting in the plane of motion. The depressors consist of the latissimus dorsi, pectoralis major (sternal head) and the teres major and minor, which insert into the proximal one fourth of the humeral shaft. Their action rotates the shaft during abduction. Paralysis of this group causes disability only in the performance of activities requiring a weight to be lifted above shoulder level.

The functional inter-relationship between the first two groups is demonstrated by the disappointing functional results noted following tendon transfer for prime-mover weakness, when there is associated paralysis of the steering muscles.[17] Saha recommends careful evaluation before they are replaced simultaneously with the transfer procedure to supplement deltoid function. Isolated replacement of deltoid function results in shoulder elevation of 90° and distortion of scapulohumeral function.[70,83]

DELTOID PARALYSIS

Transfer of the trapezius is recommended for paralysis of the deltoid. Yadav noted that the upper trapezius simulates the deltoid in shape, size, and strength and also is in the correct plane for abduction.[208] The technique of Saha is preferred.[161]

TECHNIQUE.[161] Transfer of the trapezius is suggested for paralysis of the deltoid (Fig. 4-39). The upper and middle parts of the trapezius are completely mobilized through a

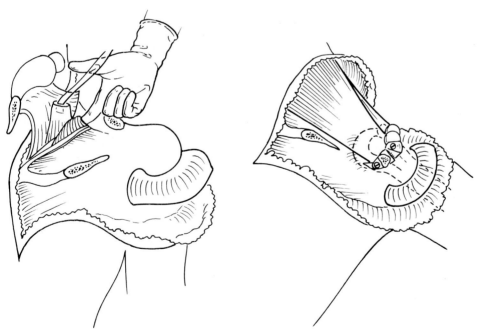

FIG 4-39. The entire insertion of the trapezius along with the attached lateral end of the clavicle, acromioclavicular joint, the acromion, and an adjoining section of the scapular spine have been anchored by two screws to the lateral aspect of the humerus distal to the tuberosities. (Saha AK: Surgery of the paralyzed and flail shoulder. Acta Orthop Scand (Suppl) 97, 1967)

sabre-cut incision. An osteotomy is performed through the clavicle lateral to the conoid ligament, as well as the acromion process and adjacent scapular spine. The remaining insertion of the upper two thirds of the trapezius is freed and the transfer rerouted to a denuded area on the lateral proximal humerus. Two screws fix the acromion and the trapezius to the humerus. Postoperatively, the limb is immobilized in a shoulder spica applied in 45° of abduction, positioning the arm in the scapular plane.

STEERING MUSCLE PARALYSIS

Paralysis of two of the three steering muscles requires a power transfer. The transferred muscle must have a direction of pull corresponding to that of the muscle it replaces, and it must have the ability to be attached to the appropriate humeral tuberosity. Rerouting should be close to the axis of the humeral head and neck, in order to restore the steering mechanism. Surgical exposure is simplified, since these procedures are carried out after the superior and middle parts of the trapezius muscle have been mobilized.

Subscapularis activity can be replaced by freeing the two superior digitations of the serratus anterior from the vertebral border of the scapula and rerouting them to the humeral lesser tuberosity. The levator scapulae is chosen to replace the supraspinatus because of its line of pull. The sternocleidomastoid can also be used for supraspinatus paralysis, but this muscle has the disadvantage of causing webbing of the neck when it contracts. A latissimus dorsi or teres major transfer can be substituted for paralysis of the subscapularis or infraspinatus. (The reader is referred to the original paper by Saha for technical details of these infrequently performed procedures.) Ober uses the short head of the biceps and the long head of the triceps for deltoid paralysis.[136,139]

Complete paralysis of the girdle muscles controlling the scapula is comparatively rare, possibly because of their multisegmental innervation.[109] Serratus anterior paralysis allows the scapula to protrude posteriorly and rotate laterally, due to the weight of the upper extremity. The lack of scapulothoracic fixation results in marked limitation of abduction and elevation of the extremity. Both Chaves and Rapp recommend posterior transfer of the pectoralis minor insertion to the middle third of the vertebral edge of the scapula to replace the serratus anterior.[31,154]

ARTHRODESIS OF THE SHOULDER

Arthrodesis of the shoulder may be indicated when extensive paralysis of the scapulohumeral muscles leads to a symptomatic shoulder subluxation or dislocation. Strong trapezius and serratus anterior muscles are necessary to allow increased functional scapulothoracic movement to compensate for that lost by fusion of the glenohumeral joint.[7] Normal function of the forearm and hand is a prerequisite.

Rowe lists the important standards for satisfactory function following shoulder arthrodesis: (1) the hand should be able to reach the face, head, and midline of the body, anteriorly and posteriorly; (2) the arms should be in a position of maximum strength for lifting, pushing, and pulling; and (3) the shoulders should be comfortable when the arm is at the side of the body, and the scapula should not be prominent in this position.[158]

Charnley and Rowe recommend that the angle of abduction should be determined on the basis of the clinical presentation of the arm's position in relation to the body.[28,30] The angle of abduction traditionally obtained by measuring an angle between the vertebral border of the scapula and the humerus is frequently difficult to determine in preoperative and operative roentgenograms. Rowe recommends that the position of the arm in shoulder arthrodesis should be established with the arm at the side of the body, with enough clinically determined abduction of the arm from side of the body (15° to 20°) to clear the axilla, and enough forward flexion (25° to 30°) and internal rotation (40° to 50°) to bring the hand to the midline of the body. An additional 10° of abduction should be used in shoulder fusion in the child with poliomyelitis when no internal fixation is used. Makin recommends that the position of arthrodesis for flail shoulder in a young child includes 80° to 90° abduction, 25° flexion, and 25° external rotation.[119] Care must be taken to preserve the proximal humeral growth plate in the skeletally immature patient.

Several forms of shoulder arthrodesis have proven effective in poliomyelitis, including those by Brittain, Charnley, Gill, and Watson-

Jones.[16,30,56,200] All of these procedures require internal fixation and postoperative immobilization in a modified plaster Velpeau spica cast for 8 weeks.

The Elbow

PARALYSIS OF ELBOW FLEXION

Loss of elbow flexion, a common upper-extremity deficit in poliomyelitis, results from paralysis of the biceps brachii and the brachialis muscles. The patient is unable to bring his hand to the mouth, trunk, or head. Restoration of active elbow flexion is a critical part of reconstruction of the upper limb, but it should not be performed until hand function has been restored by appropriate tendon transfers. An accurate assessment must be made of the motor strength of the remaining upper-extremity muscles before deciding on a particular transfer, since weakness of muscles of the shoulder, forearm, and hand frequently accompanies loss of elbow flexion.[166]

The Steindler flexorplasty, which substitutes the intact wrist flexors for the paralyzed elbow flexors, has been the most effective procedure for restoring active flexion (Fig. 4-40).[128,130,189] The flexor carpi radialis, palmaris longus, pronator teres, flexor digitorum sublimis, and flexor carpi ulnaris are transferred from their common origin on the medial humeral epicondyle to a more proximal level on the humerus. The lever effect and the muscle tension of the transposed muscle group are enhanced by the increased distance between the mechanical axis of the transfer and the center of motion of the elbow joint. The major disadvantage is the frequent development of a fixed pronator deformity, which may limit the position of an otherwise functional hand.

Flexorplasty is indicated in the patient with a functional hand who has paralysis of the elbow flexors and in whom the muscles to be transferred are rated fair or better in strength. The best functional results are found in the patient whose elbow flexors are only partially paralyzed and whose fingers and wrist flexors are normal.

A prerequisite is careful examination of the strength of the muscles to be transferred. The examination is performed with the upper extremity held at a right angle to the body to eliminate the effect of gravity. The ability of the muscles to flex the elbow in this position is determined. Inability to flex in this position dooms the Steindler flexorplasty to failure, and an alternate solution should be sought. Steindler stresses the need for full passive supination. Shoulder stability is important, since glenohumeral abduction assists elbow flexion and decreases the amount of strength necessary for flexion. The presence of a flail shoulder may require preliminary arthrodesis.

TECHNIQUE.[188] The common origin of the flexor muscles of the wrist are detached en

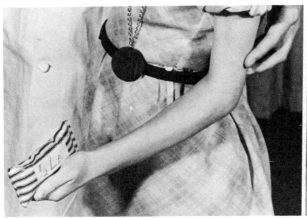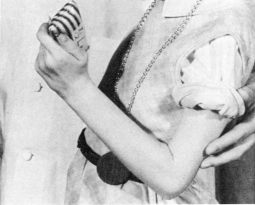

FIG. 4-40. This patient, having undergone a Steindler flexorplasty, demonstrates full range of motion of the elbow and the ability to lift weight. (Courtesy of Newington Children's Hospital)

bloc. The ulnar nerve is isolated posterior to the medial epicondyle. The muscles are freed distally one-and-one-half inches along the ulnar side of the muscle mass because the flexors receive their motor supply from the radial side. Their common origin is transferred proximally and attached through drill holes to a site 2 inches above the medial humeral epicondyle.

Kettelkamp and Larson evaluated the long-term results of the Steindler flexorplasty in 15 patients.[106] Strength was greatest with a flexion contracture of 30° or more developing in patients whose triceps brachii motor strength was less than fair. Nine patients were able to lift a 1-lb weight to 110° of flexion. Kettelkamp noted that the extent of supination and pronation had no effect on the strength of flexorplasty and that a fixed pronator deformity did not develop when the supinators were rated good. The major causes for failure were overestimation of the strength of the muscles to be transferred and an insecure fixation of the transfer.

Bunnell eliminated the pronator deformity by attaching the muscle origin to the lateral humeral border (Fig. 4-41).[21] Additional length was gained by using a free graft of fascia lata and the transfer attached 2 inches above the elbow joint. Both procedures require immobilization in a long arm cast with the elbow flexed above 90° in full supination for 4 weeks.

TRANSFER OF PART OF THE PECTORALIS MAJOR MUSCLE. Clark transferred the sternal head of the pectoralis major to restore elbow flexion.[34] This part of the muscle has a separate neurovascular supply, and it may still be active when the clavicular portion of the pectoralis major is paralyzed. The detached sternal head is passed subcutaneously and is sutured to the biceps tendon, with the elbow flexed 120°. The major indication for the Clark procedure is paralysis resulting from a traction injury to the brachial plexus.

TRANSFER OF THE PECTORALIS MAJOR TENDON. Brooks and Seddon use the entire pectoralis major muscle to restore active elbow flexion.[19] This transfer should be employed only when the biceps brachii is completely paralyzed.[170] This procedure is recommended when the Steindler flexorplasty is not applicable, or when the sternal portion of the pec-

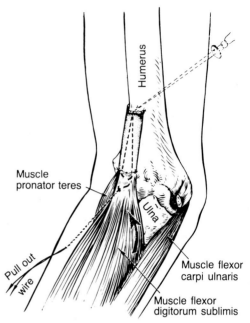

FIG. 4-41. The common muscle origin is transferred laterally on the humerus by means of a fascia lata graft. (Bunnell S: Restoring flexion to the paralytic elbow. J Bone Joint Surg 33A:566, 1951)

toralis major is too weak for the Clark transfer.[169]

The Brooks–Seddon transfer allows the pectoralis major muscle to act both on the shoulder and the elbow joints. Active flexion of the elbow may be accompanied by undesirable movements of the shoulder, resulting in, for example, the hand hitting the chest wall, thus impairing the functional results of the operation. Muscle control of the shoulder and scapula must be good, or a shoulder arthrodesis may be required to limit the pectoralis major activity to flexion of the elbow.[20] The transfer rarely limits the full extension of the elbow. The effect of the transfer can be enhanced by a Steindler flexorplasty performed with muscles of less than fair strength.

TECHNIQUE.[20] An incision is made from the lower end of the deltopectoral groove distally to the junction of the proximal and middle thirds of the arm. The pectoralis major is detached from the humerus and the muscle mobilized by blunt dissection from the chest wall. The long head of the biceps is exposed by retraction of the deltoid laterally and is severed at the upper end of the bicapital groove. All vessels entering into the long head of the biceps are ligated, converting their structure into fibrotic tissue that will be used as a bridge between the distal end of the pectoralis tendon and the radial tuberosity.

A second incision in the antecubital fossa exposes the biceps insertion. The severed long head of the biceps is mobilized distally to the radial tuberosity and drawn into this field. The tendon is passed through two slits in the pectoralis major and looped on itself so that the proximal tendon is brought into the distal incision and sutured through a slit in its distal tendon. The elbow is flexed acutely and held in immobilization for 3 weeks before gentle mobilization is begun. Two or 3 months may be required before full extension is achieved.

TRANSFER OF THE PECTORALIS MINOR. Spira transferred the pectoralis minor to restore elbow flexion in patients with complete paralysis of the pectoralis major, biceps brachii, and deltoid.[182,183] A fascia lata graft is necessary to bridge the gap between the detached origin of the pectoralis minor and the site of insertion into the biceps tendon, near the radial tuberosity.

TRANSFER OF THE STERNOCLEIDOMASTOID MUSCLE. Bunnell devised an operation in which the sternoclavicular insertion of the sternocleidomastoid muscle is detached and sutured to a long tube of fascia lata, which is passed subcutaneously to the elbow, where it is inserted under maximum tension into the tuberosity of the radius (Fig. 4-42).[21] The strength of this elbow flexion transfer is excellent, but the grotesque webbing of the active sternocleidomastoid on the lateral neck limits the cosmetic acceptance of this procedure.

TRANSFER OF THE LATTISIMUS DORSI. Hovnanian transferred the latissimus dorsi muscle to restore elbow flexion (Fig. 4-43).[92] His technique for this procedure is discussed under the section describing muscle transfers for triceps brachii paralysis. Active elbow flexion is regained by attaching the origin of the latissimus dorsi muscle into the biceps tendon near the radial tuberosity. Zancolli stresses that the anatomical features of the latissimus dorsi are better adjusted for placement in the arm than in the pectoralis major.[211]

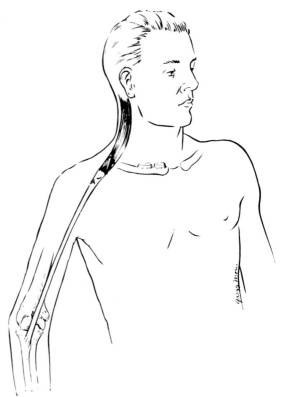

FIG. 4-42. The transfer of the sternocleidomastoid muscle may be considered when there is paralysis of the biceps and brachialis muscles. Obvious webbing limits the cosmetic acceptance of the functional transfer. (Bunnell S: Restoring flexion to the paralytic elbow. J Bone Joint Surg 33A:566, 1951)

ANTERIOR TRANSFER OF THE TRICEPS. The triceps brachii may be transferred anteriorly around the lateral aspect of the humerus to the radial tuberosity to restore elbow flexion. It is indicated when the Steindler flexorplasty cannot be used and other muscles are not available for transfer. Carroll reported a series of 15 patients with poliomyelitis or arthrogryposis who, prior to surgery, were unable to flex the elbow against gravity or to bring the hand to the mouth.[26] He reported 10 successes in this series. Loss of active extension against gravity may be a major disadvantage to the patient with poliomyelitis who requires active extension in some activities of daily living.

TECHNIQUE.[26] An incision is made in the midline of the posterior aspect of the lower arm and is carried laterally to the olecranon

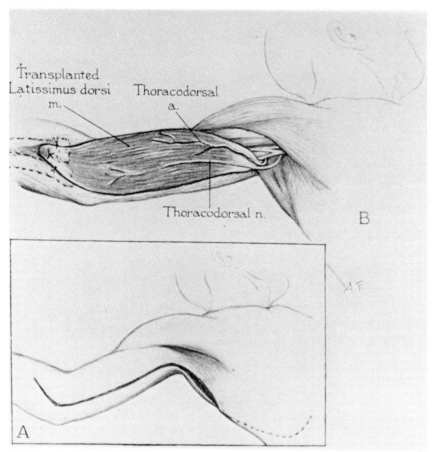

FIG. 4-43. This transfer is possible because the neurovascular bundle of the muscle is long and easily mobilized. (Hovnanian AP: Latissimus dorsi transplantation for loss of flexion or extension at the elbow. Ann Surg 143:493, 1956)

along the subcutaneous border of the ulna. The ulnar nerve is mobilized immediately. The triceps insertion is detached with a long tail of ulnar periosteum and the muscle mobilized from the distal third of the humeral shaft. The interval between the brachial radialis and pronator teres is developed through an incision in the antecubital fossa. The triceps tendon is passed subcutaneously and superficial to the radial nerve and anchored to either the biceps tendon or to the radial tuberosity by a suture through a drill hole. A long arm cast holds the elbow in 90° of flexion with the forearm in full supination for 4 weeks before active motion is begun.

POSTERIOR BONE BLOCK. This procedure stops elbow extension at 90°, when the olecranon impinges against the lower humerus. This rarely performed procedure may be indicated to assist a Steindler flexorplasty or to prevent weakened elbow flexors from becoming overstretched, with subsequent further loss of strength.

Boyd modified the original Putti bone block procedure by using an onlay tibial graft attached with one or two screws to the posterior distal humerus.[13] The distal end of the graft blocks the elbow extension at 90°.

PARALYSIS OF THE TRICEPS
BRACHII MUSCLE

Triceps paralysis seldom interferes with function, since gravity passively extends the elbow. Good triceps function is necessary for reaching over the head. The triceps is essential in activities where the body weight is shifted to the hands, such as in transferring from bed to wheelchair or in crutch walking. The patient with good shoulder depressors who requires crutches can compensate by adding a triceps band to the crutch, enabling the elbow to be locked in slight hyperextension.

Ober and Barr transferred the muscle belly of the brachioradialis from the lateral to the posterior elbow.[139,140] This allows the brachioradialis to change its function from an elbow flexor to an elbow extensor. Additional power can be obtained by including the extensor carpi radialis longus in the transfer.

TRANSFER OF THE LATISSIMUS DORSI. Transfer of the origin and muscle belly of the latissimus dorsi into the arm, a technique developed by Hovnanian (Fig. 4-44), is possible because the thoracodorsal nerve and artery are long and can be mobilized easily.[92] The exposure extends from the flank upward, follows the lateral border of the muscle to the axilla, proceeds distally along the medial aspect of the arm to the medial humeral epicondyle, and then proceeds laterally to the posterior ulnar shaft. The origin of the muscle is freed by dividing the musculofascial portion inferiorly and the muscle fibers superiorly. Care must be taken to preserve the muscle

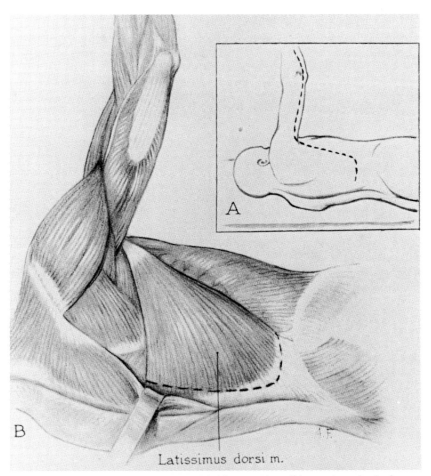

Latissimus dorsi m.

FIG. 4-44. A strong triceps is essential for crutch walking or transfer techniques. The origin of the latissimus dorsi is transferred to the olecranon leaving its insertion intact in this procedure. (Hovnanian, AP: Latissimus dorsi transplantation for loss of flexion or extension at the elbow. Ann Surg 143:493, 1956)

fascia and to mobilize the entire muscle. The neurovascular bundle enters the superior third of the muscle, and it must be protected during transfer. A bed is prepared on the posterior aspect of the arm and elbow, and the aponeurosis of the lumbodorsal origin is sutured to the triceps tendon and the olecranon. The limb is bandaged to the body with the elbow in extension. Active and passive exercises are begun 3 to 4 weeks later. Latissimus dorsi transfer can also be used to restore active elbow flexion by anchoring the aponeurosis of the latissimus dorsi into the biceps tendon near the radial tuberosity.

The Forearm

Fixed deformity of the forearm seldom creates a major functional disability. Pronation and supination contractures may develop, limiting the positioning of an otherwise functional hand. Pronation contracture, the more common disability, develops when the active forearm pronators and wrist flexors are unopposed. Function can be improved by combining pronation contracture correction with a flexor carpi ulnaris transfer.

SUPINATION CONTRACTURE

Fixed supination develops when finger flexors and pronators arising from the medial humeral epicondyle are weak, and the biceps brachii and wrist extensors are strong. Contracture of the interosseous membrane and secondary bone deformities in the forearm may develop. The radius becomes markedly bowed, and the radioulnar joints may sublux. A fixed supination deformity combined with a weak shoulder that will abduct yields marked limitation of an otherwise functional hand.

Blount recommends closed osteoclasis of the middle third of both bones in the patient under age 12 who has insufficient muscle power for tendon transfer.[12] Overcorrection is required, since further growth may cause the supination deformity to recur.

TECHNIQUE. The shoulder is abducted and externally rotated to bring the wrist near the shoulder. The forearm is placed in midpronation with the dorsum toward the table, a position with no important structures between the bones. The forearm is held on each side of the wedge and, with a quick thrust, both bones are fractured. The force is then reversed to complete the fracture, bending the midforearm backward and forward several times to be certain that the fractures are complete. A long arm cast is applied, extending from the axilla to the knuckles, with the forearm held in 45° to 90° of pronation and the elbow at a right angle.

Zaoussis performed a formal osteotomy near the radial tuberosity to correct this type of deformity.[212] Almost no forearm motion is retained, in contrast to the Blount procedure. Zaoussis believes that the surgically created synostosis between the proximal radius and the ulna does not impair the functional result.

For a developing deformity, Zancolli recommends physical therapy and pronation casts worn at night.[210] A fixed deformity is corrected by releasing the interosseous membrane, throughout its length, close to the ulna. In addition, a release of the radioulnar joints may be necessary if the radius has become deformed. The biceps is lengthened by a Z-plasty, and the distal segment is rerouted to a new insertion on the radial aspect of the radial neck.

Acute Idiopathic Postinfectious Polyneuropathy (Guillain–Barré–Strohl Syndrome)

Acute polyradiculoneuritis is characterized by the rapid onset of symmetrical motor paresis of the extremities and in some cases, of the trunk. Although the etiology is unknown, an acute demyelinating process of the anterior ramus of the spinal cord may take place.[1] More than one half of the patients gives a history of a viral infection 2 to 4 weeks prior to the onset of the syndrome. The mode of onset is variable. The patient may present with diffuse weakness or paresis beginning distally in the lower extremities and spreading proximally to involve the upper limbs, the respiratory muscles, and then the bulbar muscles in the most severe cases.[147] Many patients have moderately severe pain, especially in the back and limbs, which may resemble the clinical picture of poliomyelitis. Sensory loss is usually slight.[27] The syndrome progresses for 1 to 2 weeks with maximum paresis developing in 1 to 4 weeks.

Cerebrospinal fluid analysis demonstrates a normal cell count with a disproportionate elevation of protein and cytoalbumin which reaches its maximum level in 2 to 4 weeks before subsiding to normal.[67,68] The maximum rise occurs between the tenth and twentieth day and the protein level may rise to 1,800 mg per 100 ml. The involved nerves show marked delay in both motor and sensory conduction.[147] A peripheral nerve biopsy is rarely indicated, but when it is done, it demonstrates inflammatory cells, predominantly lymphocytes, infiltrating the perivascular spaces and the interstitium.

Paradoxically, patients with mild symptoms wait longer for the onset of recovery than those more severely involved. The convalescent period may extend for 3 to 6 months. Patients with the acute syndrome have a good prognosis for recovery while those with subacute and chronic forms have a worse prognosis.[79] A long interval from the time of greatest weakness to the time of beginning improvement augurs for ultimate incomplete recovery as does the initial absence of the deep-tendon reflexes. Berman feels that a plateau of motor return has been established when there is at least 16 months without improvement.[9] Eighty percent of muscle strength can be expected to return by 9 months in most muscle groups with the quadriceps and gluteus maximus taking slightly longer.[123] Probable permanent loss in the foot evertors and dorsiflexors is expected if they have not improved by 4 months. This residual muscle imbalance of the foot and ankle may require tendon transfers or may cause bony deformity that requires corrective bony procedures, such as a triple arthrodesis, before orthotic control can be achieved. In the occasional chronic case,

paralytic scoliosis develops which requires spinal fusion.

Those who are severely paralyzed have a worse prognosis. Bradley recommends a trial of one week of corticosteroids when the condition is deteriorating or severe.[14] If no improvement appears, cytotoxic immunosuppressive therapy is added for the second week. General support remains the most important treatment including the possible need for tracheostomy.[204] There is a 10% mortality rate in most series.[78,156] Eighteen percent of patients—those with onset in childhood—have a greater risk for residua when followed for more than 3 years.[14]

Gordon has carefully outlined the medical and orthopaedic management of these patients.[59] He emphasizes the need for constant observation during the acute phase because of the threat of respiratory impairment. Bulbar involvement may require nasogastric feedings or a gastrostomy. If bilateral facial palsies occur, the corneas must be protected from excessive drying to prevent corneal ulcers. Proper positioning in bed, turning the patient every 2 hours, and using a protective mattress help avoid pressure decubiti. The temporary use of intermittent catheterization and the development of a routine bowel training program with the use of stool softeners and suppositories is recommended.

Gordon emphasizes the need for an exercise program in the early course of treatment which will prevent unnecessary contractures and complications.[59] Full range of motion of all joints is carried out at least twice a day. When the acute phase has subsided and the patient shows neurologic improvement, an active rehabilitation program is instituted. As in poliomyelitis, the program is changed from passive to active therapy with active resistive exercises introduced for muscles rating fair or better. Overfatigue must be avoided. Gordon recommends the use of the Hubbard tank during the early stages of muscle recovery. Potential positional hypotension is avoided by the use of elastic stockings, ace bandages, an abdominal binder, and a tilt-table. When trunk stability and control are regained, a wheelchair is used. If motor function of the lower extremities returns, the patient can use parallel bars, a walker, crutches, or canes. Adaptive equipment for the upper extremities may help the patient to feed and dress himself, and even to type. This inpatient program lasts 4 to 6 months, until the patient is sufficiently ambulatory to be able to be handled by parents at home. Follow-up as an outpatient may be necessary for 2 years. Since residual weakness usually affects the distal part of the extremities, most of the patients eventually are able to walk without assistive devices.

Amyotrophic Lateral Sclerosis (Motor Neuron Disease)

Amyotrophic lateral sclerosis is a chronic progressive disease of unknown etiology. This condition is one of the few diseases in which muscle spasticity is present with muscle atrophy. It represents the combined degeneration of motor cells of the spinal cord and medulla oblongata. Motor neuron disease is relatively common and occurs more frequently in males. It generally presents in the fifth and sixth decades of life. Mulder suggested that a forme fruste of amyotrophic lateral sclerosis might be demonstrated in a group of patients with progressive muscle weakness which occurred many years after an episode of acute poliomyelitis.[133]

Initially, weakness may have a patchy distribution. Commonly, the distal muscles are affected first. The patient may present with loss of hand coordination and function. The initial weakness occurs with equal frequency in the upper and lower extremities while 20% of the patients present with primary bulbar symptoms. Within weeks to months, the disease spreads to involve all muscles of the other extremities and trunk with distal involvement greater than proximal. Rapid progressive wasting and weakness of the involved muscles is coupled with spasticity. Usually weakness of the muscles is proportional to the degree of atrophy. Initially, deep-tendon reflexes are brisk and the Babinski generally positive. As the process continues and causes complete wasting of muscles, the deep-tendon reflexes may disappear. Two additional symptoms which may precede actual clinical muscle weakness are an aching sensation in muscle groups, which disappears with the advance of the motor paralysis, and cramps, which occur at night after stretching. If isolated spinal cord lateral tracts become involved, spasticity results which may precede atrophy as the first symptom.

Clinical diagnosis is made when weakness, wasting, and fasciculations associated with hyper-reflexia are found in three or more limbs. There is weakness in the hands as well as atrophy of the thenar eminence. Muscles of the upper extremities, including the deltoid and muscles of the neck, show considerable atrophy. No sensory complaints or findings are present. The absence of gross fasciculations is associated with slow progression of the disease, whereas in patients with widespread fasciculations, the disease progresses more rapidly. Also the disease has a more rapid course when there are bulbar symptoms, which indicate involvement of the medulla oblongata. Although mastication is rarely affected, deglutition is difficult because the tongue cannot control the movement of food and the pharyngeal muscles are weak. Terminally, gross tongue fasciculations are seen.

On an electromyogram there is widespread fibrillation associated with giant polyphasic potentials and fasciculations. Nerve conduction studies, serum enzymes, and muscle biopsy are generally nonspecific. There may be a moderate increase in protein in the cerebrospinal fluid. If bulbar symptoms are present, myelography may be needed to differentiate motor neuron disease from cervical spine disease with cord compression.

Usually adults are confined to the wheelchair within 12 to 18 months of clinical onset. Their mind remains alert, and they are acutely aware of the inexorable progression of the disease. Speech becomes thick and monotonous due to weakness of the tongue, palate, and lips. Swallowing is made easier by taking neostigmine bromide 30 to 45 minutes before meals and by pureeing solid foods.[178] Eventually a nasogastric tube, cricopharyngeal myotomy, or cervical esophagostomy, may be required. Lack of tongue control may lead to choking and require the use of amitriptyline HCl (Elavil), portable suction, or a transtympanic neurectomy. Death, generally due to pneumonia, occurs in one half of these patients within 3 years of onset. Rosen reports that in terms of a 5-year survival period, younger patients had a better prognosis than those who were diagnosed after age 50.[157] Chances for surviving 5 years were 3 times higher for those with the spinal form of the disease than for those with bulbar involvement. Mean age of diagnosis was 56.

The orthopaedist is confronted with several problems as he seeks to improve the quality of life for these patients. Better head control can be obtained when the patient uses an occipital collar or orthosis to support the sterno-occipitomandibular muscles.

When the upper extremities are involved, the patient may need a functional wrist splint and occasionally a page-turner. A polypropylene ankle–foot orthosis controls dropfoot in patients who retain ambulation. Canes may also be necessary, but a wheelchair is likely to be needed within 18 months of onset of the disease. Frequent but brief periods of physical therapy may minimize the rapid onset of disuse atrophy and prevent contracture. Night cramps may be temporarily controlled by quinine or diazepam (Valium).

A rare form of motor neuron disease may present in childhood. The pattern of this disease is symmetrical atrophy and spasticity of the extremities that results in muscle weakness. There is weakness in the hands and atrophy of the thenar eminence. The course is more similar to childhood spinal muscular atrophy than to the motor neuron disease seen in adulthood. Patients with this disease should not be given spinal anesthesia or succinylcholine chloride because of the possibility of cardiac arrest.[178]

REFERENCES

1. Asbury AK, Arnason BG, Adams RD: The inflammatory lesion in idiopathic polyneuritis. Its role in pathogenesis. Medicine 48:173, 1969
2. Ashley RK, Larsen LJ, James PM: Reduction of dislocation of the hip in older children. J Bone Joint Surg 54A:545, 1972
3. Axer A: Transposition of gluteus maximus, tensor fasciae latae and ilio-tibial band for paralysis of lateral abdominal muscles in children after poliomyelitis. A preliminary report. J Bone Joint Surg 40B:644, 1958
4. Axer A: Into-talus transposition of tendons for correction of paralytic valgus foot after poliomyelitis in children. J Bone Joint Surg 42A:1119, 1960
5. Baker AB, Cornwell S: Poliomyelitis, the spinal cord. AMA Archives of Pathology 61:185, 1956
6. Barr JS: Poliomyelitic hip deformity and the erector spinae transplant. JAMA 144:813, 1950
7. Barr JS, Freiberg JA, Colonna PC, Pemberton PA: A survey of end-results on stabilization of the paralytic shoulder. Report of the research committee of the American Orthopaedic Association. J Bone Joint Surg 24:699, 1942
8. Bentzon PGK: Pes cavus and the musculi peroneus longus. Acta Orthop Scand 4:50, 1933
9. Berman AT, Tom L: The Guillain–Barré syndrome in children. Orthopedic management and pattern of recovery. Clin Orthop 116:61, 1976
10. Bernau A: Long-term results following Lambrinudi Arthrodesis. J Bone Joint Surg 59A:473, 1977
11. Bickel WH, Moe JH: Translocation of the peroneus longus tendon for paralytic calcaneus deformity of the foot. Surg Gynecol Obstet 78:627, 1944
12. Blount WP: Osteoclasis for supination deformities in children. J Bone Joint Surg 22:300, 1940
13. Boyd HB: Posterior bone block of the elbow. In Crenshaw AH (ed): Campbell's Operative Orthopaedics, ed. 3. St Louis, Mosby, 1956
14. Bradley WG: Disorders of Peripheral Nerves. Oxford, Blackwell Scientific Publications, 1974
15. Brewster AH: Countersinking the astragalus in paralytic feet. N Engl J Med 209:71, 1933
16. Brittain HA: Architectural Principles in Arthrodesis, ed. 2. Edinburgh, Churchill Livingstone, 1952
17. Brockway A: An operation to improve abduction power of the shoulder in poliomyelitis. J Bone Joint Surg 21:451, 1939
18. Broderick TF, Reidy JA, Barr JS: Tendon transplantations in the lower extremity. A review of end results in poliomyelitis, II. Tendon transplantations at the knee. J Bone Joint Surg 34A:909, 1952
19. Brooks DM, Seddon HJ: Pectoral transplantation for paralysis of the flexors of the elbow. A new technique. J Bone Joint Surg 41B:36, 1959
20. Brooks DM, Zaoussis A: Arthrodesis of the shoulder in reconstructive surgery of paralysis of the upper limb. J Bone Joint Surg 41B:207, 1959
21. Bunnell S: Restoring flexion to the paralytic elbow. J Bone Joint Surg 33A:566, 1951
22. Caldwell GD: Correction of paralytic footdrop by hemi gastrosoleus transplant. Clin Orthop 11:81, 1958
23. Campbell WC: An operation for the correction of "drop-foot." J Bone Joint Surg 5:815, 1923
24. Carayon A, Bourrel M, Touze M: Dual transfer of the posterior tibial and flexor digitorum longus tendons for drop foot. Report of thirty-one cases. J Bone Joint Surg 49A:144, 1967
25. Carmack JC, Hallock H: Tibiotarsal arthrodesis after astragalectomy, a report of eight cases. J Bone Joint Surg 29:476, 1947

26. Carroll RF, Hill NA: Triceps transfer to restore elbow flexion. J Bone Joint Surg 52A:239, 1970

27. Casamajor L, Lapert GR: Guillain–Barré syndrome in children. Am J Dis Child 61:99, 1941

28. Charnley J: Compression arthrodesis of the ankle and shoulder. J Bone Joint Surg 33B:180, 1951

29. Charnley J: Compression Arthrodesis. London, Churchill Livingstone, 1953

30. Charnley J, Houston JK: Compression arthrodesis of the shoulder. J Bone Joint Surg 46B:614, 1964

31. Chaves JP: Pectoralis minor transplant for paralysis of the serratus anterior. J Bone Joint Surg 33B:228, 1951

32. Cholmeley JA: Elmslie's operation for the calcaneus foot. J Bone Joint Surg 35B:46, 1953

33. Chuinard EG, Peterson RE: Distraction-compression bone-graft arthrodesis of the ankle. A method especially applicable for children. J Bone Joint Surg 45A:481, 1963

34. Clark JMP: Reconstruction of biceps brachii by pectoral muscle transplantation. Br J Surg 34:180, 1946

35. Cole WH: The treatment of claw-foot. J Bone Joint Surg 22:895, 1940

36. Conner AN: The treatment of flexion contractures of the knee in poliomyelitis. J Bone Joint Surg 52B:138, 1970

37. Cravener EK: Device for overcoming non-bony flexion contractures of the knee. J Bone Joint Surg 12:437, 1930

38. Crego CH Jr, Fischer FJ: Transplantation of the biceps femoris for the relief of quadriceps femoris paralysis in residual poliomyelitis. J Bone Joint Surg 13:515, 1931

39. Crego CH Jr, McCarroll HR: Recurrent deformities in stabilized paralytic feet. A report of 1100 consecutive stabilizations in poliomyelitis. J Bone Joint Surg 20:609, 1938

40. Dekel S, Weissman SL: Osteotomy of the calcaneus and concomitant plantar stripping in children with talipes cavo-varus. J Bone Joint Surg 55B:802, 1973

41. Dennyson WG, Fulford GE: Subtalar arthrodesis by cancellous grafts and metallic internal fixation. J Bone Joint Surg 58B:507, 1976

42. Dewar FP, Harris RI: Restoration of function of the shoulder following paralysis of the trapezius by fascial sling fixation and transplantation of the levator scapulae. Clin Orthop 108:4, 1975

43. Dickson FD: An operation for stabilizing paralytic hips; a preliminary report. J Bone Joint Surg 9:1, 1927

44. Dickson FD: Fascial transplants in paralytic and other conditions. J Bone Joint Surg 19:405, 1937

45. Dickson FD, Diveley RL: Operation for correction of mild claw foot, the result of infantile paralysis. JAMA 87:1275, 1926

46. Dunn J: Stabilizing operations in the treatment of paralytic deformities of the foot. Proceedings of the Royal Society of Medicine [Section on Orthopaedics], 15:15, 1922

47. Dwyer FC: Osteotomy of the calcaneum for pes cavus. J Bone Joint Surg 41B:80, 1959

48. Elmslie RI: In Turner GG (ed): Modern Operative Surgery, ed. 2. London, Cassell, 1934

49. Emmel HE, LeCocq JF: Hamstring transplant for the prevention of calcaneocavus foot in poliomyelitis. J Bone Joint Surg 40A:911, 1958

50. Evans D: Calcaneo-Valgus Deformity. J Bone Joint Surg 57B:270, 1975

51. Fitzgerald FP, Seddon HJ: Lambrinudi's operation for drop-foot. Br J Surg 25:283, 1937

52. Flint MH, MacKenzie IC: Anterior laxity of the ankle. A cause of recurrent paralytic drop foot deformity. J Bone Joint Surg 44B:377, 1962

53. Forbes AM: The tensor fasciae femoris as a cause of deformity. J Bone Joint Surg 10:579, 1928

54. Fried A, Hendel C: Paralytic valgus deformity of the ankle. Replacement of the paralyzed tibialis posterior by the peroneus longus. J Bone Joint Surg 39A:921, 1957

55. Garceau GJ, Brahms MA: A preliminary study of selective plantar-muscle denervation for pes cavus. J Bone Joint Surg 38A:553, 1956

56. Gill AB: A new operation for arthrodesis of the shoulder. J Bone Joint Surg 13:287, 1931

57. Goldner JI, Irwin CE: Paralytic deformities of the foot. American Academy of Orthopaedic Surgeons Instructional Course Lectures 5:190, 1948

58. Goldthwait JE: Tendon transplantation in the treatment of deformities resulting from infantile paralysis. Boston Medical and Surgical Journal, 133:447, 1895

59. Gordon SL, Morris WT, Stoner MA, Greer RB III: Residua of Guillain–Barré polyneuritis in children. J Bone Joint Surg 59A:193, 1977

60. Green WT, Grice DS: The treatment of poliomyelitis: Acute and convalescent stages. American Academy of Orthopaedic Surgeons Instructional Course Lectures 8:261, 1951

61. Green WT, Grice DS: The management of chronic poliomyelitis. American Academy of Orthopaedic Surgeons Instructional Course Lectures 9:85, 1952

62. Green WT, Grice DS: The surgical correction of the paralytic foot. American Academy of Orthopaedic Surgeons Instructional Course Lectures 10:343. 1953

63. Green WT, Grice DS: The management of calcaneus deformity. American Academy of Orthopaedic Surgeons Instructional Course Lectures 13:135, 1956

64. Grice DS: An extra-articular arthrodesis of the subastragalar joint for correction of paralytic flat feet in children. J Bone Joint Surg 34A:927, 1952

65. Grice DS: The role of subtalar fusion in the treatment of valgus deformities of the feet. American Academy of Orthopaedic Surgeons Instructional Course Lectures 16:127, 1959

66. Groves EWH: Some contributions to the reconstructive surgery of the hip. Br J Surg, 14:486, 1926-1927

67. Guillain G: Radiculoneuritis with acellular hyperalbuminosis of the cerebrospinal fluid. Archives of Neurology and Psychiatry 36:975, 1936

68. Guillain G, Barré JA, Strohl A: Sur un syndrome de radiculonévrite avec hyperalbuminose du liquide céphalorachidien sans réaction cellulaire. Bulletin et Memoires de la Société Medicale des Hospitaux de Paris 40:1462, 1916

69. Gunn DR, Molesworth BD: The use of tibialis posterior as a dorsiflexor. J Bone Joint Surg 39B:674, 1957

70. Haas SL: The treatment of permanent paralysis of the deltoid muscle. JAMA 104:99, 1935

71. Haas SL: Correction of extreme flexion contracture of the knee joint. J Bone Joint Surg 20:839, 1938

72. Hallgrimsson S: Studies on reconstructive and stabilizing operations on the skeleton of the foot, with special reference to subastragalar arthrodesis in treatment of foot deformities following infantile paralysis Acta Chir Scand [Suppl 78] 88:1, 1943

73. Hallock H: Arthrodesis of the hip for instability and pain in poliomyelitis. J Bone Joint Surg 32A:904, 1950

74. Hamsa WR: Panastragaloid arthrodesis. A study of end-results in eighty-five cases. J Bone Joint Surg 18:732, 1936

75. Harandi BA, Zahir A: Severe hypertension following correction of flexion contracture of the knee. J Bone Joint Surg 56A:1733, 1974

76. Hart VL: Corrective cast for flexion-contracture deformity of the knee. J Bone Joint Surg 16:970, 1934

77. Hart VL: Lambrinudi operation for drop-foot. J Bone Joint Surg 22:937, 1940

78. Haymaker W, Kernohan JW: The Landry–Guillain–Barré syndrome, a clinicopathologic report of 50 fatal cases and a critique of the literature. Medicine 28:59, 1949

79. Heller GL, Dejong RN: Treatment of the Guillain–Barré syndrome. Arch Neurol 8:179, 1963

80. Henderson MS: Reconstructive surgery in paralytic deformities of the lower leg. J Bone Joint Surg 11:810, 1929

81. Herndon CH: Tendon transplantation at the knee and foot. American Academy of Orthopaedic Surgeons Instructional Course Lectures 18:145, 1961

82. Herndon CH, Strong JM, Heyman CH: Transposition of the tibialis anterior in the treatment of paralytic talipes calcaneus. J Bone Joint Surg 38A:751, 1956

83. Herzmark MH: Traumatic paralysis of the serratus anterior relieved by transplantation of the rhomboidei. J Bone Joint Surg 33A:235, 1951

84. Heyman CH: A method for the correction of paralytic genu recurvatum. Report of a bilateral case. J Bone Joint Surg 6:689, 1924

85. Heyman CH: Operative treatment of paralytic genu recurvatum. J Bone Joint Surg 29:644, 1947

86. Heyman CH: Operative treatment of paralytic genu recurvatum. J Bone Joint Surg 44A:1246, 1962

87. Heyman CH: Long-term results following a bone-shelf operation for congenital and some other dislocations of the hip in children. J Bone Joint Surg 45A:1113, 1963

88. Hogshead HP, Ponseti IV: Fascia lata transfer to the erector spinae for the treatment of flexion abduction contractures of the hip in patients with poliomyelitis and meningomyelocele. Evaluation of results. J Bone Joint Surg 46A:1389, 1964

89. Hoke M: An operation for stabilizing paralytic feet. American Journal of Orthopaedic Surgery 3:494, 1921

90. Holmdahl HC: Astragalectomy as a stabilizing operation for foot paralysis following poliomyelitis: results of a follow-up investigation of 153 cases. Acta Orthop Scand 25:207, 1956

91. Horstmann DM: Need for monitoring vaccinated populations for immunity levels. Prog Med Virol 16:215, 1973

92. Hovnanian AP: Latissimus dorsi transplantation for loss of flexion or extension at the elbow. Ann Surg 143:493, 1956

93. Hsu LCS, O'Brien JP, Yau ACMC, Hodgson AK: Batchelor's extra-articular subtalar arthrodesis. A report on sixty-four procedures in patients with poliomyelitic deformities. J Bone Joint Surg 58A:243, 1976

94. Hughes RE: Knee-flexion deformity following poliomyelitis. Its correction by operative procedures. J Bone Joint Surg 17:627, 1935

95. Hunt JC, Brooks AI: Subtalar extraarticular arthrodesis for correction of paralytic valgus deformity of the foot. Evaluation of forty-four procedures with particular reference to associated tendon transference. J Bone Joint Surg 47A:1310, 1965

96. Inclan A: End results in physiological blocking of flail joints. J Bone Joint Surg 31A:748, 1949

97. Ingersoll RE: Transplantation of peroneus longus to anterior tibial insertion in poliomyelitis. Surg Gynecol Obstet 86:717, 1948

98. Ingram AJ, Hundley JM: Posterior bone block of the ankle for paralytic equinus. An end-result study. J Bone Joint Surg 33A:679, 1951

99. Irwin CE: Genu recurvatum following poliomyelitis; controlled method of operative correction. JAMA 120:277, 1942

100. Irwin CE: The iliotibial band, its role in producing deformity in poliomyelitis. J Bone Joint Surg 31A:141, 1949

101. Johnson EW Jr: Results of modern methods of treatment of poliomyelitis. J Bone Joint Surg 27:223, 1945

102. Johnson EW Jr: Contractures of the iliotibial band. Surg Gynecol Obstet 96:599, 1953

103. Jones GB: Paralytic dislocation of the hip. J Bone Joint Surg 36B:375, 1954

104. Jones GB: Paralytic dislocation of the hip. J Bone Joint Surg 44B:573, 1962

105. Jones R: The soldier's foot and the treatment of common deformities of the foot. Br Med J 1(2891):749, 1916

106. Kettelkamp DB, Larson CB: Evaluation of the Steindler flexorplasty. J Bone Joint Surg 45A:513, 1963

107. Kuhlmann RF, Bell JF: A clinical evaluation of tendon transplantations for poliomyelitis affecting the lower extremities. J Bone Joint Surg 34A:915, 1952

108. Lambrinudi C: New operation on drop-foot. Br J Surg, 15:193, 1927

109. Langerskiöld A, Ryöppy S: Treatment of paralysis of trapezius muscle by the Eden–Lang operation. Acta Orthop Scand 44:383, 1973

110. Legg AT: Tensor fasciae femoris transplantation in cases of weakened gluteus medius. N Engl J Med 209:61, 1933

111. Leikkonen O: Astragalectomy as ankle stabilizing operation in infantile paralysis sequelae. Acta Chir Scand 100:668, 1950

112. Leibolt FL: Pantalar arthrodesis in poliomyelitis. Surgery 6:31, 1939

113. Lipscomb PR, and Sanchez JJ: Anterior transplantation of the posterior tibial tendon for persistent palsy of the common peroneal nerve. J Bone Joint Surg 43A:60, 1961

114. Lowman CL: Fascial transplants in paralysis of abdominal and shoulder girdle muscles American Academy of Orthopaedic Surgeons Instructional Course Lectures, 14:300, 1957

115. Lowman CL: Fascial transplants in relation to muscle function. J Bone Joint Surg 45A:199, 1963

116. MacAusland WR, MacAusland AR: Astragalectomy

(the Whitman operation) in paralytic deformities of the foot. Ann Surg 80:861, 1924

117. McFarland, B: Paralytic instability of the foot (editorial) J Bone Joint Surg 33B:493, 1951

118. MacKenzie IG: Lambrinudi's arthrodesis. J Bone Joint Surg 41B:738, 1959

119. Makin M: Early arthrodesis for a flail shoulder in young children. J Bone Joint Surg 59A:317, 1977

120. Makin M: Tibiofibular relationship in paralyzed limbs. J Bone Joint Surg 47B:500, 1965

121. Makin M, Yossipovitch A: Translocation of the peroneus longus in the treatment of paralytic pes calcaneus. A follow-up study of thirty-three cases. J Bone Joint Surg 48A:1541, 1966

122. Marek FM, Schein AJ: Aseptic necrosis of the astragalus following arthrodesing procedures of the tarsus. J Bone Joint Surg 27:587, 1945

123. Marshall J: The Landry–Guillain–Barré syndrome. Brain 86:55, 1963

124. Mayer L: The physiological method of tendon transplantation. I. Historical: anatomy and physiology of tendons. Surg Gynecol Obstet 22:182, 1916

125. Mayer L: The physiological method of tendon transplantation. II. Operative technique. Surg Gynecol Obstet 22:298, 1916

126. Mayer L: The physiological method of tendon transplantation. III. Experimental and clinical experiences. Surg Gynecol Obstet 22:472, 1916

127. Mayer L: Fixed paralytic obliquity of the pelvis. J Bone Joint Surg 13:1, 1931

128. Mayer L: Operative reconstruction of the paralyzed upper extremity. J Bone Joint Surg 21:377, 1939

129. Mayer L: The physiologic method of tendon transplants. Reviewed after forty years. American Academy of Orthopaedic Surgeons Instructional Course Lectures 13:116, 1956

130. Mayer L, Green W: Experiences with the Steindler flexorplasty at the elbow. J Bone Joint Surg 36A:775, 1954

131. Mitchell GP: Posterior displacement osteotomy of the calcaneus. J Bone Joint Surg 59B:233, 1977

132. Mortens J, Pilcher MF: Tendon transplantation in the prevention of foot deformities after poliomyelitis in children. J Bone Joint Surg 38B:633, 1956

133. Mulder DW, Rosenbaum RA, Layton DD Jr: Late progression of poliomyelitis or forme fruste amyotrophic lateral sclerosis? Mayo Clin Proc 47:756, 1972

134. Mustard WT: Iliopsoas transfer for weakness of the hip abductors; preliminary report. J Bone Joint Surg 34A:647, 1952

135. Mustard WT: A follow-up study of iliopsoas transfer for hip instability. J Bone Joint Surg 41B:289, 1959

136. Ober FR: An operation to relieve paralysis of the deltoid muscle. JAMA, 99:2182, 1932

137. Ober FR: Tendon transplantation in the lower extremity. N Engl J Med 209:52, 1933

138. Ober FR: The role of the iliotibial band and fascia lata as a factor in the causation of lowback disabilities and sciatica. J Bone Joint Surg 18:105, 1936

139. Ober FR: Transplantation to improve the function of the shoulder joint and extensor function of the elbow joint. American Academy of Orthopaedic Surgeons Instructional Course Lectures on Reconstruction Surgery 2:244, 1944

140. Ober FR, Barr JS: Brachioradialis muscle transposition for triceps weakness. Surg Gynecol Obstet 67:105, 1938

141. O'Brien JP, Dwyer AP, Hodgson AR: Paralytic pelvic obliquity. Its prognosis and management and the development of a technique for full correction of the deformity. J Bone Joint Surg 57A:626, 1975

142. Ogra PL, Karzon DT: The role of immunoglobulins in the mechanism of mucosal immunity to virus infection. Pediatr Clin North Am 17:385, 1970

143. Paluska DJ, Blount WP: Ankle valgus after the Grice subtalar stabilization: the late evaluation of a personal series with a modified technic. Clin Orthop 59:137, 1968

144. Parsons DW, Seddon HJ: The results of operations for disorders of the hip caused by poliomyelitis. J Bone Joint Surg 50B:266, 1968

145. Patterson RI, Parrish FF, Hathaway EN: Stabilizing operations on the foot. A study of the indications, techniques used, and end results. J Bone Joint Surg 32A:1, 1950

146. Pauker E: Correction of the outwardly rotated leg from poliomyelitis. J Bone Joint Surg 41B:70, 1959

147. Paulson GW: The Landry–Guillain–Barré–Strohl syndrome in childhood. Dev Med Child Neurol 12:604, 1970

148. Peabody CW: Tendon transposition: and end-result study. J Bone Joint Surg 20:193, 1938

149. Peabody CW: Tendon transposition in the paralytic foot. American Academy of Orthopaedic Surgeons Instructional Course Lectures 6:179, 1949

150. Perry J, O'Brien JP, Hodgson AR: Triple tenodesis of the knee. A soft-tissue operation for the correction of paralytic genu recurvatum. J Bone Joint Surg 58A:978, 1976

151. Phemister DB: Operative arrestment of longitudinal growth of bones in the treatment of deformities. J Bone Joint Surg 15:1, 1933

152. Pollock JH, Carrell B: Subtalar extraarticular arthrodesis in the treatment of paralytic valgus deformities. A review of 112 procedures in 100 patients. J Bone Joint Surg 46A:533, 1964

153. Pyka RA, Coventry MB, Moe JH: Anterior subluxation of the talus following triple arthrodesis. J Bone Joint Surg 46A:6, 1964

154. Rapp IH: Serratus anterior paralysis treated by transplantation of pectoralis minor. J Bone Joint Surg 36A:852, 1954

155. Ratliff AHC: The short leg in poliomyelitis. J Bone Joint Surg 41B:56, 1959

156. Ravn H: The Landry–Guillain–Barré syndrome—a survey and a clinical report of 127 cases. Acta Neurol Scand 43:1, 1967

157. Rosen AD: Amyotrophic lateral sclerosis. Clinical features and prognosis. Arch Neurol 35:638, 1978

158. Rowe CR: Re-evaluation of the position of the arm in arthrodesis of the shoulder in the adult. J Bone Joint Surg 56A:913, 1974

159. Ryerson EW: Arthrodesing operations on the feet. J Bone Joint Surg 5:453, 1923

160. Sabin AB: Oral poliovirus vaccine. History of its development and prospects. Eradication of poliomyelitis. JAMA 194:872, 1965

161. Saha AK: Surgery of the paralyzed and flail shoulder. Acta Orthop Scand [Suppl 97], 1967

162. Salk JE: Studies in human subjects on active im-

munization against poliomyelitis. JAMA 151:1081, 1953

163. Salter RB, Dubos JP: The first fifteen years' personal experience with innominate osteotomy in the treatment of congenital dislocation and subluxation of the hip. Clin Orthop 98:72, 1974

164. Scheer GE, Crego CH Jr: A two-stage stabilization procedure for correction of calcaneocavus. J Bone Joint Surg 38A:1247, 1956

165. Schottsdaedt ER, Larsen LJ, Bost FC: Complete muscle transposition. J Bone Joint Surg 37A:897, 1955

166. Schottsdaedt ER, Larsen LJ, Bost FC: The surgical reconstruction of the upper extremity paralyzed by poliomyelitis. J Bone Joint Surg 40A:633, 1958

167. Schuch CP, Farmer TW: Physical therapy in acute infectious polyneuritis. Physical Therapy Review 35:238, 1955

168. Schwartzmann JR, Crego CH Jr: Hamstring–tendon transplantation for the relief of quadriceps femoris paralysis in residual poliomyelitis. A follow-up study of 134 cases. J Bone Joint Surg 30A:541, 1948

169. Seddon HJ: Transplantation of pectoralis major for paralysis of the flexors of the elbow. Proceedings of the Royal Society of Medicine 42:837, 1949

170. Segal A, Seddon HJ, Brooks DM: Treatment of paralysis of the flexors of the elbow. J Bone Joint Surg 41B:44, 1959

171. Seymour N, Evans DK: A modification of the Grice subtalar arthrodesis. J Bone Joint Surg 50B:372, 1968

172. Sharp NN, Guhl JF, Sorensen RI, Voshell AF: Hip fusion in poliomyelitis in children. A preliminary report. J Bone Joint Surg 46A:121, 1964

173. Sharrard WJW: Muscle recovery in poliomyelitis. J Bone Joint Surg 37B:63, 1955

174. Sharrard WJW: The distribution of the permanent paralysis in the lower limb in poliomyelitis. J Bone Joint Surg 37B:540, 1955

175. Sharrard WJW: Posterior iliopsoas transplantation in the treatment of paralytic dislocation of the hip. J Bone Joint Surg 46B:426, 1964

176. Sharrard WJW: The segmental innervation of the lower limb muscles in man. Ann R Coll Surg Engl 35:106, 1964

177. Smith JB, Westin GW: Subtalar extraarticular arthrodesis. J Bone Joint Surg 50A:1027, 1968

178. Smith RA, Norris FH Jr: Symptomatic care of patients with amyotrophic lateral sclerosis. JAMA 234:715, 1975

179. Somerville EW: Paralytic dislocation of the hip. J Bone Joint Surg 41B:279, 1959

180. Somerville EW: Flexion contractures of the knee. J Bone Joint Surg 42B:730, 1960

181. Soutter R: A new operation for hip contractures in poliomyelitis. Boston Medical and Surgical Journal 170:380, 1914

182. Spira E: The treatment of dropped shoulder, a new operative technique. J Bone Joint Surg 30A:229, 1948

183. Spira E: Replacement of biceps brachii by pectoralis minor transplant. Report of a case. J Bone Joint Surg 39B:126, 1957

184. Staples OS: Posterior arthrodesis of the ankle and subtalar joints. J Bone Joint Surg 38A:50, 1956

185. Steindler A: Stripping of the os calcis. Journal of Orthopaedic Surgery 2:8, 1920

186. Steindler A: Reconstructive Surgery of the Upper Extremity. New York, D Appleton Co, 1923

187. Steindler A: The treatment of the flail ankle; pan-astragaloid arthrodesis. J Bone Joint Surg 5:284, 1923

188. Steindler A: Orthopedic Operations. Indications, Technique, and End Results. Springfield, Charles C Thomas, 1940

189. Steindler A: Muscle and tendon transplantation at the elbow. American Academy of Orthopaedic Surgeons Instructional Course Lectures on Reconstruction Surgery, 276, 1944

190. Straub LR, Harvey JP Jr, Fuerst CE: A clinical evaluation of tendon transplantation in the paralytic foot. J Bone Joint Surg 39A:1, 1957

191. Stubbins SG, Riordan DC, Graham WC: Posterior tibial transfer for drop-foot. Proceedings of the Western Orthopaedic Association. J Bone Joint Surg 37A:396, 1955

192. Sutherland DH, Bost FC, Schottstaedt ER: Electromyographic study of transplanted muscles about the knee in poliomyelitic patients. J Bone Joint Surg 42A:919, 1960

193. Taylor RG: The treatment of claw toes by multiple transfers of flexors into extensor tendons. J Bone Joint Surg 33B:539, 1951

194. Thomas CI, Thompson TC, Straub CR: Transplantation of the external oblique muscle for abduction paralysis. J Bone Joint Surg 32A:207, 1950

195. Thompson TC: Astragalectomy and the treatment of calcaneovalgus. J Bone Joint Surg 21:627, 1939

196. Tuck WH: The Stanmore cosmetic caliper. J Bone Joint Surg 56B:115, 1974

197. Wagner LC: Modified bone block (Campbell) of ankle for paralytic drop foot with report of twenty-seven cases. J Bone Joint Surg 13:142, 1931

198. Wang CJ, Tambakis AP, Fielding JW: An evaluation of ankle fusion in children. Clin Orthop 98:233, 1974

199. Watkins MB, Jones JB, Ryder CT Jr, Brown TH Jr: Transplantation of the posterior tibial tendon. J Bone Joint Surg 36A:1181, 1954

200. Watson-Jones R: Extra-articular arthrodesis of the shoulder. J Bone Joint Surg 15:862, 1933

201. Waugh TR, Wagner J, Stinchfield FE: An evaluation of pantalar arthrodesis. A follow-up study of one hundred and sixteen operations. J Bone Joint Surg 47A:1315, 1965

202. Weissman SL: Capsular arthroplasty in paralytic dislocation of the hip. A preliminary report. J Bone Joint Surg 41A:429, 1959

203. Whitman A: Astragalectomy and backward displacement of the foot. An investigation of its practical results. J Bone Joint Surg 4:266, 1922

204. Wiederholt WC, Mulder DW, Lamber EH: The Landry–Guillain–Barré–Strohl syndrome or polyradiculoneuropathy. Historical review, report on 97 patients and present concepts. Mayo Clin Proc 39:427, 1964

205. Williams PF, Menelaus MB: Triple arthrodesis by inlay grafting—a method suitable for the undeformed or valgus foot. J Bone Joint Surg 59B:333, 1977

206. Wilson FC Jr, Fay GF, Lamotte P, Williams JC: Triple arthrodesis. A study of the factors affecting fusion after three hundred and one procedures. J Bone Joint Surg 47A:340, 1965

207. Wilson PD: Posterior capsulotomy in certain flexion contractures of the knee. J Bone Joint Surg 11:40, 1929

208. Yadav SS: Muscle transfer for abduction paralysis of the shoulder in poliomyelitis. Clin Orthop 135:121, 1978
209. Yount CC: The role of the tensor fasciae femoris in certain deformities of the lower extremities. J Bone Joint Surg 8:171, 1926
210. Zancolli EA: Paralytic supination contracture of the forearm. J Bone Joint Surg 49A:1275, 1967
211. Zancolli EA, Mitre H: Latissimus dorsi transfer to restore elbow flexion. An appraisal of eight cases. J Bone Joint Surg 55A:1265, 1973
212. Zaoussis AL: Osteotomy of the proximal end of the radius for paralytic supination deformity in children. J Bone Joint Surg 45B:523, 1963

Chapter 5

Spinal Muscular Atrophy

Spinal muscular atrophy is an autosomal recessive condition in which there is chronic, progressive degeneration of the anterior horn cells in the spinal cord, and at times, of the neurons of the bulbar motor nuclei.[21] There is marked variation in severity of the muscle weakness and the age at which muscle atrophy or weakness becomes clinically apparent. This syndrome is characterized by symmetrical hypotonia that affects the lower extremities more than the upper and the proximal muscle more than the distal.[24] No associated sensory or long-tract involvements are present.[3]

The infantile variety was first described by Werdnig (1891) and Hoffman (1893) as progressive weakness occurring during the second 6 months of life.[13,23] Beevor (1902) recognized the condition to be present at birth.[1] Wohlfart, Kugelberg, and Welander discovered a milder variety.[14,22,25] The onset of this type occurs after age 2 years and the life expectancy is longer than in the other forms.

Incidence is one in 15,000 live births. Carrier frequency is 1 in 80 for all types.[18] Most patients have a normal birthweight. In some of the more severely involved patients, a decreased fetal movement is noted in the last trimester of pregnancy. Many patients presenting during the first 2 years of life may survive with virtually no progression or weakness other than during intercurrent infection or enforced immobilization.[17,20] Male siblings tend to be more severely affected.[18]

The only practical guide to prognosis is the actual degree of clinical involvement of the disease.[6] Spinal muscular atrophy can be divided into four clinical classifications (Table 5-1).[4,8]

CLASSIFICATIONS

Group I

Group I patients are severely involved. Onset is in utero or during the first 6 months of life. Marked generalized weakness and wasting and a lack of spontaneous movement are noted at birth or during the first few weeks of life. The onset may be acute with the infant losing the ability to move his limbs. Marked axial weakness results in little or no head control. The patient is never able to raise the head, turn over, or sit without support. Residual movement may be present only in the toes. The infant tends to assume a characteristic frog-leg posture (Fig. 5-1).

Marked atrophy of the intercostal muscles causes paradoxical breathing in which the

TABLE 5-1 Functional Classification of Spinal Muscular Atrophy

GROUPS	MAXIMUM FUNCTIONAL ACHIEVEMENT
I	No sitting balance. Poor head control.
II	Sitting balance and head control.
III	Limited ability to walk, with or without orthoses.
IV	Walk, run, and climb stairs normally.

chest flattens during inspiration as the diaphragm descends. This leads to the development of a bell-shaped chest. The cry is weak. The facial expression is alert and lively, although mild facial weakness may be noted. Extraocular motor muscles are intact. Later in childhood tongue fasciculations are evident, although these may be visualized in some patients in infancy. This pattern of visibility of fasciculations may also be noted in the extremities. Contraction fasciculation trembling of the extrinsic finger muscles may be found.[16] Auscultation is important in differentiating this chronic neuropathic disorder from myopathic disorders. Auscultation with a standard stethoscope applied over the contracting muscles demonstrates a high intensity, lower-pitched "rumbling" than the low

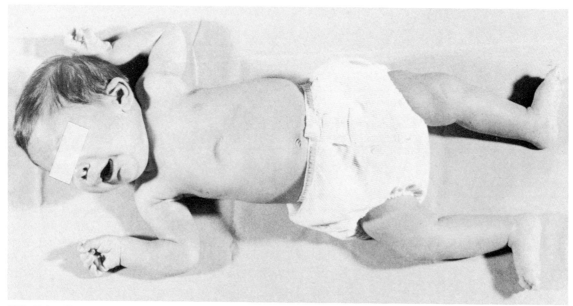

FIG. 5-1. Both upper and lower extremities are held in external rotation, flexion, and abduction. Note the bell-shaped trunk and evidence of paradoxical respirations.

intensity "hum" resulting from the synchronous firing of many normal-sized motor units.[10] Deep-tendon reflexes are absent.

The most affected patients have bulbar involvement which leads to pharyngeal muscle paresis. They are unable to swallow their saliva and may require suctioning to prevent aspiration. Tube feeding may be required because of poor ability to suck. Cardiac muscle is spared and therefore the ultimate prognosis rests on respiratory function. Most Group I patients with severe involvement will die in infancy, but the majority of those who survive to 1 year of age have a life expectancy of more than 10 years (Fig. 5-2).

Group II

Group II patients differ from patients in Group I in that they appear to achieve normal motor milestones during the first 6 months of life. The axial musculature is also less involved.

They develop independent head control, although they frequently cannot move from a lying posture to a sitting position without assistance. Approximately one third of these patients can roll over at some time. They are unable to walk even with orthotic assistance, although they may be propped up in a standing frame. Strength in the shoulder girdle and arms may allow abduction against gravity. Because the bulbar musculature is intact and the function of the intercostals is not severely altered, these patients are not seriously affected by infantile upper respiratory infections. Similarly, chewing and swallowing are not involved. Fasciculations of the extremities and tongue atrophy are common. Deep-tendon reflexes of the ankles and upper extremities are present in infancy and early childhood but are gradually lost in a centrifugal fashion. These patients can be expected to survive until early to middle adult life (Fig. 5-3) with a reduced cardiopulmonary per-

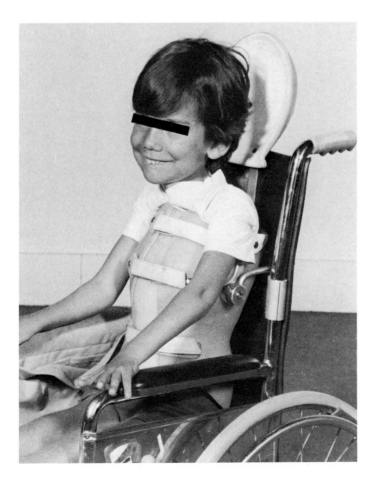

FIG. 5-2. This 10-year-old male has used a thoracic suspension orthosis for 5 years to maintain upright posture. Intermittent use of a headrest attached to the orthosis is required because of diminished neck muscle strength. Micrognathia is commonly found and may interfere with intubation required for spinal fusion.

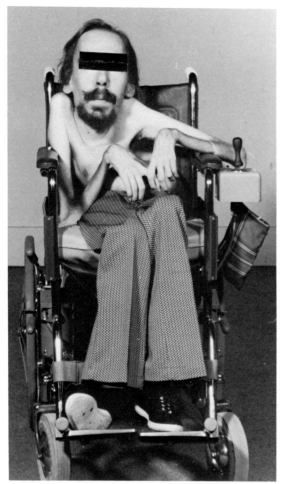

FIG. 5-3. An untreated 26-year-old male with severe kyphoscoliosis and back pain is a part-time university student and commercial artist despite obvious skeletal deformities.

formance which limits their functional ability.

Group III

Group III patients have less clinical involvement. By age 1 they are able to pull themselves to a standing position and are able to cruise on furniture. By age 2 they walk with a waddling gait, either independently or with lower-extremity orthoses, but they are never able to run or climb stairs normally (Fig. 5-4).[15] Since most patients with ambulatory potential retain adequate strength in the upper body to use crutches or a rollator, they con-

tinue to walk until after age 10 (Fig. 5-5). In the second decade of life, significant weakness of the upper extremities may develop, and in the third and fourth decades of life, neck muscles involvement is also found. Life expectancy is likely to be beyond age 45.

Group IV (Kugelberg–Welander Disease)

Group IV patients, who appear to develop normally, are able to walk, run, and climb stairs. Onset of the disease is insidious, occurring usually between ages 2 and 15. Initially there is weakness of the proximal pelvic musculature that clinically resembles Duchenne muscular dystrophy (Fig. 5-6). Occasionally there is hypertrophy of the calves. Shoulder-girdle involvement can be demonstrated by the time pelvic-girdle weakness results in a waddling gait, difficulty climbing stairs, and presence of a positive Gowers' sign. Muscles of the hand and forearm are among the last to be affected. Wrist flexors become paretic before the wrist extensors. Hand tremors and glossal fasciculations may be noted. Neck flexor and extensor weakness occurs late in the course of the disease, but facial weakness rarely develops. Although their life span is indefinite, most of these patients are in wheelchairs by their midthirties. As in the other forms of spinal muscular atrophy, this type is more severe and occurs more frequently in males.

After they have achieved maximum function, patients in Groups III and IV, and most in Group II, regress slowly. The weakness, which is greater in the lower extremities than in the upper, may become static in all groups for several years. Also, a rapid weight gain, which tends to occur in Group III patients at the end of the first decade of life, leads to decreased mobility.

LABORATORY DATA

Electromyogram results show denervation and reinnervation. Typical high-amplitude, long-duration, polyphasic potentials, in addition to fibrillation potentials at rest, are noted. Nerve conduction studies are normal. An electrocardiogram demonstrates a muscle tremor artifact, again due to the firing of large motor units.[19]

In Group I patients, histochemical eval-

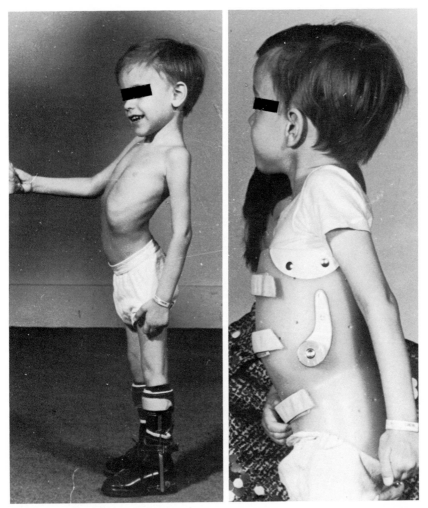

FIG. 5-4. Significant lordoscoliosis has been controlled in this 9-year-old who has worn a thoracic suspension orthosis for 6 years. He has achieved limited independent ambulation by wearing short leg braces with varus-producing T-straps which correct a severe functional talipes planovalgus.

uation of muscle biopsies demonstrates sheets of round, atrophic fibers among which are interspersed clumps of markedly hypertrophied fibers which are classified as Type 1 with ATPase stain.[5,7] Although the fibers are clustered in large groups, often whole bundles interspersed with fascicles contain hypertrophied fibers 3 to 4 times larger than normal. In Group II patients, the fibers appear in groups of the same type and Type 2 fibers are large, especially in children who survive beyond age 2. In many patients with spinal muscular

atrophy, the atrophic fibers have a unique round outline and only rarely are angulated. Neuropathological studies demonstrate a striking absence of anterior horn cells.

Serum creatine phospho kinase (CPK) levels vary among the four groups. CPK is not elevated in patients with severe involvement and little muscle mass, while approximately half of those in the Kugelberg–Welander Group (IV) have an increase in CPK 2 to 10 times the normal level. Usually elevation occurs during clinical progression of the disease.

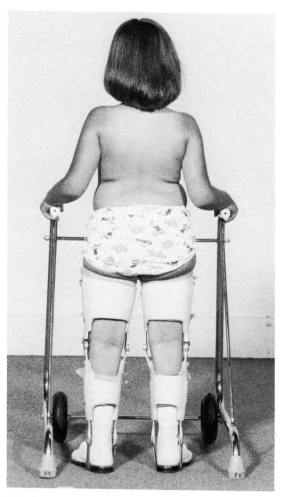

Fig. 5-5. Nearly all Group III patients require long leg braces to continue ambulation beyond the age of 5. They are household ambulators until early in the second decade.

SPINAL DEFORMITY

Spinal deformity occurs in all patients in Groups I, II, III, and in over half of those in Group IV (Table 5-2).[8] Scoliosis is most prev-

alent, but lordosis (Fig. 5-7A, B, and C) or kyphosis (Fig. 5-8A, B, and C) occasionally occurs. Spinal deformity represents a significant clinical problem for these patients because of its effect on the cardiorespiratory system.[2,12] While the cardiac muscles are spared, the primary and secondary pulmonary physiodynamics may be altered by the spinal deformity. This is reflected in the rate of morbidity and mortality among these patients. Other complications of spinal deformity include: (1) loss of independent use of the upper extremities in patients who need their arms to act as crutches to support the upright trunk (Fig. 5-9), (2) necrosis of the ischial fat pad with accompaning bursitis, (3) increasing lumbar pain, and (4) spondylosis which requires frequent change of position. Pelvic obliquity may jeopardize sitting for patients with poor head control (Fig. 5-10)

The most common deformity in spinal muscular atrophy is a thoracolumbar C-shaped curve (Fig. 5-11). The primary structural change is located at the thoracolumbar junction. Pelvic obliquity may develop as the curve gradually extends caudally.[11] The degree of axial-muscle involvement determines the cephalad extent of the curve. Severe muscle weakness causes structural changes in the upper thoracic spine while less severe involvement limits the curve to the mid-thoracic area (Fig. 5-12). The more cephalad the curve, the greater the problem in attempting orthotic control. The patient also experiences more difficulty in maintaining the head in the midline while trying to keep the eyes in a functional horizontal plane (Fig. 5-13).

Moe Subcutaneous Rodding

When fusion is contraindicated or not desired, Moe subcutaneous rodding offers an alternative to casting or bracing for correction of the collapsing spine in young children (Fig. 5-14).

TABLE 5-2 The Incidence and Distribution of Spinal Deformity

GROUP	AGE AT ONSET (YEARS)	SCOLIOSIS SINGLE CURVE	SCOLIOSIS DOUBLE CURVE	KYPHOSIS	LORDOSIS
I	<2	5	1	1	—
II	3 (1-7)	17	4	—	—
III	4.7 (2-7)	12	2	—	1
IV	8.4 (4-14)	5	1	—	1

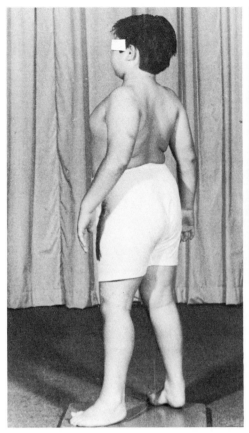

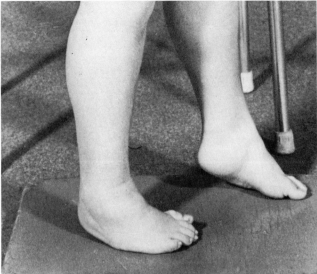

FIG. 5-6. Spinal muscular atrophy Group IV (Kugelberg–Welander syndrome.) An 11-year-old boy presented with talipes equinocavovarus and increasing lumbar lordosis. (Courtesy of Newington Children's Hospital)

TECHNIQUE.

Short incisions are made at the top and bottom of the deformity that is being corrected. Subperiosteal dissection is carried out at two or three levels on the concave aspect of the curve. A No. 1254 Harrington hook is placed under the lamina of the vertebrae at the most cephalad and caudad aspects of the curve. The longest possible Moe subcutaneous rod is selected; one nut is placed on both of the threaded ends of the rod and advanced toward the smooth central portion of the rod. The rod is passed through a subcutaneous tunnel and the threaded portion of one end is completely passed through the appropriate hook. The opposite end of the rod is inserted through the remaining hook and the nuts on the inside of each hook are advanced until the desired amount of distraction is achieved. The threads between the nut and the smooth portion of the rod are then destroyed to keep the nut from backing off. Initial laminar bone grafts may be required if the laminar bone is insuf-

ficient to permit secure fixation. Three months later a second surgical procedure is performed for proper seating of the rod. A spinal orthosis is required to complement the stability of the internal subcutaneous rod. Gillespie recommends re-exploration and hook advancement when there is a 10° loss of correction because of growth.* Each hook is advanced until the desired amount of distraction is obtained. It is again necessary to destroy the threads behind the nut as the hook is advanced. This procedure is repeated until either a longer Moe rod must be substituted or a fusion can be performed because sufficient spinal growth has occurred.

Segmental Spinal Instrumentation (Luque)

Segmental spinal instrumentation provides rigid internal spinal fixation and partial correction. Sublaminar wires are twisted over stainless steel rods at each level of the spine

---

*Gillespie R. Personal Communication.

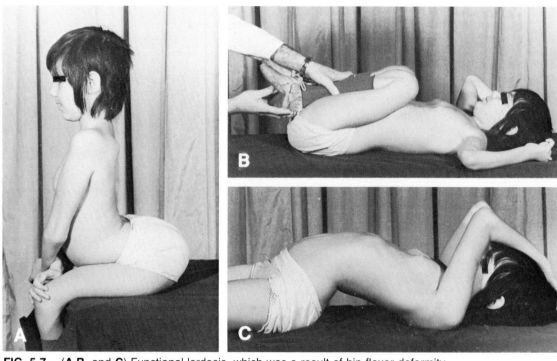

FIG. 5-7. (**A,B,** and **C**) Functional lordosis, which was a result of hip flexor deformity, has developed in this patient with spinal muscular atrophy Group III. (Courtesy of Newington Children's Hospital)

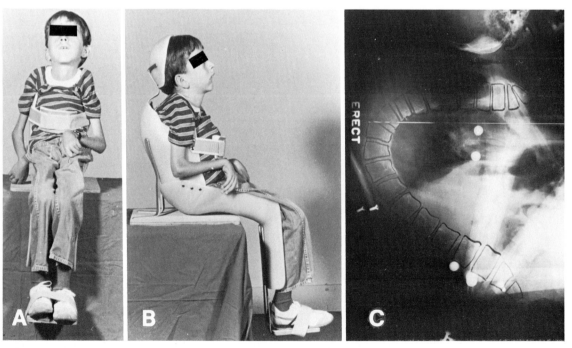

FIG. 5-8. (**A,B,** and **C**) Control laterally and posteriorly by means of a sitting orthosis permitted the anterior extrusion of the thorax in this Group I patient. This resulted in progressive, severe kyphosis with no scoliosis.

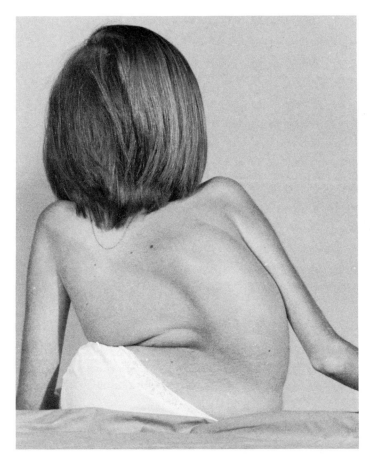

FIG. 5-9. The use of the upper extremities as crutches robs the patient of bimanual function.

to be instrumented. For patients with spinal muscular atrophy, the fusion extends from the pelvis to a level two vertebra above the most cephalad extension of the curve (Fig. 5-15).

TECHNIQUE

The laminae and spinous processes are exposed by subperiosteal dissection.[9] Decortication is not performed because it weakens the neural arch. Because the fusion must extend to the pelvis, the iliac wings are also exposed. The interspinous and flaval ligaments are sharply resected. A doubled annealed wire is passed carefully under the neural arch at each level. The wire is divided and one section is pulled to either side.

The point of entry for the short pelvic arm of the rod is usually posterior and adjacent to the sacroiliac joint at the level of the posterior inferior iliac spine. However, in these pa-

tients, underdevelopment of the posterior ilium may require the pelvic arm to be introduced through the lateral aspect of the sacrum in order to achieve proper seating along the iliopectineal line between the cortices of the ilium. French rod benders are used to carefully contour the rod to the conformation of the spine (Fig. 5-16). Both rods should lie adjacent to the laminae and abut against bone at each instrumented segment. Initially, the spine is reduced to the rod on the convex side of the curve. Beginning in the caudal portion of the curve, the wires are tightened over the rod. A similar procedure is carried out with the rod on the concave side. The surgeon can achieve greater stability by passing additional wires circumferentially around the rods in the region of the most superior and inferior twisted wires. Bone grafts are applied to the remaining exposed subperiosteal bed. No postoperative immobilization is required.

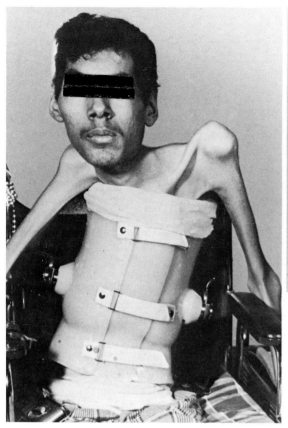

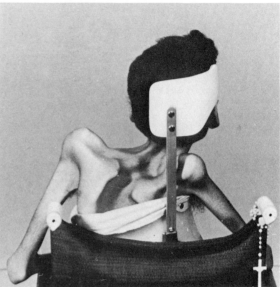

FIG. 5-10. This adolescent with spinal muscular atrophy Group II is able to sit for long periods because his head is centered over the pelvis when the spindles on a suspension jacket are placed in an eccentric pattern.

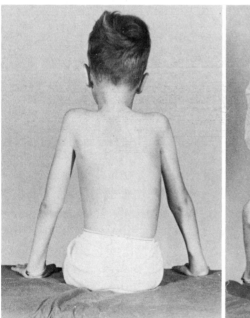

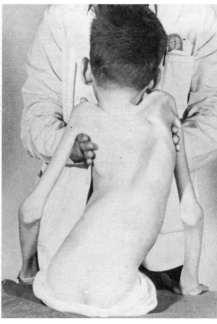

FIG. 5-11. Brothers who demonstrate a thoracolumbar paralytic scoliosis.

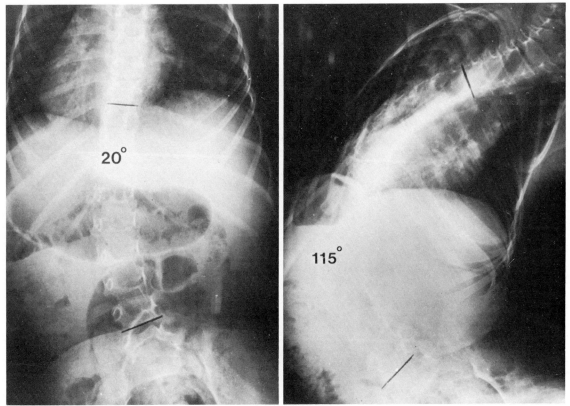

FIG. 5-12. The onset of scoliosis generally is in the thoracolumbar area. The left roentgenogram demonstrates an early structural curve in a 4-year-old Group I patient. The right roentgenogram taken 5 years later shows an increase in the length of the curve and its severity, as well as progressive rib-cage deformity.

Harrington Instrumentation

Harrington distraction instrumentation must be accompanied by posterior spinal fusion with bank bone grafts. The fusion area must include both the primary and secondary curves and the sacrum. I prefer a second short Harrington distraction rod extending to the sacrum on the contralateral side (Fig. 5-17). Decortication can be performed in a limited fashion at levels of the neural arch where seating of the distraction hooks is not planned. Postoperatively, the patient is managed in a bivalved Risser cast. The Circ-o-lectric bed can be used in the immediate postoperative period, if lower-extremity contractures do not interfere. Early mobilization following surgery is necessary to prevent a rapid increase in motor weakness in both the extremities and neck muscles. Early mobilization can most

readily be accomplished with a bivalved plastic spinal orthosis (Fig. 5-18), which is required for a minimum of 9 months following surgery.

LIMB DEFORMITY

Lower-limb contractures are most marked in the severely paralyzed. Infants with severe muscle weakness tend to assume a frog-leg posture. Generally, hip, knee, and foot deformities begin to develop in the first year of life. Contractures of the hip and knee occur at the same time and are of equal severity (Fig. 5-19). In Evans' study, 50° flexion contractures occurred in over half of the patients in Group I by age 3, while those in Group II had contractures of 30° or less at the same age.[8] By age 10, the untreated contractures of pa-

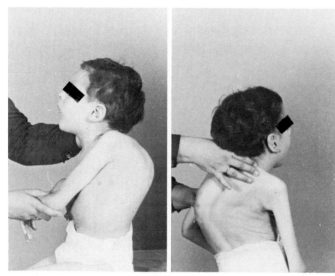

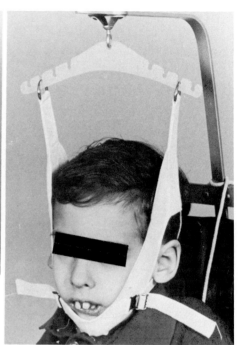

FIG. 5-13. A 7-year-old Group I patient with skin breakdown over the razor-back right rib cage and left axilla. He was able to achieve satisfactory long-term function by combining an independent head support with a T-foam contoured wheelchair insert.

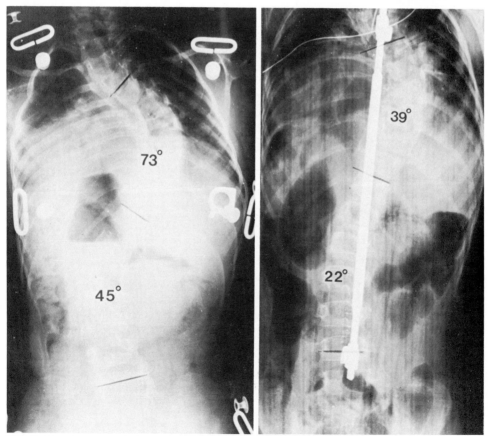

FIG. 5-14. A 7-year-old boy with rapidly progressive double major structural curve treated by Moe subcutaneous rodding. Lengthening of the apparatus will be performed when there is radiologic evidence of 10° loss of the original correction.

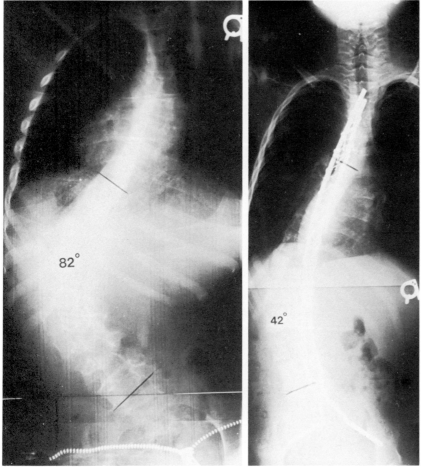

FIG. 5-15. These patients frequently have poor neural arch bone stock. Segmental wiring permits excellent fixation without overloading these fragile bony structures.

tients in both groups increased to 80° (Fig. 5-20). Patients in Group III rarely developed significant hip or knee flexion contractures before age 10. The onset of contractures in this group tended to precede, rather than follow, loss of ambulation. Group IV patients rarely developed hip or knee flexion contractures, but if they did occur, they were mild and did not interfere with independent ambulation.

Hip dislocation was found only in Groups I and II (Fig. 5-21). Bilateral dislocation was more common in Group I, whereas unilateral dislocation or subluxation was common in Group II. Hip subluxations occurred during childhood, with dislocation developing during adolescence or early adult life. Unilateral subluxation also occurred in the other two groups. These types of patients may develop pelvic obliquity and associated scoliosis.

Equinus deformity, sometimes with associated varus of valgus deformities, developed in approximately half of the patients in Groups I and II. The deformity frequently developed in patients in Group III after they had lost their ability to walk. Forefoot equinus also was noted occasionally in Group IV patients.

Although contractures of the upper extremities occurred less frequently, the elbow was the most commonly involved joint. This deformity was associated with progressive weakness in the arms and exceeded 40° only in severely involved patients in Groups I and II. Patients in Group III did not develop elbow contractures despite weakness of the upper

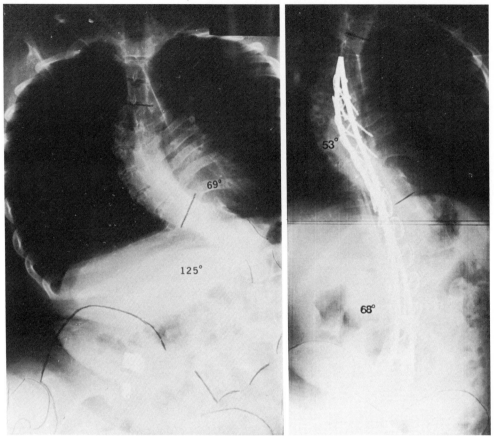

FIG. 5-16. A 19-year-old Group III patient demonstrates improvement in sitting posture following successful posterior spinal fusion complemented by segmental spinal instrumentation.

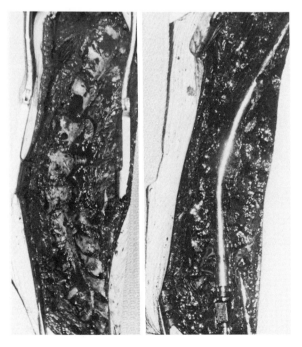

FIG. 5-17. Wide subperiosteal dissection is necessary to ensure an adequate bony bed for the fusion. Muscle tissue generally is encountered only in the upper thoracic area. The Harrington rods must be carefully contoured to accommodate the fixed element of the scoliosis.

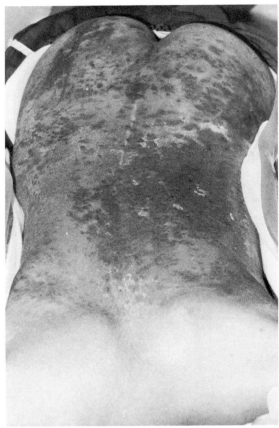

FIG. 5-18. Spinal muscular atrophy patients may have increased diapedesis. The use of a bivalved plastic spinal orthosis permits management of a heat rash which developed under a plaster body cast.

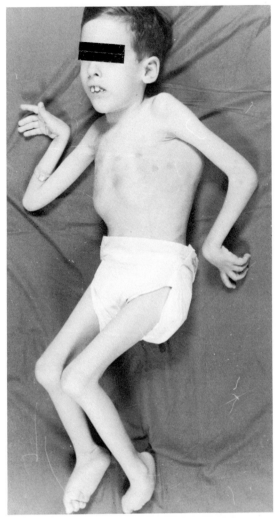

FIG. 5-19. A 7-year-old demonstrating multiple severe contractures of the upper and lower extremities.

extremities that had developed after skeletal maturation. Neck weakness and poor head control became more pronounced during the third decade of life, especially after periods of prolonged recumbency in patients in Group II and III.

Treatment

Soft-tissue surgery was effective in correcting lower-limb contractures and was well tolerated by selected patients.[4] The deformities may require correction either because they limit positioning of the patient or because of discomfort. Hip and knee flexion contractures can be released simultaneously and deformities of 60° to 80° can be reduced to 20° (Fig. 5-22).

Severe flexion-abduction contractures of the hip, if left untreated, can cause the development of hip subluxation and dislocation. A hip-flexion contracture can be corrected by releasing the fascia lata from the anterosuperior spine to the sacroiliac joint, the fascial envelope of the sartorius, and the tendons of the rectus femoris and iliopsoas. No capsular surgery is required. To release knee contractures, medial and lateral midline incisions are made. Then tenotomies of the hamstrings and iliotibial band are performed, combined with posterior capsulotomies. The incisions must be placed carefully, as the hip incision tends

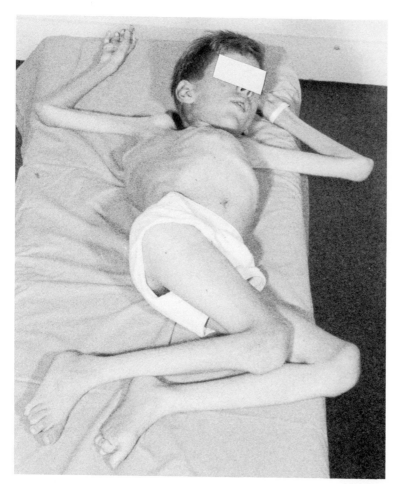

FIG. 5-20. The contractures in this 15-year-old Group I spinal muscular atrophy patient have increased because of both osseous growth and wheelchair positioning.

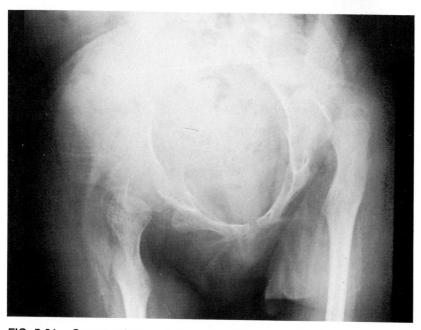

FIG. 5-21. Severe valgus and elongation of the femoral neck imply paralytic dislocations in this spinal muscular atrophy Group I patient.

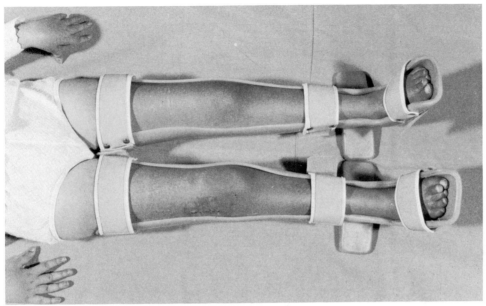

FIG. 5-22. The use of night-time long leg braces permits ongoing control of lower-extremity joints. The outriggers prevent rotation and the possibility of a windblown posture of the lower extremities.

to migrate proximally toward the bony iliac crest when the flexion contracture is released, while the knee incision migrates posteriorly as the deformity is reduced. Division of the anterior cruciate ligament may also be required. Postoperatively, serial casts or night splints may be needed to maintain or to correct minor additional contractures.

Although foot deformities rarely need surgical correction, surgery is indicated to either relieve pressure that causes skin ulcerations over the talar head or the fifth metatarsus or to allow application of footwear (Fig. 5-23). Wearing shoes improves cosmesis and also allows the foot to be placed on a footrest to avoid entangling it in the front wheels of

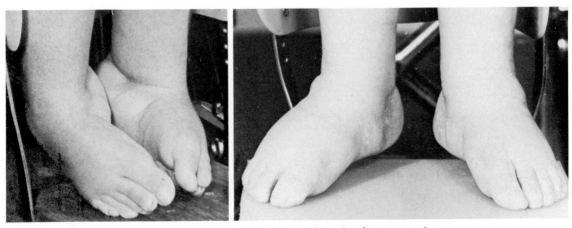

FIG. 5-23. Severe fixed talipes equinovarus may lead to ulceration from excessive pressure along the lateral forefoot in patients who cannot move their lower extremities. Long-term management with talectomy, combined with ankle-foot orthoses, is effective in correcting this problem.

a wheelchair. Talectomies, as well as soft-tissue releases, can be performed (Fig. 5-23).

REFERENCES

1. Beevor CE: A case of congenital spinal muscular atrophy (family type), and a case of haemorrhage into the spinal cord at birth, giving similar symptoms. Brain 25:85, 1902
2. Benady SG: Spinal muscular atrophy in childhood: Review of 50 cases. Dev Med Child Neurol 20:746, 1978
3. Byers RK, Banker BQ: Infantile muscular atrophy. Arch Neurol 5:140, 1961
4. Drennan JC: Skeletal deformities in spinal muscular atrophy. In Abstracts of Association of Bone and Joint Surgeons, Clin Orthop 133:266, 1978
5. Dubowitz V: Diagnostic advances in neuromuscular disease. Arch Dis Child 47:149, 1972
6. Dubowitz V: Benign infantile spinal muscular atrophy. Dev Med Child Neurol 16:672, 1974
7. Dubowitz V, Brooke MH: Muscle biopsy, A Modern Approach. London, WB Saunders, 1973
8. Evans GA, Drennan JC, Russman BS: Functional classification and orthopaedic management of spinal muscular atrophy. J Bone Joint Surg 63-B:516, 1981
9. Ferguson RL, Allen BL: Segmental spinal instrumentation for routine scoliotic curve. Contemporary Orthopaedics 2:450, 1980
10. Fredericks EJ, Russman BS: Bedside evaluation of large motor units in childhood spinal muscular atrophy. Neurology 29:398, 1979
11. Hardy JH (ed): Spinal Deformity in Neurological and Muscular Disorders. St Louis, CV Mosby, 1974
12. Hensinger RN, MacEwen, GD: Spinal deformity associated with heritable neurological conditions: Spinal muscular dystrophy, Friedreich's ataxia, familial dysautonomia, and Charcot–Marie–Tooth disease. J Bone Joint Surg 58A:13, 1976
13. Hoffman J: "Uber chronische spinale muskelatrophie im kindersalter, auf familiarer bases". Dentsche Zeitschrift fur Nervenheilkunde 3:427, 1893
14. Kugelberg E, Welander L: Heredofamilial juvenile muscular atrophy simulating muscular dystrophy. Archives of Neurology and Psychiatry 75:500, 1956
15. Letts RM, Fulford R, Hobson DA: Mobility aids for the paraplegic child. J Bone Joint Surg 58A:38, 1976
16. Moosa A, Dubowitz V: Spinal muscular atrophy in childhood. Two clues to clinical diagnosis. Arch Dis Child 48:386, 1973
17 Munsat TL, Woods R, Fowler W, Pearson CM: Neurogenic muscular atrophy of infancy with prolonged survival. Brain 92:9, 1969
18. Pearn JH, Gardner D, Wilson J: A clinical study of chronic childhood spinal muscular dystrophy. A review of 141 cases. J Neurol Sci 38:23, 1978
19. Russman BS, Fredericks EJ: Use of the ECG in the diagnosis of childhood spinal muscular atrophy. Arch Neurol 36:317, 1979
20. Schwentker EP, Gibson DA: The orthopaedic aspects of spinal muscular atrophy. J Bone Joint Surg 58A:32, 1976
21. Thieffry S, Arthuis M, Bargeton E: Werdnig–Hoffman: 40 cases with 11 autopsies. Revue Neurologique (Paris) 93:621, 1955
22. Welander L: Myopathia distalis tarda hereditaria. Acta Med Scand [Suppl] 265:1, 1951
23. Werdnig G: Zwei fruhintantile hereditäre Fälle von progressiver Muskelatrophie unter dem Bilde der Dystrophie, aber auf neurotischer Grundlage Archiv für Psychiatrie und Nervenkrankheiten 22:437, 1891
24. Wijngaarden GK van, Bethlem J: Benign infantile spinal muscular atrophy. A prospective study. Brain 96:163, 1973
25. Wohlfart G, Fex J, Eliasson S: Heredity proximal spinal muscular atrophy—a classical entity simulating progressive muscular dystrophy. Acta Psychiatrica et Neurologica Scandinavica 30:395, 1955

Chapter 6

Arthrogryposis Multiplex Congenita

Arthrogryposis multiplex congenita is a syndrome characterized by nonprogressive, multiple, congenitally rigid joints. The condition was first described by Otto in 1841.[2] Rosenkranz, in 1905, first used the term "arthrogryposis," meaning "curved joint."[23] Stern, in 1923, initiated use of the term "arthrogryposis multiplex congenita."[26] The pathophysiology of this clinical syndrome has not been established, and its name remains descriptive. The disease can be divided into neuropathic and myopathic forms and a mixed form, in which the muscle appears normal upon histologic and histochemical examination.

ETIOLOGY AND PATHOGENESIS

A diarthrodial joint is characterized by a joint cavity with a peripheral fibrous capsule between movable skeletal parts. During the third month of gestation, the joint cavity develops from clefts in the dense mesenchyme. Arey states that the joint cavity is produced when the sluggishly growing peripheral tissue resists the axial expansion of the faster growing cartilaginous center.[1] Nervous, muscular, or vascular influences do not appear to be factors in joint development.

The joint develops in arthrogryposis multiplex congenita, but the periarticular soft-tissue structures become fibrotic, leading to the development of an incomplete fibrous ankylosis. Theories as to the cause of arthrogryposis relate to abnormalities of the central nervous system, the muscles and joints, and mechanical abnormalities, as well as infection and miscellaneous causes.[3,6,15,17,20,23,25,26] A decrease in the number of anterior-horn cells, without an accompanying increase in the number of microglial cells, is the evidence supporting the theory of involvement of the central nervous system.[6,12] Drachman was able to cause fibrous ankylosis of many joints in chick embryos injected with tubocurarine.[6] He demonstrated a direct relationship between the degree of deformity and the amount of drug infused. The possibility of severe deformity increased with the age of the embryo. This study supports Jago's clinical observation of arthrogryposis in an offspring following treatment of maternal tetanus with muscle relaxants.[18] Lloyd-Roberts concludes that arthrogryposis represents an end-product of anterior-horn cell disease in utero, which arrests spontaneously.[21] Other authors have implicated intrauterine compression, increased or decreased amniotic fluid, or weak fetal movements.[13,23] A condition similar to arthrogryposis has been noted in sheep and cattle following ingestion of locoweed or lupine.[19] Whittem reported arthrogryposis associated with hydrocephalus and blindness in calves.[27]

PATHOLOGY

The involved striated muscle is pale pink and markedly shrunken. Histologic examination demonstrates a marked decrease in the number of muscle fibers, with severely involved muscles having been entirely replaced by fibrous tissue. Partially affected muscles show large well-striated fibers among those that are atrophic. The architecture of the involved fibers is altered very little, and cross-striations are retained.[22]

Gross examination of the spinal cord reveals a decrease in its diameter, especially in the cervical and lumbar areas. Microscopically there is a reduction in the number of anterior-horn cells in the cervical, thoracic, and lumbosacral segments, and no evidence of an inflammatory response.[6,12] The posterior-root and posterior-horn cell population is

intact. Associated cerebral- and corticospinal-tract atrophy also has been reported.

Pathologic changes in the myopathic form of arthrogryposis are limited to skeletal muscle. On serial muscle biopsies Banker noted steady degenerative changes closely resembling those of progressive muscular dystrophy.[2] These include loss of muscle fibers, with evidence of degeneration, and marked variation in the size of the remaining fibers. There was also an increased amount of fibro-fatty tissue, with no evidence of inflammation or regeneration. Peripheral nerve endings and anterior-horn cells were all normal, and no associated brain abnormalities were found.

Electromyography demonstrates fibrillation potential in the neuropathic form of arthrogryposis.

CLINICAL FEATURES

Limb involvement is usually quadrimelic. The joint changes are limited to the lower limbs when only two extremities are involved. The frequency of joint involvement in both the upper and lower extremities increases from the proximal to the distal segments and usually is symmetric. Marked limitation of active and passive motion is present, but at least a few degrees of painless free motion in the major joints is retained, which is stopped by a firm inelastic block. Joints may be fixed in flexion or extension (Fig. 6-1).

The muscle mass is diminished, making the joints appear large and fusiform. Normal skin creases are absent; the skin is tense and glossy, with scant subcutaneous tissue and muscle volume. Webbing frequently is present (Fig. 6-2) with knee and elbow flexion contractures. Dimpling may be noted in the involved elbows, hips, knees, and wrists. Sensation is intact, but deep-tendon reflexes are decreased or absent. Intelligence usually is normal. The most frequent orthopaedic deformities in the newborn are talipes equinovarus, dislocated hip, and dislocated patella (Fig. 6-3). Scoliosis may develop in childhood from involvement of the erector spinae muscles.[24] Port wine stains of the forehead, congenital heart disease, and renal anomalies have been reported.[13]

The classic arthrogrypotic deformities are present at birth (Fig. 6-4). The shoulders are adducted and internally rotated, the elbows

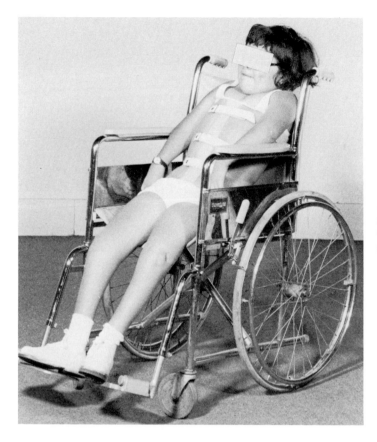

FIG. 6-1. Fixed extension of major lower extremity joints makes a wheelchair level of activity precarious. The visible knee dimpling is associated with a dislocated patella.

are fixed in flexion or extension (Fig. 6-5), and the wrists are in flexion and ulnar deviation. The fingers are very slender, held close together (Fig. 6-6), and waxy in appearance. The hips usually are flexed, externally rotated and abducted. Knee flexion often occurs, as well as hyperextension. Clubfeet are common.

MANAGEMENT

The orthopaedist caring for the patient with arthrogryposis must be realistic about long-term goals and expectations. The overall goal is achievement of a maximal degree of function. Minimum requirements include independent walking, self-care, and eventually, the physical ability to be gainfully employed.[22]

Arthrogryposis generally leads to very stiff and deformed joints with limited range-of-motion, which will not increase with aggressive therapy. However, the joints can be changed and maintained in a more advantageous functional position. Recurrence of a corrected deformity is common as the limb grows and the inelastic periarticular structures fail to stretch.

The orthopaedist's concerns should be the correction of the disabling deformity and the achievement of range-of-motion in the major joints sufficient for the patient's needs. This objective is accomplished in the young child by the use of serial casts, with or without soft-tissue surgical procedures.[14] Williams reports improved results with aggressive surgical treatment in infancy and early childhood.[29] Long-term orthotic control maintains the correction (Fig. 6-7).[13] Osteotomy of long bones should be reserved for the patient nearing skeletal maturity. Osteotomy performed on immature bone results in recurrence of the deformity, if the pericapsular structures remain intact. The more distal the surgery from the individual joint, the less likely it is that a lasting improvement is achieved.

Newborn Period

The diagnosis must be formally established in the newborn period, and active orthopaedic

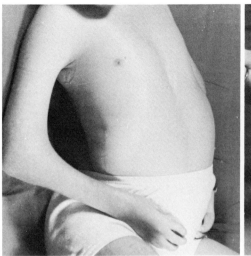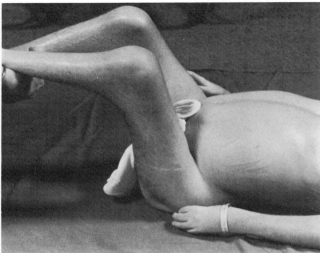

FIG. 6-2. Webbing of the shoulders, elbows, and knees is associated with muscle aplasia and extreme restriction in joint motion.

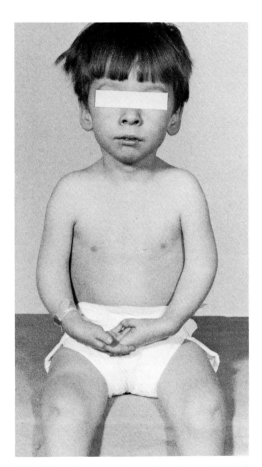

FIG. 6-3. Dislocated patellae are associated with bilateral dimpling. Arthrogrypotic patellae may be hypoplastic but are present in the displaced quadriceps mechanism.

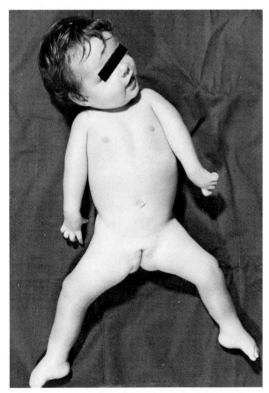

FIG. 6-4. Deformities that present in the newborn period include internally rotated and adducted shoulders and extended elbows and wrists. The hips are flexed, externally rotated, and abducted, and the feet demonstrate talipes equinocavus. Dimpling is evident over the extensor surfaces of the knees and wrists. (Courtesy of Newington Children's Hospital)

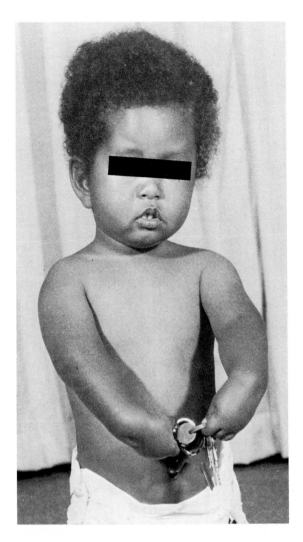

management begun. A thorough search should rule out other more common congenital abnormalities. The back and neck are examined for evidence of spinal dysrhaphism, and motor and sensory evaluations of the head, trunk, and extremities should be performed. Roentgenograms may be necessary to rule out spinal dysrhaphism or a congenital hip dislocation.

The establishment of rapport between the orthopaedist and the patient's family is very important. The child's normal intelligence should be stressed and his family reassured of the favorable long-term functional prognosis and the nonprogressive nature of the disease. The long-term plan for total, ongoing orthopaedic management should be outlined for the family. The continuing dedication of the family is essential if the physical handicaps of the child are to be alleviated.

Neonatal contractures, especially of the hands, feet, and knees, should be corrected by serial manipulation and casting.[14] Physical therapy, splinting, and bracing maintain correction and are important in avoiding the development of postural deformity.

FIG. 6-5. Bilateral manual function and dexterity are gained despite upper extremity contractures which include wrist flexion and ulnar deviation. Surgery to correct these deformities is contraindicated because of potential loss of function.

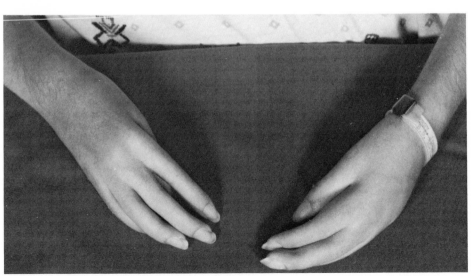

FIG. 6-6. These functionless hands demonstrate an absence of interphalangeal skin creases which are associated with rigid joints.

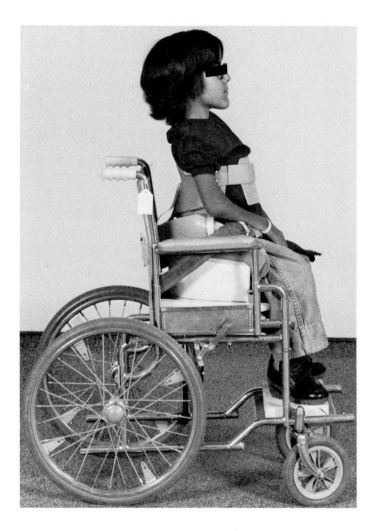

FIG. 6-7. Orthoses frequently must be individualized. This trunk orthosis is combined with a rocker-type of wheel-chair sitting orthosis. It permits upright activity while it relieves the patient of excessive ischial discomfort.

Surgical Management of Extremities

The goal is to correct, before the age of 2 years, all lower-extremity deformities that might delay the patient's ability to walk. Management of an individual deformity must be considered in relation to the total handicap. Surgery in a young child should be limited to soft-tissue procedures. Full-time bracing may be required until at least 6 years of age, and night splints should be used until skeletal maturity is reached. Delaying surgery on the upper extremities for several years allows time for a more complete functional assessment and reduces the possibility of surgical interference with acquired function.[21]

THE FOOT

Talipes equinovarus is the most common deformity. Usually it is severe and is associated with limited ankle and tarsal motion. The untreated clubfoot results in difficulty in walking and fitting shoes as well as in pain and ulceration. Serial manipulation and casting in the newborn may partially correct the condition, but recurrence of the deformity will promptly result when the nonoperative treatment is interrupted.

Surgical correction should be performed before the young child begins to walk. The objective is to convert the stiff, deformed foot into a stiff, plantigrade foot. Posteromedial release, tendon transfer, and tenotomy are ineffective. Talipes equinovarus is most effectively managed by talectomy performed at 12-18 months of age, which results in a satisfactory long-term plantigrade foot (Fig. 6-8).[10,14,21] An excisional tenotomy of the tendo Achillis to allow positioning of the calcaneus under the tibia is required (Fig. 6-9). It may be

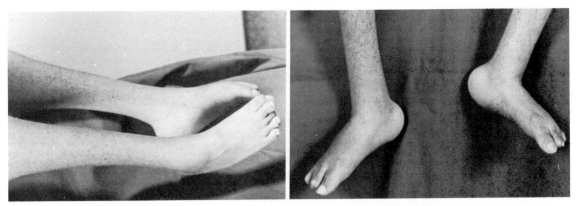

FIG. 6-8. A talectomy performed on the 11-year-old patient in Figure 6-7 permitted the use of ankle-foot orthoses, regular shoes, and prevented recurrent entanglement of her feet with the front wheels of the wheelchair.

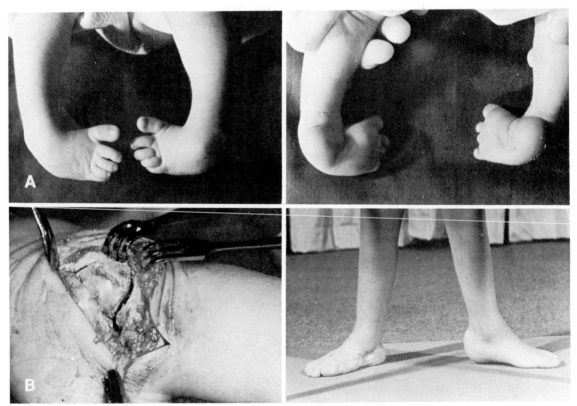

FIG. 6-9. (*A*) Talipes equinovarus. (*B*) Meticulous dissection is necessary to open the narrow fibrotic joints to permit talectomy. Definitive correction by talectomy must be accompanied by ablation of all muscle forces across the angle plus long-term use of an ankle-foot orthosis. The best results achieve a functional ankle ankylosis.

necessary to excise the navicula to obtain satisfactory posterior displacement of the foot.[5,8]

TECHNIQUE.   Exposure is gained through an anterolateral incision. Identification of the individual joints by means of a fine-tipped hemostat is made more difficult by the narrowing of the joint and the relative capsular thickening. The ankle joint should be identified first. The entire bone is completely enucleated. Meticulous technique is required because small, cartilaginous fragments left behind eventually ossify and may reproduce the original deformity. Anterior subluxation of the os calcis will recur if the posterior soft-tissue structures are not adequately released. Occasionally, it is also necessary to remove the navicula to gain satisfactory correction. The tendo Achillis is tenotomized through a short posterior incision. The fibula or calcaneus occasionally require careful shaving and remodeling to allow a satisfactory calcaneal alignment in the ankle mortise. The calcaneus must be aligned with the ankle joint. A Kirschner wire passed through the heel into the tibia is maintained for 3 weeks. Astragalectomy requires plaster immobilization for 3 months. The corrected foot is held in a right-angle brace for an indefinite period.

FOOT SURGERY IN THE OLDER CHILD

Triple arthrodesis with limited bone resection is the procedure of choice in children over age 10 with talipes equinovarus. Residual equinovarus in the skeletally mature patient can be managed by a supramaleolar closing-wedge osteotomy, with the wedge posteriorly and laterally. Pantalar arthrodesis also has been employed in the skeletally mature patient, as the recurrence of the deformity following triple arthrodesis usually is at the ankle. Occasionally, forefoot equinus develops, causing a significant cavus. This may require a limited midfoot, closing dorsal wedge osteotomy.

The calcaneovalgus foot occasionally seen in the child with arthrogryposis often presents no management problem and should be left alone.

CONGENITAL CONVEX PES VALGUS

Two separate types of congenital vertical talus are recognizable, depending on whether the calcaneocuboid joint is involved.[7] Calcaneocuboid joint subluxation or dislocation makes management more difficult (Fig. 6-10).

TECHNIQUE.   I prefer a one-stage procedure, using two incisions. The surgery should be performed before the patient begins walking. Correction must be complete, or the deformity will recur.

A complete posteromedial release is combined with a limited dorsolateral release. The tibialis posterior is carefully preserved. Correction of the medial longitudinal arch is buttressed by a proximal advancement of an inverted-V flap, created from the superficial deltoid ligament and deep fascia of the distal medial tibia. The flap is begun 1 inch proximal to the tip of the medial malleolus and is developed posteriorly toward the os calcis, while its distal limb extends to the first cuneiform bone. Tendo-Achillis lengthening is delayed until all other soft tissues have been released, thereby allowing the surgeon to maintain control over the hindfoot. Peroneal tenotomies and capsulotomies of the subluxated, or dislocated, calcaneocuboid joint and the lateral aspect of the subtalar joint are made through a short lateral incision. No tendon transfers are performed.

The completely mobilized hindfoot bones require Kirschner wire fixation for stability. The first pin is passed through the heel into the os calcis, the talus, and the tibia to control the correction of the hindfoot valgus and equinus. The forefoot alignment is then reassessed. The second Kirschner wire fixes the talonavicular joint. It is passed retrograde through the first metatarsal and the navicula into the talus, or, conversely, through the posterior talus into the navicula and the first metatarsal. The third wire stabilizes the calcaneocuboid joint and prevents eversion of the forefoot. This correction is maintained in a nonweight-bearing long leg cast for 6 months. A medial longitudinal arch support should be added to the lower-limb orthosis.

Forefoot abduction deformities can occur in the younger child and can be managed by excision of the navicula.

KNEE JOINT

FLEXION CONTRACTURE.   The goal is to straighten the knee and to maintain correc-

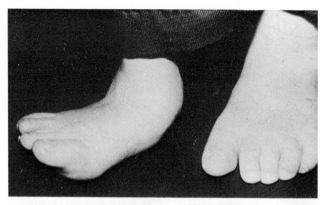

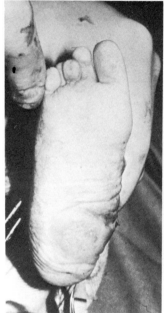
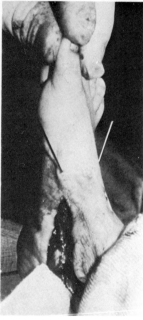

FIG. 6-10. A 6-year-old boy with an uncorrected congenital convex pes valgus. Preoperatively the talar head is the only weight-bearing component of the foot. A medial longitudinal arch is created and proper weight-bearing is achieved by one-stage surgical correction. (Courtesy of Newington Children's Hospital)

tion by bracing (Fig. 6-11). Recurrence of the deformity in a corrected knee is less common than in other joints, if prolonged bracing is employed. The range-of-motion is not increased, but the knee is changed to a more functional position. The extension gained allows most patients to walk, but they frequently find it difficult to cope with shoes and socks. Management in the newborn requires a long leg spica, with appropriate corrective wedging.

Posterior Capsulotomy. A posterior capsulotomy combined with hamstring division may be required in the young child having a fixed deformity of as little as 30°. Two midaxial longitudinal incisions are used; the neurovas-

cular structures are identified and protected. The joint capsule should be identified medially and laterally, to prevent unnecessary proximal dissection in the popliteal space. A thorough capsulotomy is performed. Division of the cruciate and collateral ligaments may be required to gain adequate posterior release. Tension in the neurovascular structures may limit the final amount of correction until after the second or third cast change. Posterior subluxation of the tibia can develop as the flexion deformity is corrected (Fig. 6-12). It is caused by the adaptive changes in the distal femur and posterior tibial plateau, as well as by the tethering effects of the scarred remnants of the hamstrings. This tendency is controlled postoperatively by using the Quengel cast

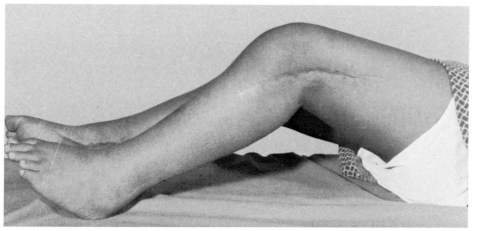

FIG. 6-11. Correction of this recurrent knee deformity required division of all soft tissues about the knee, with the exception of the posterior neurovascular bundle and the patellar tendon. Postoperative use of a Quengel cast was required to gain full extension and permit long leg brace application.

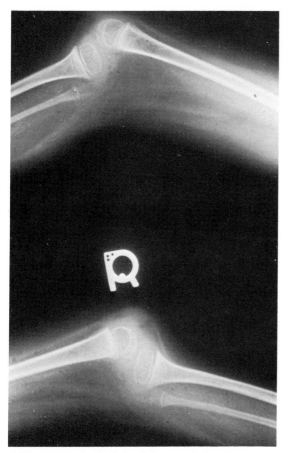

FIG. 6-12. Posterior tibial subluxation may develop when correction of the knee flexion deformity by casting is not monitored by roentgenograms. (Courtesy of Newington Children's Hospital)

technique (Fig. 6-13). A second method employs a short leg cast with tibial pins. The first Kirschner wire is placed in the distal tibia and is used for longitudinal traction. A second wire inserted into the anterior proximal tibia gives vertical traction and lifts the tibia upward and forward, as the knee joint is distracted by the longitudinal traction. Long-term use of a Hessing-type lower-limb orthosis has proven helpful to me. Initially, no orthotic knee joint is used, but, when stability has been achieved, the knee joint can be added to the brace to use the available range-of-motion.

A supracondylar osteotomy does not release the rigid periarticular soft tissue. It should be reserved until the child nears skeletal maturity and no recurrence is anticipated. Osteotomies done earlier in life result in diaphyseal angulation as the femur lengthens. This not only leads to problems in bracing, but also creates a grotesque iatrogenic cosmetic deformity.[21] The osteotomy is performed at the junction of the femoral diaphysis and metaphysis. Extension of the distal limb forces the diaphysis into the metaphysis, correcting the deformity and affording stability.

EXTENSION DEFORMITY. A knee fixed in extension does not benefit from attempted correction. Hyperextension requires quadriceps lengthening and anterior capsulotomy, including freeing of the patella and the suprapatellar pouch.[10,14] The hypoplastic patella may be dislocated laterally, but can be reduced

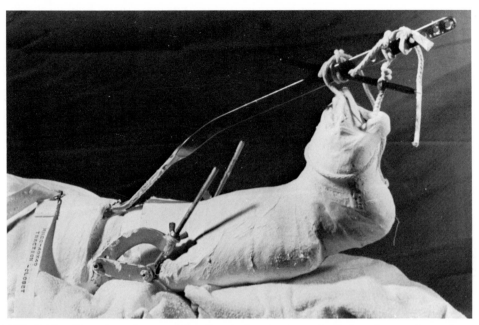

FIG. 6-13. The minute forces of the Quengel cast act constantly in a three-point system of corrective forces. A Spanish windlass toggle is used to shorten the cords. (Courtesy of Newington Children's Hospital)

when the quadriceps have been lengthened. This necessitates a release of the lateral patellar retinaculum, combined with a Roux procedure, and advancement of the remaining oblique fibers of the vastus medialis. Satisfactory tracking of the patella must be determined at the time of surgery. The surgeon is urged to be aggressive in obtaining as much correction as is possible with both the flexion and extension releases, since these patients will require long-term orthotic management.

HIP JOINT

The hip in the newborn frequently is fixed in flexion, abduction, and external rotation, and it may be dislocated. Arthrography may be necessary to establish the hip position. Mobile hips in the infant with arthrogryposis are treated in a manner similar to the typical congenital hip dislocation.[14,15] Lloyd-Roberts recommends accepting the dislocated position when both hips are dislocated and the range-of-motion is severely limited.[21] The dislocations tend to be stable and high, and usually are symmetrical, with the pelvis balanced. This is consistent with a satisfactory gait. Open reduction is contraindicated with bilateral

dislocation, since only a unilateral reduction may be achieved.

A high unilateral dislocation can lead to severe pelvic obliquity and secondary scoliosis.[10] Open reduction should be performed when the child is approximately 1 year old, and after control of the knee flexion contracture has been accomplished. Excessive delay makes the reduction more difficult. Concern about the possibility of pelvic obliquity and leg length inequality outweighs the risk of possible stiffness. Most experienced orthopaedic surgeons feel that if both hips are not reduced by 2 years of age, their position should be accepted.[14,22] Increased risk of unilateral failure of relocation, myositis ossificans, and increased scarring about the hip joint all contraindicate heroic surgical efforts in the older child.

Hip contracture presents a greater functional problem than does dislocation, and it compromises walking. A mild flexion contracture can be compensated for by a supple spine, but a flexion contracture exceeding 35° leads to the development of lumbar lordosis, difficult ambulation, and, eventually, pain from degenerative problems. These severe deformities invariably are associated with a knee

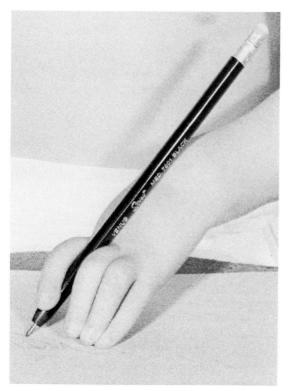

FIG. 6-14. Despite intrinsic atrophy, this 4-year-old demonstrates satisfactory fine motor skills for many activities of daily living.

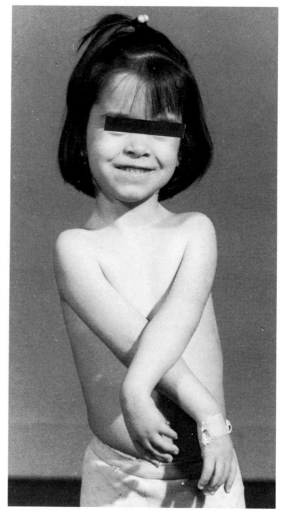

FIG. 6-15. Bimanual upper extremity functional activity must be analyzed before surgery is undertaken. (Courtesy of Newington Children's Hospital)

flexion contracture. Correction of the knee must be carried out first, and at a young age. The hip contracture can then be managed by incorporating the corrected knee into a long leg plaster cast with a crossbar, and maintaining the patient in a prone position. Surgical release is generally unsatisfactory, since the periarticular structures also are rigid, and a total capsulectomy may result in avascular necrosis of the femoral head. The most definitive correction is obtained by a subtrochanteric osteotomy when the child nears skeletal maturation.

UPPER EXTREMITY

Upper extremity surgery in the majority of cases is designed to increase hand function. Goals include independence in feeding, attention to toilet, and handling of objects (Fig. 6-14). Upper-extremity surgery should be postponed for several years to allow full analysis of the function of the individual hand and the mutual dependence of the hands, which frequently work effectively as a functional unit (Fig. 6-15).[10] Despite severe physical handicaps, these patients often exhibit great dexterity, and, while the appearance may be distressing, the functional result can be surprisingly good. A patient's adaptability in the performance of specific functions quite commonly has made surgical intervention both unnecessary and unwise.

THE HAND. The upper limbs are dominated by the hand and especially by the position of the fingers. Good finger mobility and power demand an agressive approach to associated upper-extremity contractures. Stiff, spidery, weak fingers offer little hope for improved hand function, despite extensive surgical attempts. This type of hand is best left alone. The accompanying palmar fixed flexion deformity at the wrist can be used to create a functional hook.

The most frequent deformity is flexed fingers, particularly of the proximal interphalangeal and metacarpal phalangeal joints, which interfere with the handling of objects. Soft-tissue procedures including capsulotomies and tendon transfers are disappointing. The thumb-in-palm deformity can be managed by Z-plasty, combined with release of the adductor hallucis.[10] A metacarpophalangeal fusion of the thumb may increase stability of grip in selected cases.

THE WRIST JOINT. The wrist frequently is in a flexed pronated position, with ulnar deviation. This deformity is accepted when the hand is stiff, because it enables the forearm radial borders to oppose one another, thereby producing a pincer grip.

A fixed flexion deformity is a severe handicap to a patient with a functional hand. Initial serial casts in infancy may ameliorate but not correct this deformity. The young child may benefit from an anterior wrist capsulotomy, which places the wrist in a position of neutral or slight dorsiflexion. Long-term protective splinting is required. The most satisfactory long-term results are achieved with carpectomy, combined with wrist fusion.[10,14]

THE ELBOW AND SHOULDER JOINTS. The elbow and shoulder joints should be considered in combination, because correction of the deformity and restoration of elbow mobility is dependent upon the position and mobility of the other joint. Functional use of the hands is largely determined by the position in which the elbow–shoulder unit allows them to be placed. Correction of elbow- and shoulder-joint deformity is directed toward restoring the ability to lift the hand to the mouth, in order to make use of the limited function of the disabled hand. Correction of one side should be completed and the results assessed before the other side is corrected. Better long-term funciton may result when one elbow is left in extension to allow toilet independence or use

of long arm crutch, or to allow the patient to make the required push off when rising from a chair.

The Shoulder. Shoulder range-of-motion usually is adequate for self-care, and surgery is seldom required. Internal rotation deformity of the shoulder should be corrected before any effort is made to perform muscle transfers to gain elbow flexion. Failure to correct internal rotation would direct the flexed elbow and hand toward the opposite shoulder, rather than toward the mouth.

Lloyd-Roberts recommends an external rotation osteotomy, performed at the junction of the proximal and midhumerus and stabilized by an intramedullary nail.[21] Postopera-

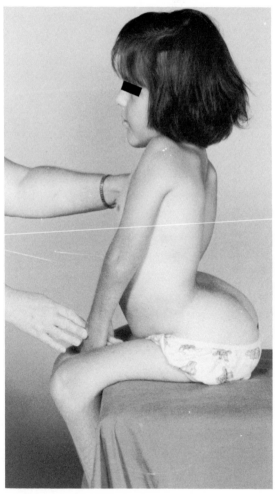

FIG. 6-16. Severe lordoscoliosis compromises the wheelchair posture of this adolescent.

tively, a shoulder spica is used. There is risk of possible radial nerve palsy when the osteotomy is performed in the proximal one third of the humerus.

The Extended Elbow. Fixed bilateral elbow extension is common, and it severely handicaps the child with arthrogryposis. Surgical correction on one side is necessary to allow the patient's hand to reach the mouth. Extension is preserved on the other side for hygienic needs. Fixed deformity is corrected by a posterior elbow capsulotomy, combined with elongation of the fibrotic triceps.[10,13]

Williams stressed that the involved joint has normal articulations at birth and urged early capsular-release tendon transfer to replace the absent or ineffective muscles combined with prolonged physical therapy or splinting to maintain correction of the fixed extension.[28] Posterior release of the elbow should permit 90° of flexion and still allow useful triceps action. A muscle imbalance will determine whether the triceps are lengthened or transferred at the time of posterior elbow release. Elbows that have a flexion contracture usually have a useful range-of-motion and good function; thus, surgery is not indicated.

Passive elbow flexion to a right angle is a prerequisite for attempting to introduce active elbow flexion. Transfer of the triceps brachii and pectoralis major has been used.[4,21,28] Use of the pectoralis major requires that the portion of the rectus sheath to the level of the umbilicus also be freed to allow sufficient length to attach the transfer subcutaneously to the radius, thereby increasing the mechanical advantage of the transfer. The Steindler flexorplasty can be used in those rare cases in which some active biceps function can be demonstrated.

SCOLIOSIS. Scoliosis may develop at birth or in early childhood.[24] The curves are progressive and become rigid and fixed at an early age. They frequently are associated with pelvic obliquity and lumbar lordosis, as well as significant contractures about the hip (Fig. 6-

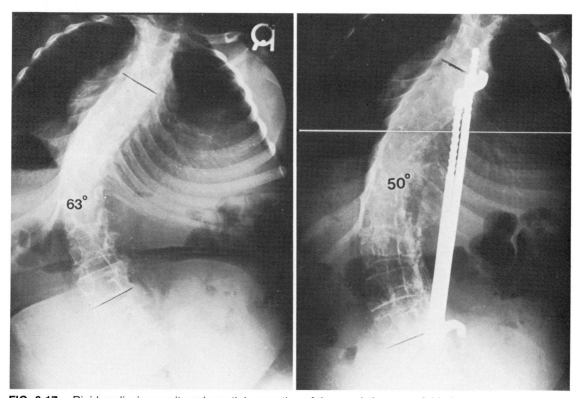

FIG. 6-17. Rigid scoliosis permits only partial correction of the paralytic curve. A Lindseth bilateral posterior iliac osteotomy corrected residual pelvic obliquity.

16). Congenital scoliosis has also been reported.[9]

A Milwaukee brace may be used for temporary control of mild curves. Spinal arthrodesis should be considered when the curve exceed 40° because little correction can be expected due to the marked scarring of the connective tissue. Posterior spinal fusion with Harrington instrumentation is the preferred method of treatment (Fig. 6-17). A high incidence of pseudarthrosis and progression of the scoliosis have been reported.[16]

MYOPATHIC ARTHROGRYPOSIS

This rare condition, first described by Banker, may present in the newborn period with hypotonia, hyporeflexia, and muscle weakness, with or without joint contracture.[2] The distal limb musculature may be larger than the proximal. The disease is limited to males. Paralytic scoliosis, additional chest deformities, torticollis, and a fixed position of the lower extremities, including flexion adduction of the hips and flexion of the knees, are commonly noted. A furrowed and curved tongue is characteristic. There is a strong hereditary or familial tendency. This disease is now considered to be a variant of congenital muscular dystrophy.[11]

REFERENCES

1. Arey LB: Developmental Anatomy: A Textbook and Laboratory Manual of Embryology, ed 7. Philadelphia, WB Saunders, 1974
2. Banker BQ, Victor M, Adams RD: Arthrogryposis multiplex due to congenital muscular dystrophy. Brain 80:319, 1957
3. Brown LM, Robson, MJ, Sharrard WJW: The pathophysiology of arthrogryposis multiplex congenita neurologica. J Bone Joint Surg 62B:291, 1980
4. Carroll RF, Hill NA: Triceps transfer to restore elbow flexion. J Bone Joint Surg 52A:239, 1970
5. Clark WM, D'Ambrosia RD, Ferguson AB: Congenital vertical talus. Treatment by open reduction and navicular excision. J Bone Joint Surg 58A:816, 1977
6. Drachman DB, Banker BQ: Arthrogryposis multiplex congenita. A case due to disease of the anterior horn cells. Arch Neurol 5:77, 1961
7. Drennan JC, Sharrard WJW: The pathological anatomy of convex pes valgus. J Bone Joint Surg 53B:455, 1971
8. Drummond DS, Cruess RL: The management of the foot and ankle in arthrogryposis multiplex congenita. J Bone Joint Surg 60B:96, 1978
9. Drummond DS, Mackenzie DA: Scoliosis in arthrogryposis multiplex congenita. Spine 3(2):146, 1978
10. Drummond DS, Siller TM, Cruess RL: Management of arthrogryposis multiplex congenita. The American Academy of Orthopaedic Surgeons Instructional Course Lectures 23:79, 1974
11. Dubowitz V, Brooke MH: Muscle biopsy: A modern approach. London, Saunders, 1973
12. Fowler M: A case of arthrogryposis multiplex congenita with lesions in the nervous system. Arch Dis Child, 34:505, 1959
13. Friedlander HL, Westin GW, Wood WL Jr: Arthrogryposis multiplex congenita. J Bone Joint Surg 50A:89, 1968
14. Gibson DA, Urs, NDK: Arthrogryposis multiplex congenita. J Bone Joint Surg 52B:483, 1970
15. Hansen OM: Surgical anatomy and treatment of patients with arthrogryposis. J Bone Joint Surg 43B:855, 1961
16. Herron LD, Westin GW, Dawson EG: Scoliosis in arthrogryposis multiplex congenita. J Bone Joint Surg 60A:293, 1978
17. Hillman JW, Johnson JTH: Arthrogryposis multiplex congenita in twins. J Bone Joint Surg 34A:211, 1952
18. Jago RH: Arthrogryposis following treatment of maternal tetanus with muscle relaxants. Arch Dis Child 45:277, 1970
19. James LF, Shupe JL, Binns W: Abortive and teratogenic effects of locoweed on sheep and cattle. Am J Vet Res 28:1379, 1967
20. Lipton FL, Morgenstern SA: Arthrogryposis multiplex congenita in identical twins. Am J Dis Child 89:233, 1955
21. Lloyd-Roberts GC, Lettin AWF: Arthrogryposis multiplex congenita. J Bone Joint Surg 52B:494, 1970
22. Mead NG, Lithgow WC, Sweeney HJ: Arthrogryposis multiplex congenita. J Bone Joint Surg 40A:1285, 1958
23. Rosenkranz E: Ueber kongenitale Kontrakturen der oberen extremitäten: im Anschluss an die Mitteilung eines einschlägigen Falles. Z Orthop 14:905, 1905
24. Siebold RM, Winter RB, Moe JH: The treatment of scoliosis in arthrogryposis multiplex congenita. Clin Orthop 103:191, 1974
25. Smith EM, Bender LF, Stover CM: Lower motor neutron deficit in arthrogryposis. Arch Neurol 8:97, 1963
26. Stern WG: Arthrogryposis multiplex congenita. JAMA 81:1507, 1923
27. Whitten JH: Congenital abnormalities in calves: Arthrogryposis and hydrancephaly. Journal of Pathology and Bacteriology 73:357, 1957
28. Williams PF: The elbow in arthrogryposis. J Bone Joint Surg 55B:834, 1973
29. Williams P: The management of arthrogryposis. Orthop Clin North Am 9(1):67, 1978

Peripheral Neuropathies, Hereditary Spinal and Cerebellar Ataxia, and Congenital Indifference to Pain

Hereditary Neuropathies and Peripheral Nerve Lesions

PERIPHERAL NEUROPATHIES

Patients with peripheral neuropathies comprise a large segment of the neuromuscular disorder population. Included are those who were previously classified as having peroneal muscular atrophy (Charcot–Marie–Tooth disease) or familial interstitial hypertrophic neuritis (Déjérine–Sottas disease).[5,7,45] Patients with these neuropathies have slow progression of weakness, with minor sensory abnormalities. There frequently is a positive family history but within a given family there may be great variability. Females tend to have a more severe form (Fig. 7-1). Life expectancy is

normal. Dyck developed a classification of peripheral neuropathies in which peroneal muscular atrophy and weakness were prominent features early in the course of the disease.[13]

Dyck's Classification

Type I consists of the hypertrophic neuropathy of Charcot–Marie–Tooth disease, as well as hereditary areflexic dystaxia (Roussy–Lévy syndrome).[39,40] Type I is characterized by an autosomal dominant pattern of inheritance, although sporadic cases have been reported. It usually presents during the second decade

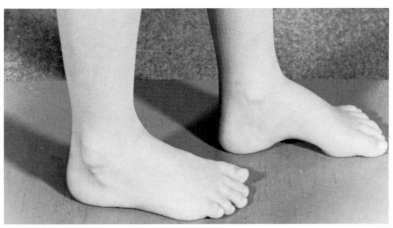

FIG. 7-1. A 10-year-old girl's feet show early fixed deformity. More pronounced muscle weakness and pedal shortening occur in females within a given family

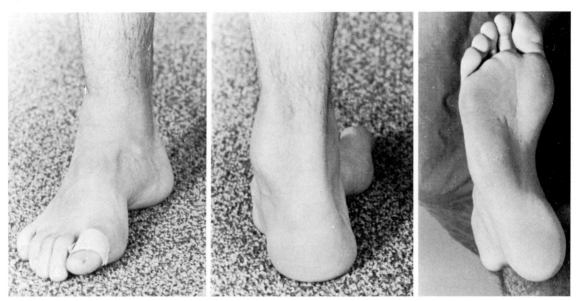

FIG. 7-2. Rigid equinocavovarus deformity results from peroneal and intrinsic paresis and creates a marked overload along the lateral aspect of the forefoot.

of life with a mild cavus or clawing of the toes. The first complaint may be abnormal shoe wear or muscle cramps. Initially, the foot deformity is flexible but with increasing involvement of the peroneals an equinocavovarus deformity gradually develops (Fig. 7-2). This may lead to discomfort beneath the lateral metatarsal heads during walking. The patient has difficulty running, especially on uneven ground. A physical examination at this point in the course of the disease would demonstrate wasting and weakness of the peroneals and dorsiflexors and, in particular, the extensor digitorum brevis. Initially, the sensory examination may be normal, but eventually slight diminution of vibration, proprioception, and light touch sensation will be noted in the distal aspect of the limbs. Nerves are hypertrophic and palpable in one quarter of the cases.

Eventually the patient will develop a clumsy gait, trip frequently, and develop a propensity for ankle sprains (Fig 7-3). Motor weakness spreads proximally, and frequently

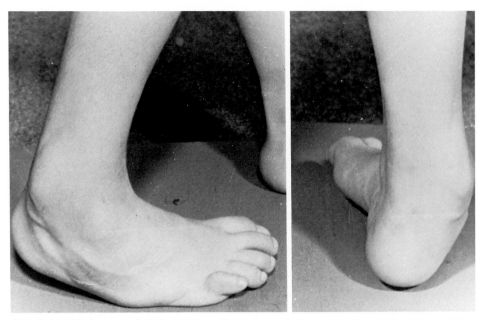

FIG. 7-3. Displacement of the heel medial to the weight-bearing line of the limb and the inability to dorsiflex and evert the foot create an unstable weight-bearing platform. Heel strike does not occur, further decreasing the weight-bearing area.

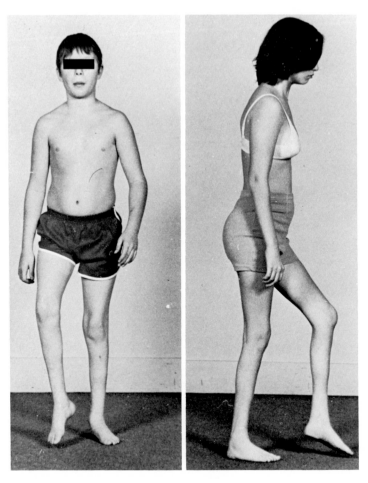

FIG. 7-4. This brother and sister are able to compensate for the drop-foot gait by increased flexion of the hip and knee during swing-phase.

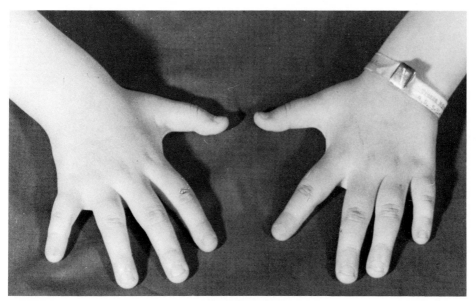

FIG. 7-5. Marked atrophy of the volar and dorsal intrinsic muscles is demonstrated. (Courtesy of Newington Children's Hospital)

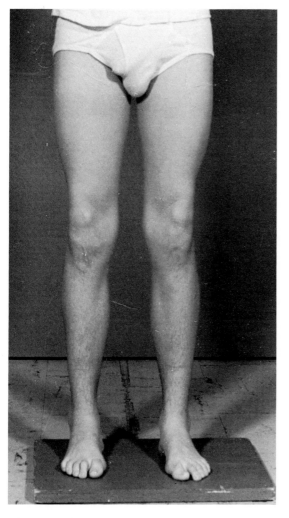

FIG. 7-6. Atrophy of the thigh musculature is limited to the distal one-third of these muscle groups, creating the stork-leg appearance. (Courtesy of Newington Children's Hospital)

involves the plantar flexors as well as more proximal muscles. The classic stork-leg configuration caused by wasting of the distal one third of the thigh musculature is not seen in Type I. Loss of deep-tendon reflexes begins with the ankle jerk and spreads centripetally to the knee. Even though the patient may develop a dramatic slap-foot gait later in the course of the disease, this weakness will not lead to wheelchair confinement (Fig. 7-4). Upper-extremity involvement, although delayed, begins with atrophy of the intrinsic muscles (Fig. 7-5), spreads later to the radially innervated muscles of the forearm, and causes progressive difficulty with fine motor activities. Eventually upper-extremity reflexes diminish as individual muscles become weakened.

Nerve conduction velocities are reduced even when clinical findings are minimal. Later, motor conduction velocities may be only half the normal value. The distal latency of response may be three times normal and may be a valuable adjunct in identifying latent carriers among relatives of the patient. A muscle biopsy demonstrates changes in fiber-type groupings, as well as other mild changes of denervation and reinnervation. A biopsy of the lateral sural nerve reveals an increase in the fascicular cross-sectional area and evidence of repetitive demyelinization and remyelinization that results in the formation of the "onion bulb" structures. Cerebrospinal fluid protein is normal.

Type II is equivalent to the neuronal form of Charcot–Marie–Tooth disease. Inheritance is by an autosomal dominant pattern. The histopathology is dominated by neuronal changes versus desegmental demyelinization or hypertrophic changes of the previous variety. Conduction velocities are either slightly reduced or may be normal. Onset is generally in the third or fourth decade of life. Distal lower-extremity weakness is more pronounced than in Type I, and the characteristic stork-leg appearance is seen frequently (Fig. 7-6). Weakness of the plantar flexors is common and results in a hindfoot calcaneus deformity (Fig. 7-7). Because intrinsic hand weakness is less serious and sensory changes even less marked, these patients retain the ability to perform most activities of daily living despite marked lower-extremity atrophy.

Type III includes the hypertrophic neuropathy of infancy (Déjérine–Sottas disease). The symptoms of this autosomal recessive disease are first noted in infants or in young children.[2] Walking is delayed and weakness and atrophy of the foot and calf muscles lead to the development of pes cavus (Fig. 7-8) and drop-foot deformities. Atrophy and weakness is more marked in the lower extremities than in the upper limbs. The enlarged peroneals and ulnar peripheral nerves can be felt when

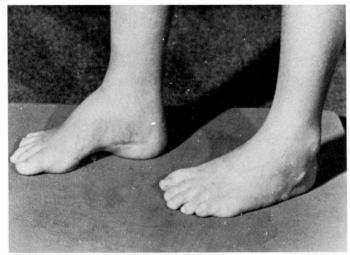

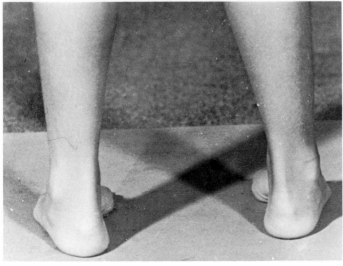

FIG. 7-7. Calcaneus deformity is associated with an absence of the heel prominence, as well as the development of a progressive cavus deformity.

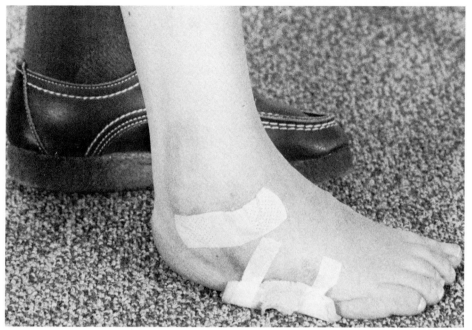

FIG. 7-8. Muscle imbalance creates a dynamic foot deformity which cannot be controlled by standard orthotic means.

palpated. Sensory modalities are lost in a stocking-glove type of distribution. Subjective sensory complaints, such as a deep, sharp pain or a lightning type of pain, may interfere with the gait pattern. Deep-tendon reflexes are lost. Truncal ataxia and spasmodic finger movements may be noted. The patient is confined to a wheelchair during the third or fourth decade of life.

All Type III patients have markedly slow conduction times. A biopsy of a sensory nerve, usually the lateral sural nerve, (Fig. 7-9) may be indicated to establish the diagnosis. Concentric proliferation of Schwann cells about the nerve fibers, the "onion bulb" formation, is found with frequent segmental demyelinization. However, complications of the biopsy may occur, such as a slight loss of sensation and the possible development of painful dysesthesia during the period of recovery of sensation. Therefore, it is recommended that only one fascicle of the nerve be removed and that the remainder be left intact. The cerebrospinal fluid protein content usually is elevated.

Type IV (Refsum's disease) is a rare condition.[34,35,42] It is inherited as an autosomal recessive disease and has its onset in childhood or puberty. It can be differentiated from Friedreich's ataxia by its clinical course, which is characterized by remissions and relapses. Its course is unpredictable, the patient returning to a nearly normal state between the early attacks. Repeated attacks and remissions of distal sensory and motor loss in the hands and feet are typical. Initial findings are frequently anosmia, progressive deafness, and night blindness caused by retinitis pigmentosa. Ichthyosis, cardiac abnormalities, and cerebellar abnormalities of ataxia and nystagmus also develop. Hypertrophic neuropathy and areflexia are common. The Babinski sign and spasticity are absent. Orthopaedic complications include scoliosis, pes cavus, and pes equinus. The prognosis is grave.

Serum elevation of phytanic acid is pathognomic of Refsum's disease. A phytol-loading test is useful in detecting carriers. Cerebrospinal fluid protein levels usually are markedly elevated. Nerve conduction velocity is slow. Nerve biopsy shows hypertrophic nerves with fat deposits, increased endomesium, and "onion bulb" formation.

Treatment has been attempted by dietary reduction of phytol from which phytanic acid is derived.[14,23] Although this may result in considerable improvement, death generally

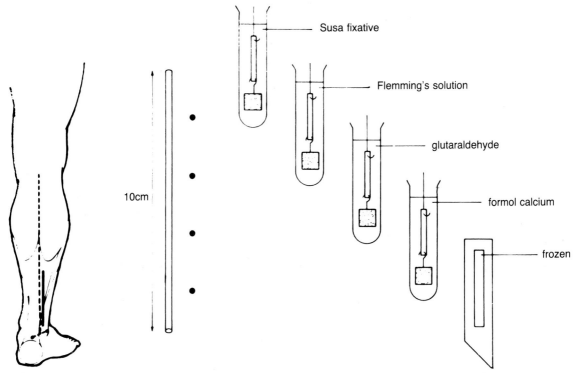

FIG. 7-9. These are surface markings for the sural nerve. 8–10 cm. of a fascicle are biopsied and then divided to permit appropriate fixation for histologic and electron microscopic evaluation. (Bradley, W.G.: Disorders of peripheral nerves. Oxford, Blackwell Scientific Publications, 1974)

results from pulmonary infection or cardiac disease occurring during exacerbation of the disease. Orthopaedic management of foot and spine problems follows the principles outlined in the section on Friedreich's ataxia.

The remaining three types are rare and have infrequent orthopaedic ramifications. Type V is a condition inherited as an autosomal dominant disease in which the major problem is spastic paraplegia. Evidence of peripheral neuropathy may be demonstrated on electromyographic or pathologic studies. Occasionally it may be clinically obvious.

Type VI includes patients who combine the clinical characteristics of Type I with optic atrophy (Fig. 7-10), while patients with Type VII disease have retinitis pigmentosa.

General Clinical Features

Loss of balance is a major problem for nearly all patients regardless of the type of hereditary motor and sensory neuropathies (HMSN). They experience difficulty walking on uneven ground, climbing stairs, or walking with their eyes closed. Diffuse weakness, as well as foot deformity, combines with decreased proprioception to create a lack of balance. In addition, a decrease in the size of the feet diminishes the standing base (Fig. 7-11). Patients with early structural foot deformity first become aware of the loss of balance when proprioception becomes decreased in the toes. When proprioception becomes decreased at the ankle level, patients can no longer keep their balance without shifting their feet or without touching a stationary object with their hands in order to ensure their position in space.[24] Therefore, they become fearful of being isolated in crowds where they are unable to shift their feet or in areas with numerous moving objects. Patients with decreased proprioception levels to the knees, coupled with profound weakness, stabilize themselves by either touching a stationary object or bending their knees, thereby activating the proprioceptive sensation of the knee joint itself.

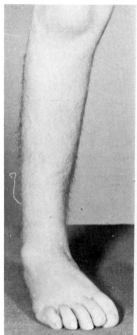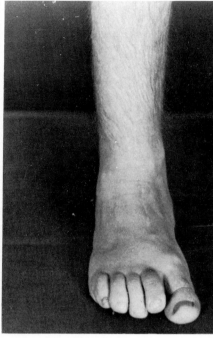

FIG. 7-10. Type VI HMSN in a 4-year-old with progressive equinovarus. This resulted from marked weakness of the peroneals and intrinsics. The deformity was corrected by calcaneal osteotomy, posterior tibial lengthening, and split anterior tibial transfer.

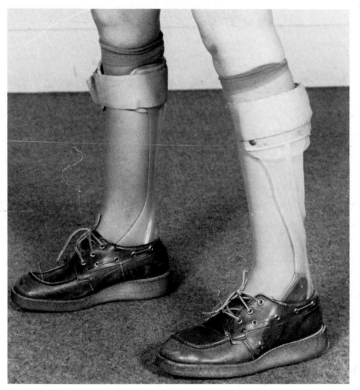

FIG. 7-11. Crepe sole shoes act as shock absorbers. The introduction of the polypropylene brace into the shoe artificially widens the heel and makes it necessary for this girl to wear shoes that are three sizes too large to accommodate both her foot and the brace.

Balance can be improved when the foot is made plantigrade and lateral-flexor instability is eliminated. This can be achieved by surgical or nonsurgical techniques. For example, the young child who presents with tight heel cords or persistent toe-walking can be successfully managed by stretching exercises, manipulations, or applications of serial walking casts followed by the use of short leg, night splints. Later in the first decade of life, patients may present with a calcaneocavovarus (Fig. 7-12) or equinocavus deformity. When this is not associated with significant bony deformity in the skeletally immature child, repeated manipulations and serial walking plasters help the patient to regain normal alignment of the foot. Maintenance of the correct position is accomplished with a short leg, double upright orthosis with a wide, valgus-producing T-strap and a 90° plantar-flexion stop. A polypropylene ankle–foot orthosis

with a lateral heel extension to prevent recurrent varus of the heel may also be used. Similarly the flail dangle foot may also benefit from an ankle–foot orthosis when it is combined with an oxford-style shoe with a crepe sole.

For mild equinovarus deformity with early cavus, Washington recommends performing a Dwyer calcaneal osteotomy (Fig. 7-13).[46] This usually is combined with a plantar fascial release or, occasionally, with a tendon transfer. He states that when the Dwyer procedure is performed before there is a fixed forefoot deformity, the osteotomy effectively corrects the hindfoot varus and avoids the need for toe surgery. When the tibialis anterior muscle becomes weak before the tibialis posterior, the latter muscle should be transferred to the dorsum in combination with the Dwyer osteotomy.

Tendon transfers (Fig. 7-14), particularly

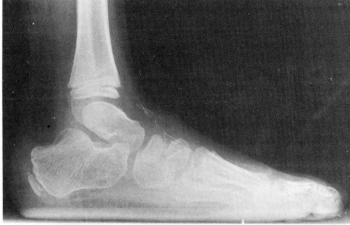

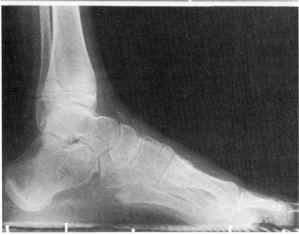

FIG. 7-12. Roentgenograms 3 years apart demonstrate the rapid progression of a calcaneal deformity during the first decade.

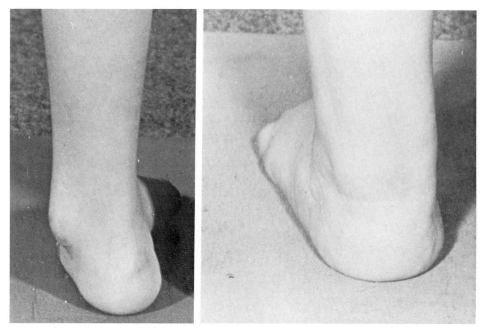

FIG. 7-13. Plantar fascial release and closing calcaneal osteotomy create a neutral hindfoot in a 9-year-old boy.

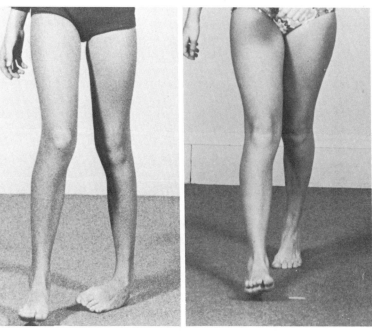

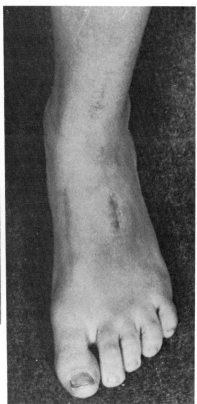

FIG. 7-14. Unstable stance posture can be corrected by appropriate tendon transfers. The ideal transfer enables the patient to become brace-free, but critical, long-term follow-up is required in patients with progressive peripheral neuropathies.

the transfer of the tibialis posterior through the interosseous membrane to the third cuneiform, have been used in young children to prevent equinovarus deformity. When they are performed in adolescents to improve the standing base and relieve deformity (Fig. 7-15), an ankle–foot orthosis generally is necessary to prevent recurrent deformity. Posterior tibial tendons have also been transferred in conjunction with triple arthrodeses. Tenotomies have limited application but may be necessary in order to make feet braceable and to relieve claw-toe deformities in adolescents. A Steindler plantar release by itself, is not an effective procedure but may be useful when combined with a variety of bony procedures.

Foot stabilization by triple arthrodesis remains the definitive procedure for long-term surgical management and may be performed at the age of skeletal maturity (Figs. 7-16,17).[20] By displacing the calcaneus posteriorly, the weakened triceps surae is augmented and the weight-bearing forces are brought closer to the center of the axis of the foot (Fig. 7-18). Levitt reported better results in patients who had

the procedure combined with posterior tibial transfer.[25] However, the experience at Newington Children's Hospital suggests that patients with muscle balance do equally well without the transfer.[24] The triple arthrodesis may also be combined with a first metatarsal osteotomy (Fig. 7-19). Major complications, such as talonavicular nonunion, are related primarily to poor surgical technique (Fig. 7-20).

Claw-toe deformities may be corrected either by simple tenotomy or transfer of the long toe extensors and flexors. A combination of the Jones procedure (placing the extensor hallucis longus into the first metatarsal head) with arthrodesis of the interphalangeal joint is recommended.[22] The Hibbs procedure (placing the common extensors into the third cuneiform bone) may also be indicated for toe deformity.[19] These procedures give good results by permanently relieving dorsal bunions, excessive pressure on the tips of the toes, and excessive plantar pressure beneath the metatarsal heads.

The second most common complaint is

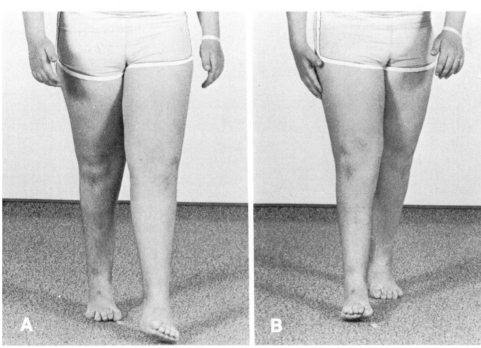

FIG. 7-15. (A) The advantage of a posterior tibial transfer is demonstrated in a boy who presented with bilateral swing-phase equinovarus. (B) A normal foot position has been achieved in the operated limb. Unilateral procedures followed by limb rehabilitation may be necessary to ensure optimal ambulation in these patients.

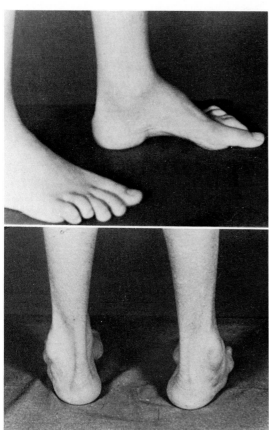

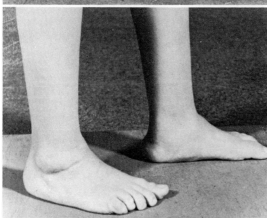

FIG. 7-16. Triple arthrodesis remains the definitive approach in skeletally mature patients with hindfoot deformity. (Courtesy of Newington Children's Hospital)

weakness in the lower extremities, which prevents the patient from running or participating in vigorous sporting activities. Almost all patients over age 20 who do not participate in vigorous exercise have, in addition to their muscle paresis, functional weakness of the quadriceps, hamstrings, and hip muscles. Their adaptive gait pattern interferes with the normal function of these muscles and, as might be expected from muscles that retain normal innervation, a return to normal strength can be anticipated. This has a significant positive impact on the patient's balance. Balance also may be improved by wearing low-heeled, broad-based shoes with a firm counter; by wearing high-top shoes; maintaining the heel in good repair; and by using an ankle-foot orthosis, cane, or crutch. Most patients noted that their instability was increased either when they were shoeless or when they wore shoes without heels.

Upper-extremity weakness interferes with the fine motor control necessary for sewing, writing, buttoning shirts, and using zippers (Fig. 7-21). Frequently, children are unable to write fast enough to complete school assignments and may have difficulty with physical education classes. Weakness of wrist flexors may interfere with carrying objects, especially in the kitchen or at work.

Opponensplasty, with or without intrinsic reconstruction, is a useful procedure only in Type I disease, in which the substituted motor muscles remain strong. Patients who do not require this procedure until after age 20 can expect good, long-term results with a strong pinch persisting.

Scoliosis has occasionally been noted in patients with Types I, II, and IV disease. The majority of Type III patients develop a spinal deformity that may require fusion in early adolescence (Fig. 7-22). The use of a Milwaukee brace may be indicated for curves of a lesser degree.

These patients may encounter a lack of appropriate genetic counseling. There may be a great variability in the manifestations of the disease in a single family (Fig. 7-23) and thus it is not possible to predict the progression of the disease in a younger family member based on the disease in a parent or older sibling. Women, frequently, have a more severe form of the disease in terms of earlier onset of weakness and functional disability. Most pa-

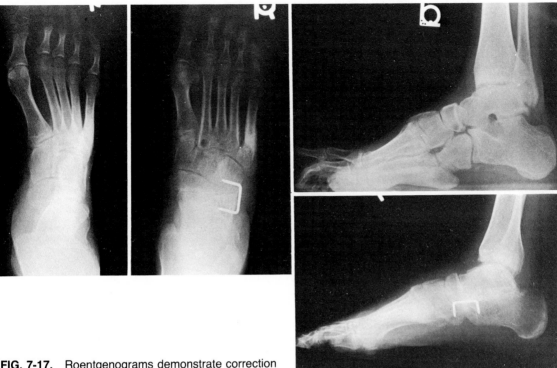

FIG. 7-17. Roentgenograms demonstrate correction obtained by triple arthrodesis.

tients receive no vocational guidance and may choose an inappropriate life-time occupation, since they lack knowledge about the progression of the disease.

Kling has identified a subclassification of Type II which differs from that described by Dyck and Lambert.[24] This disease is transmitted as an autosomal dominant trait. Onset is in the first decade of life. Equinocavovarus foot deformity is present early in the disease (Fig. 7-24). All functional muscle power below the knee is absent by the second decade of life. Marked intrinsic atrophy presents concomitantly or shortly after foot deformity presents. Forearm muscular atrophy and weakness are prominent features and lead to a severely deformed or functionless hand by the second decade of life (Fig. 7-25). Results of laboratory studies, similar to those in Type II, show normal or slightly low nerve conduction velocities, normal cerebrospinal fluid protein, and nerve biopsies that are consistent with those seen in the Type II form.

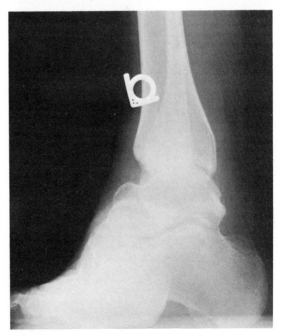

FIG. 7-18. Many patients have posterior displacement of the lateral malleolus. With triple arthrodesis the foot must be aligned with the ankle joint. This lateral ankle roentgenogram demonstrates the amount of true forefoot varus deformity.

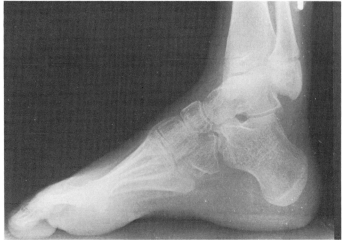

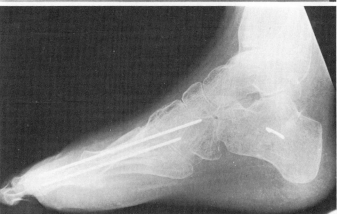

FIG. 7-19. Patients with excessively short feet cannot afford a further reduction in foot length which might result from triple arthrodesis. A calcaneal osteotomy combined with metatarsal osteotomies offers an alternative management of the calcaneocavus foot.

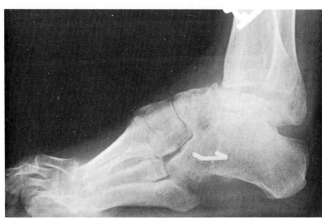

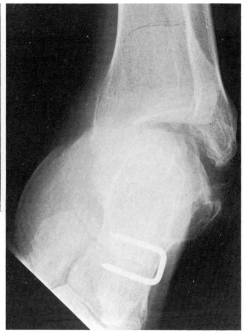

FIG. 7-20. Progression of peripheral weakness following an unprotected triple arthrodesis will eventually lead to degenerative ankle arthritis in the young adult. Ankle fusion may further decrease proprioception and aggravate the diminished standing balance. Therefore, orthotic control is preferred.

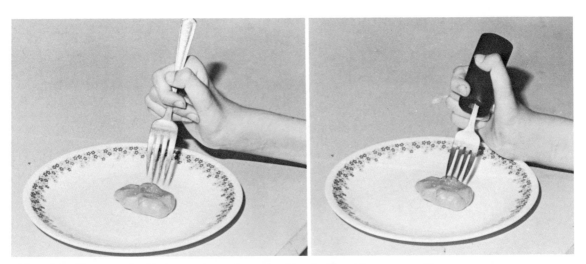

FIG. 7-21. The use of adaptive equipment may lead to significant improvement in specific activities of daily living.

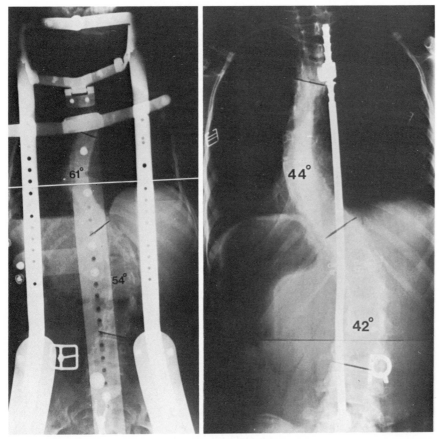

FIG. 7-22. Despite a Milwaukee brace, scoliosis progressed in this Type III adolescent and required posterior spinal fusion with Harrington instrumentation.

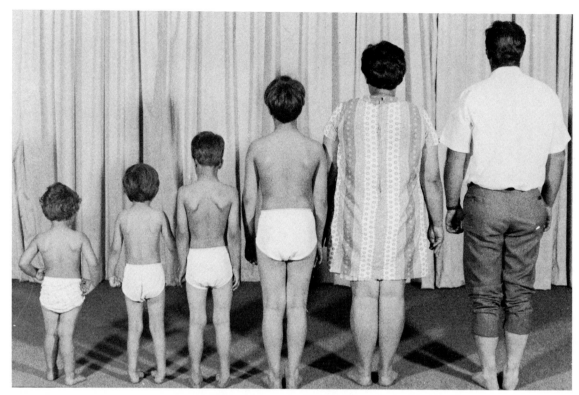

FIG. 7-23. The father demonstrates mild peripheral muscle weakness. Two of his children have obvious foot deformities secondary to muscle involvement.

Hereditary Spinal and Cerebellar Degenerative Disease

Hereditary spinal and cerebellar degenerative diseases are a group of genetically determined diseases characterized by lesions in multiple areas of the central nervous system. Frequently, both the peripheral and central nervous system may be involved simultaneously. The orthopaedic surgeon seeing the patient for a cavus foot may make the initial diagnosis of the spinal cerebellar degenerative condition. This disease tends to show similar characteristics in all affected relatives, but it may differ markedly from a second family with the same established diagnosis. Considerable clinical overlap occurs in the spinal cerebellar degenerative diseases. These conditions generally are transmitted by autosomal dominant inheritance and are slowly progressive over decades.

HEREDITARY SPINAL CEREBELLAR ATAXIA (FRIEDREICH'S ATAXIA)

Freidreich's ataxia is the most common form of spinal cerebellar degenerative disease. Both sexes are equally involved. The autosomal recessive form is more common than the autosomal dominant variety which has its onset between ages 8 and 22.[4] An unsteady gait, the first clinical sign of the recessive form, is usu-

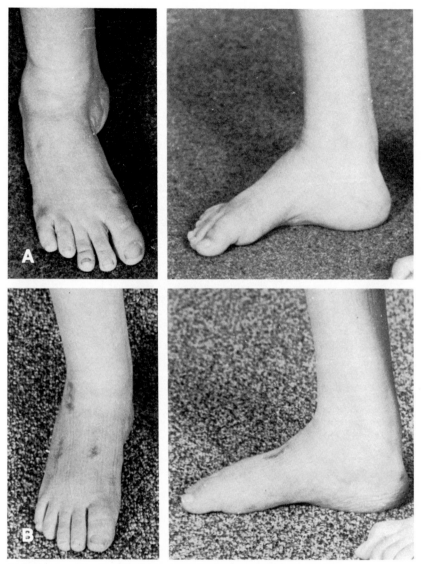

FIG. 7-24. (*A*) Intrinsic and peroneal weakness leads to inversion of both the hindfoot and forefoot. (*B*) Correction by calcaneal and metatarsal osteotomies is demonstrated.

ally apparent before age 10. The parents usually know the exact age of the child when the disease starts. They notice that the child is clumsy while playing certain games and has difficulty walking (Fig. 7-26), especially in the dark. The disease may present unilaterally but soon becomes bilateral. Intercurrent infection may aggravate existing symptoms or unmask new deficiencies.

A physical examination performed early in the course of the disease demonstrates a positive Romberg sign, an unsteady wide-based gait, especially with the eyes closed; decreased vibration and position sense; and depressed or absent lower-extremity deep-tendon reflexes. Later, when upper-extremity ataxia develops, new problems with writing and eating with a fork or spoon occur. Finger-to-nose and heel-to-knee tests are positive. Many patients have pes cavus (Fig. 7-27), which may be present before any neurologic signs or symptoms.

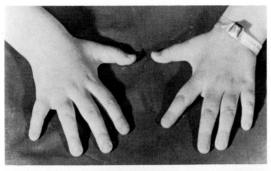

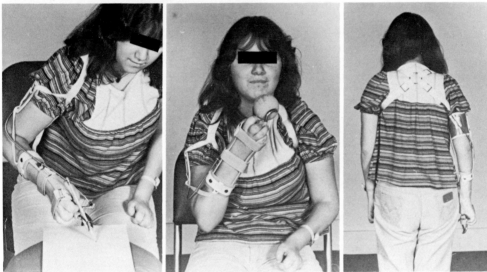

FIG. 7-25. An 8-year-old girl with marked intrinsic atrophy has been treated as a below-elbow amputee to permit retention of limited activities. A Northwestern shoulder ring is used and the prosthesis is activated by shoulder shrug.

Later, lateral nystagmus, intention tremor, and explosive dysarthria are found. Plantar responses are usually extensor. Muscle atrophy in the lower extremities may occur. Distal weakness of the lower extremities and wasting of the intrinsic muscles of the feet and hands is out of proportion to the degree of severity of the disease. The cavus deformity is symmetric and progressive.[25] Initially, it is flexible, but soon it becomes fixed and may develop a heel varus component. Intrinsic muscle wasting adds to the extrinsic muscle imbalance and contributes to the developing cavus (Fig. 7-28). Pain, paresthesia, and foot cramps are common.

Mental deficiency or deterioration may occur. Bladder and bowel function may be impaired. Optic atrophy may appear late in the course of the disease.

Remissions and stable periods are uncommon in Friedreich's ataxia. The age at onset and the rate of progression are similar among siblings. Younger children show only progressive ataxia and depressed deep-tendon reflexes with minimal peripheral sensory loss. Older children and adults demonstrate the more classic picture with skeletal deformities, cardiomyopathies, and extensor plantar responses. By 20 years of age, the patient may be severely ataxic and by 30 years, confined to a wheelchair. The majority develop scoliosis, which increases with the progression of the disease (Fig. 7-29).[17] Occasionally the symptoms of Friedreich's ataxia and hereditary motor and sensory neuropathies overlap. There is a greater incidence of diabetes mellitus in patients with Friedreich's ataxia than in the normal population.

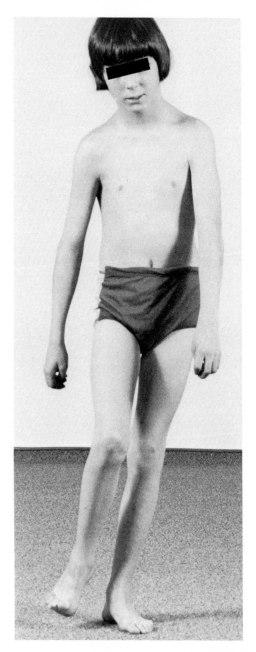

FIG. 7-26. Note the absence of trunk and upper extremity equilibrium responses in this 10-year-old boy with gross ataxia.

Laboratory Data

Nerve conduction studies show a markedly decreased sensory action potential and a slight decrease in motor fiber conduction velocity. The conduction studies distinguish Friedreich's ataxia from the hereditary motor and sensory neuropathies, in which the decrease is most marked in the motor fiber conduction velocity. Frequently, cardiac involvement is demonstrated by electrocardiographic changes which include T-wave inversion, signs of left ventricular hypertrophy, extra systole, and congenital heart block.[43] Also, a muscle biopsy reveals the presence of small or large fiber group atrophy, which is pathognomonic of denervation.[11] Cerebrospinal fluid analysis is normal.

Management

Scoliosis (Fig. 7-30) and cavus deformity of the foot, the major orthopaedic problems, are unrelentingly progressive.[15] Pes cavus, present in nearly all patients, may be present from infancy but in most cases seem to develop during the course of the disease. Forefoot equinus is best seen with the foot in the dependent position. As the disease progesses, the deformity becomes fixed and the feet assume

FIG. 7-27. Dependency accentuates the developing cavus. Standing or pressure under the metatarsal heads lessens the deformity if it has not become fixed. (Courtesy of Newington Children's Hospital)

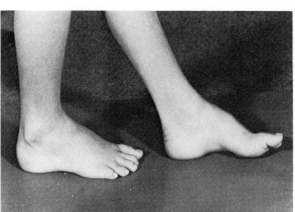

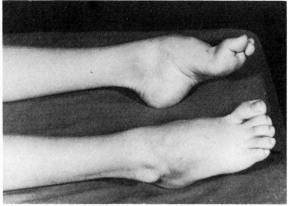

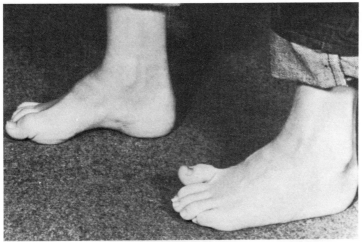

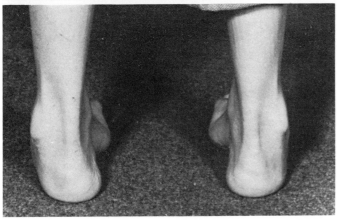

FIG. 7-28. In adolescence, the early onset of toe deformities may accompany the rapidly progressive cavus.

a broad, stumpy, foreshortened, high-arched appearance. Secondarily, overactivity of the long toe dorsiflexors may lead to subluxation of the metatarsal phalangeal joints.

The flexible cavus deformity can be corrected by combining a Dwyer calcaneal closing wedge osteotomy with a plantar intrinsic release (Fig. 7-31).[8,12] The use of an ankle–foot orthosis that entends the length of the foot, is recommended. When this orthosis is used, the height of the shoe heel must be carefully titrated in an effort to improve the patient's standing balance. Eventually a triple arthrodesis may be required for stabilization.[25] A variety of tendon transfers, generally involving either the tibialis posterior or tibialis anterior, may be used to complement either the triple arthrodesis or the tendon transfers. A combination of Jones and Hibbs procedures with arthrodeses of the imterphalangeal joints may be necessary for claw toes.[28] Ambulant patients benefit from the use of weighted walkers or rollators. Occasionally a talectomy may be necessary because of the development of a grotesque foot deformity (Fig. 7-32) that prevents wearing shoes and positioning of the foot on a wheelchair footrest.

Over 80% of patients with Friedreich's ataxia develop scoliosis.[17] They do not tolerate a Milwaukee brace and are unable to perform the exercise regimen which accompanies the use of this type of orthosis. Initially, a total contact orthosis is recommended. These curves are difficult to control with bracing, and progression does not stop with maturation. As the scoliosis progresses, a posterior fusion may be needed, using either Harrington rod instrumentation (Fig. 7-33) or segmental spinal stabilization.[26] The latter method may permit continuation of sitting and makes transferring and sitting less fatiguing for the patient.

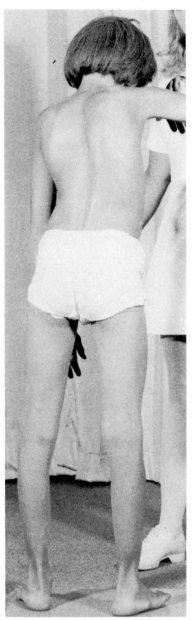

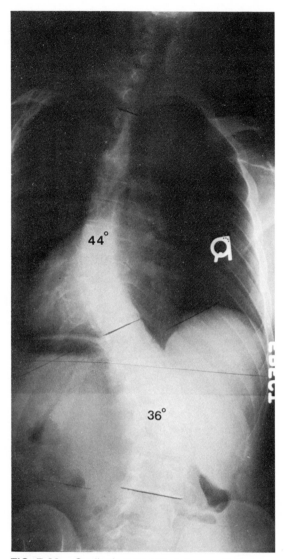

FIG. 7-30. Scoliosis generally follows a thoraco-lumbar pattern although double structural curves may also be encountered.

FIG. 7-29. Orthotic management in the ambulatory patient is difficult because it removes any compensatory trunk movement.

Prognosis

This disease is progressive. Death, generally occurring before age 40, may be due to dysfunction of the bulbar centers which leads to dysphagia, aspiration pneumonia, or myocar-dial failure secondary to interstitial myocarditis. The bedridden patient may die of inanition.

Postmortem examination of the spinal cord reveals atrophy in both the dorsal ventral cerebellar tracts and the posterior column.[18] A decreased number of normal appearing anterior-horn cells are present. Atrophy of the Purkinje's cells and dentate nucleus are also found.

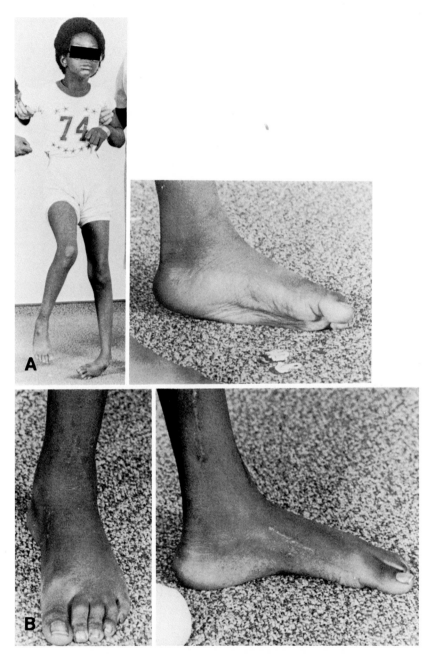

FIG. 7-31. (*A*) The desire to avoid excessive postoperative morbidity in a marginal ambulator may dictate unique surgical approaches. (*B*) A calcaneal osteotomy, lengthening of the tibialis posterior, and a split anterior tibial transfer create a plantigrade foot.

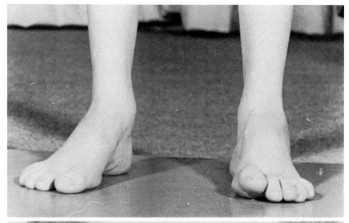

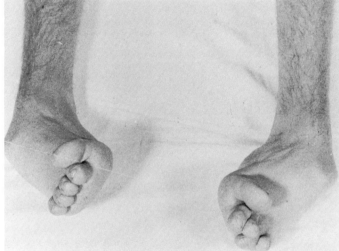

FIG. 7-32. For this adolescent a dramatic change in foot deformity over 18 months was associated with loss of ambulation and inability to wear shoes.

Congenital Indifference to Pain

Disorders which exhibit congenital or hereditary indifference to pain are classified by their clinical presentation in Table 7-1.

CONGENITAL INSENSITIVITY TO PAIN

Congenital insensitivity to pain is a rare condition in which the threshold for perception of ordinary painful stimuli is normal. However, these stimuli are not considered noxious, and the patient fails to demonstrate the usual objective and subjective responses.

Dearborn first described this condition in a carnival performer who called himself the "human pincushion."[6] Physical examination was normal, except for the absence of pain sensation.[3,44]

The patient usually presents late in infancy, after evidence of nonreaction to repeated minor skin trauma or burns. Acute surgical abdominal disorders or fractures may be undetected for long periods.[27] Anhidrosis and mental deficiency may be associated findings. No physiologic or anatomic lesions of

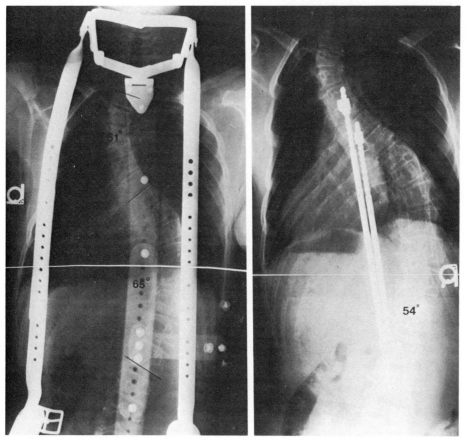

FIG. 7-33. This demonstrates correction and posterior spinal arthrodesis.

the central and peripheral nervous systems have been demonstrated at autopsy.

CONGENITAL SENSORY NEUROPATHY

Congenital sensory neuropathy is nonprogressive and is an inherited autosomal recessive trait. It becomes clinically apparent in late infancy, when the child mutilates his fingers, resulting in the progressive loss of digits (Fig. 7-34).[30,48] All sensory modalities are affected, with the distal portion of the limbs being more severely involved than the proximal (Fig. 7-35).[31] Minor injury causes local tissue damage in the anesthetic area, which the patient cannot appreciate. Normal care is not given to these minor injuries, which heal at a normal rate when appropriate care is given. Deep-tendon reflexes are hypoactive or absent. Autonomic function is normal. Anhidrosis occasionally is present and may be manifested by a recurrent fever. Mental re-

tardation, deafness, and retinitis pigmentosa also may be present. The normal axon reflex response to histamine is lost. The skin biopsy shows no myelinated fibers. Sensory nerve conduction is grossly abnormal. It is postulated that the dorsal root ganglion cells are absent or defective.

Congenital sensory neuropathy must be differentiated from Lesch–Nyhan syndrome, Hansen's disease, infantile autism, familial dysautonomia, and congenital insensitivity to pain. Characteristics of Lesch–Nyhan syndrome include mental retardation, choreoathetosis with lower-extremity scissoring, self-destructive biting of fingers and lips, and the overproduction of uric acid. The disease is transmitted as a sex-linked recessive trait. The self-mutilation is not the result of inability to feel pain but is the product of an uncontrollable aggressive impulse that can be directed against others as well as the self. Absence of hypoxanthineguanine–phosphoribosyltrans-

TABLE 7-1. Comparison of Congenital or Hereditary Causes of Insensitivity to Pain

PARAMETER	CONGENITAL INDIFFERENCE	CONGENITAL SENSORY NEUROPATHY	HEREDITARY SENSORY RADICULAR NEUROPATHY	FAMILIAL DYSAUTONOMIA	FAMILIAL SENSORY NEUROPATHY WITH ANHIDROSIS
Intelligence	Normal	Dull to normal	Normal	Dull to normal	Defective
Heredity	None D-trisomy mosaicism	Mostly sporadic; occ. dominant			
Age at onset	Birth	Birth	Late childhood	Birth	Birth
Distribution of sensory loss	Universal	Incomplete	Predominantly distal extremities	Incomplete	?Incomplete
Temperature perception	Normal	Absent	Absent	Reduced	Reduced
Touch perception	Normal	Lost	Lost	Present	Present
Axon reflex	Normal	None	None	None*	None
Physiologic pain reactions	Present	None	None	None†	None
Sensory nervous system anatomy	Normal	No myelinated fibers or dermal nerve networks	No myelinated fibers	Absence of fungiform papillae and taste buds on tongue	Absence of Lissauer's tract and small dorsal root axon; myelinated fibers and dermal nerve networks present

*Avon reflex is restored during intravenous infusion of mecholyl.
†No response to cold pressor test.
(Pinsky L, DiGeorge AM: Congenital familial sensory neuropathy with anhidrosis. J Pediatr 68:9, 1966).

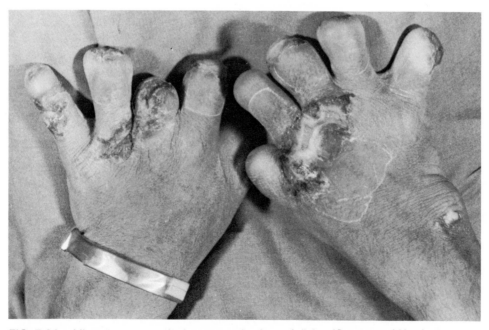

FIG. 7-34. Minor trauma results in progressive loss of digits. (Courtesy of Newington Children's Hospital)

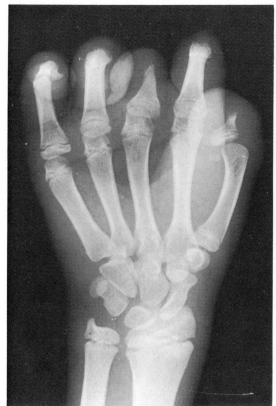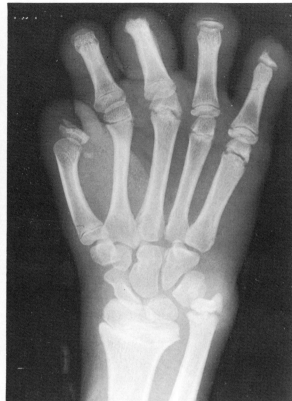

FIG. 7-35. Soft-tissue infections frequently spread to involve bone and this contributes to progressive osseous shortening.

ferase activity interferes with normal urate metabolism and results in hyperuricemia.

HEREDITARY SENSORY RADICULAR NEUROPATHY

Hereditary sensory radicular neuropathy is a slowly progressive disorder with onset in late childhood. This condition affects all sensory modalities. It begins distally in the lower extremity and slowly progresses proximally, but rarely extends above the knee. Late involvement of the upper extremities has been reported. The deep-tendon reflexes and the axon reflex response are lost in the affected areas. Sweating is normal. Denny-Brown postulates that this autosomal dominant disease is due to a primary degeneration of the dorsal root ganglia.[9]

FAMILIAL DYSAUTONOMIA (RILEY–DAY SYNDROME)

Familial dysautonomia, a rare disease found only in patients with Ashkenazic Jewish ancestry, is transmitted as an autosomal recessive trait. The diagnostic criteria are: a history suggesting neurologic abnormality, including feeding difficulty from birth onward; failure to regularly produce overflow tears; absence of the corneal reflex; postural hypotension; emotional liability; relative indifference to pain; absence of glossal fungiform papillae; and absence of a normal axon reflex response to histamine.[36,37,47] Sensory loss is incomplete. The major orthopaedic complication is the development of a progressive, rigid scoliosis.[17,49] Abnormal temperature control and excessive sweating complicate surgical management.

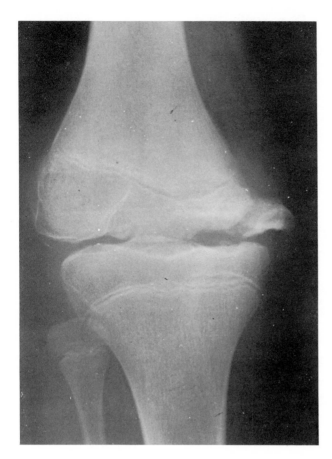

FIG. 7-36. Lack of protective sensation results in repeated trauma to the weight-bearing joints.

FAMILIAL SENSORY NEUROPATHY WITH ANHIDROSIS

Familial sensory neuropathy with anhidrosis is a congenital defect usually associated with low intelligence.[16,33] Temperature perception is reduced, while the touch sensation is intact. The axon reflex response to histamine is absent. The disorder is thought to be autosomal recessive.

Orthopaedic Complications

Many patients with various forms of congenital indifference to pain develop Charcot changes in the weight-bearing joints (Fig. 7-36).[1,21,32,38,41] These joints, in the absence of the normal protective mechanism of pain, are subjected to repeated abnormal stresses and trauma and cause hemarthrosis, synovial thickening, and secondary ligamentous laxity. This, along with hyperemia and the resulting bone resorption and atrophy, establishes a vicious cycle, and complete joint destruction is inevitable. The unstable joint requires an appropriate lower-extremity protective orthosis and, occasionally, arthrodesis (Fig. 7-37). Long-term follow-up of an initially successful major joint fusion may reveal the delayed development of pseudarthrosis.

Orthopaedic complications include unsuspected dislocations, fractures (Fig. 7-38), and chronic osteomyelitis of the long bones.[10,27,29] Whenever the clinical examination reveals the presence of erythema, warmth, or swelling, appropriate roentgenograms of the involved limb should be obtained.

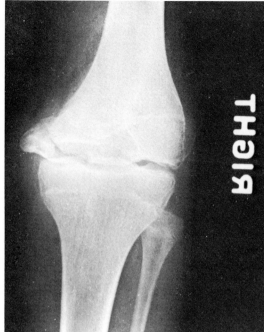

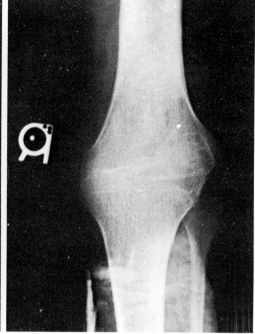

FIG. 7-37. Arthrodesis can be accomplished by employing the Charnley technique. Union may be delayed and the apparent solid fusion may be subject to later fracture.

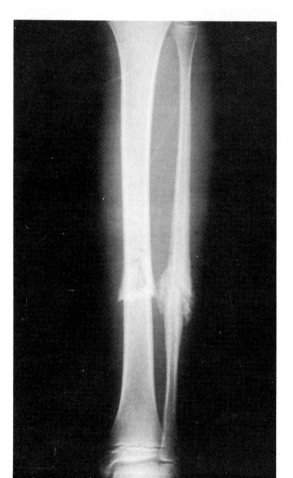

FIG. 7-38. A 10-year-old boy presented with obvious trauma and physical findings of tibial fracture. An unsuspected healing fibular fracture can also be seen on this radiograph.

REFERENCES

1. Abell JM Jr, Hayes JT: Charcot knee due to congenital insensitivity to pain. J Bone Joint Surg 46A:1287, 1964
2. Anderson RM, Dennett X, Hopkins IJ, Shield LK: Hypertrophic interstitial polyneuropathy in infancy. Clinical and pathologic features in two cases. J Pediatr 82:619, 1973
3. Baxter DW, Olszewski J: Congenital universal insensitivity to pain. Brain 83:381, 1960
4. Bradley WG: Disorders of Peripheral Nerves. Oxford, Blackwell Scientific Publications, 1974
5. Charcot J, Marie P: Sur une forme particuliére d'atrophic musculaire progressive, souvent familiale, débutant par les pieds et les jambes et atteignant plus tard les mains. Revue de Medicine (Paris) 6:97, 1886
6. Dearborn GV: A case of congenital pure analgesia. J Nerv Ment Dis 75:612, 1932
7. Déjérine J, Sottas J: Sur la néurite interstitielle hypertrophique et progressive de l'enfance. C R Soc Biol (Paris) 45:63, 1893
8. Dekel S, Weissman SL: Osteotomy of the calcaneus and concomitant plantar stripping in children with talipes cavo-varus. J Bone Joint Surg 55B:802, 1973
9. Denny-Brown D: Hereditary sensory radicular neuropathy. J Neurol Neurosurg Psychiatry 14:237, 1954
10. Dimon JH, Funk FJ Jr, Wells RE: Congenital indifference to pain with associated orthopedic abnormalities. South Med J, 58:524, 1965
11. Dubowitz V, Brooke MH: Muscle Biopsy: A Modern Approach. London, W B Saunders, 1973
12. Dwyer FC: Osteotomy of the calcaneum for pes cavus. J Bone Joint Surg 41B:80, 1959
13. Dyck PJ, Lambert EH: Lower motor and primary sensory neuron diseases with peroneal muscular atrophy. Part I. Neurologic, genetic and electrophysiologic findings in hereditary poly-neuropathies. Arch Neurol 18:603, 1968 Part II. Neurologic, genetic, and electrophysiologic findings in various neuronae degenerations. Arch Neurol 18:619, 1968
14. Eldjarn L, Try K, Stokke O, Munthe-Kaas AW, Refsum S, Steinberg D, Avigan J, Mize C: Dietary effects on serum-phytanic-acid levels and on clinical manifestations in heredopathia atactica poly-neuritiformis. Lancet 1:691, 1966
15. Fogan L, Munsat TL: Spinocerebellar degenerative diseases. In Hardy JH (ed): Spinal Deformity in Neurological and Muscular Disorders, p 38. Saint Louis, C V Mosby, 1974
16. Gillespie JB, Perucca LG: Congenital generalized indifference to pain. Am J Dis Child 100:124, 1960
17. Hensinger RN, MacEwen GD: Spinal deformity associated with heritable neurological conditions: Spinal muscular atrophy, Friedreich's ataxia, familial dysautonomia, and Charcot–Marie–Tooth disease. J Bone Joint Surg 58A:13, 1976
18. Hewer RL: Study of fatal cases of Friedreich's ataxia. British Medical Journal 3:649, 1968
19. Hibbs RA: An operation for "claw-foot." JAMA 73:1583, 1919
20. Jacobs JE, Carr CR: Progressive muscular atrophy of the peroneal type (Charcot–Marie–Tooth disease), orthopedic management and end-result study. J Bone Joint Surg 32A:27, 1950
21. Johnson JTH: Neuropathic fractures and joint injuries. J Bone Joint Surg 49A:1, 1967
22. Jones R: The soldier's foot and the treatment of common deformities of the foot. Br Med J 1(2891):749, 1916
23. Kahlke W, Wagener H: Conversion of H3-phytol to phytanic acid and its incorporation into plasma lipid fractions in heredopathia atactica polyneuritiformis. Metabolism 15:687, 1966
24. Kling TF Jr, Drennan JC: Orthopaedic management of hereditary motor and sensory neuropathies. Presented at the Thirty-fourth Annual Meeting of the American Academy for Cerebral Palsy and Developmental Medicine, Oct 1980
25. Levitt RL, Canale ST, Cooke AJ Jr, Gartland JJ: The role of foot surgery in progressive neuromuscular disorders in children. J Bone Joint Surg 55A:1396, 1973
26. Luque ED, Cardoso A: Sequential correction of scoliosis with rigid internal fixation. Orthopaedic Transactions 1:136, 1977
27. MacEwen GD, Floyd GC: Congenital insensitivity to pain and its orthopedic implications. Clin Orthop 68:100, 1970
28. Makin M: The surgical treatment of Friedreich's ataxia. J Bone Joint Surg 35A:425, 1953
29. Mazar A, Herold HZ, Vardy PA: Congenital sensory neuropathy with anhidrosis. Orthopedic complication and management. Clin Orthop 118:184, 1976
30. Murray RO: Congenital indifference to pain with special reference to skeletal changes. Br J Radiol 30:2, 1957
31. Murray TJ: Congenital sensory neuropathy. Brain 96:387, 1973
32. Petrie JG: A case of progressive joint disorders caused by insensitivity to pain. J Bone Joint Surg 35B:399, 1953
33. Pinsky L, DiGeorge AM: Congenital familial sensory neuropathy with anhidrosis. J Pediatr 68:1, 1966
34. Refsum S: Heredopathia atactica polyneuritiformis: A familial syndrome not hitherto described. Acta Psychiatrica El neurologica (Suppl 38), 1946
35. Refsum S, Salmonsen L, Skatvedt M: heredopathia atactica polyneuritiformis in children. J Pediatr 35:335, 1949
36. Riley CM, Day RL, Greeley, DM, Langford WS: Central autonomic dysfunction with defective lacrimation. Pediatrics 3:468, 1949
37. Riley, CM, Moore RH: Familial dysautonomia differentiated from related disorders. Pediatrics 37:435, 1966
38. Rose GK: Arthropathy of the ankle in congenital indifference to pain. J Bone Joint Surg, 35B:408, 1953
39. Roussy G, Lévy G: A propos de la dystasie aréflexique héréditaire. Rev Neurol (Paris) 62:763, 1934
40. Roussy G, Lévy G: Sept cas d'une amladie familiale particulaire: Troubles de la marche, pieds, bots er aréfléxie tendineuse généralisée, avec accessoirement, légère maladresse des mains. Rev Neurol (Paris) 54:427, 1926
41. Siegelman SS, Heimann WG, Manin MC: Congenital indifference to pain. American Journal of Roentgenology 97:242, 1966
42. Steinberg D, Vroom FQ, Engel WK, Cammermeyer J, Mize CE, et al: Refsum's disease—a recently characterized lipidosis involving the nervous system. Ann Intern Med 66:365, 1967

43. Thilenius OG, Grossman BJ: Friedreich's ataxia with heart disease in children. Pediatrics 27:246, 1961

44. Thrush DC: Congential insensitivity to pain: A clinical, genetic, and neurophysiological study of four children from the same family. Brain 96:369, 1973

45. Tooth HH: The Peroneal Type of Progressive Muscular Atrophy. London, H K Lewis & Co, 1886

46. Washington R, Scranton PE Jr, Martinez AJ: Charcot–Marie–Tooth disease: Clinical presentation, histopathology, and treatment. Orthopedic Survey 2:314, 1979

47. Welton W, Clayson D, Axelrod FB, Levine DB: Intellectual development and familial dysautonomia. Pediatrics 63:708, 1979

48. Winkelmann RK, Lambert EH, Hayles AB: Congenital absence of pain. Arch Dermatol 85:325, 1962

49. Yoslow W, Becker MH, Bartels J, Thompson WAL: Familial dysautonomia. Review of sixty-five cases. J Bone Joint Surg 53A:1541, 1971

Chapter **8**

Myasthenia Gravis

CHARACTERISTICS

Myasthenia gravis is a chronic disease characterized by the insidious development of an abnormal amount of muscle fatigability in voluntary muscles following repetitive activity or prolonged tension. There is partial or complete restoration of function following rest, or treatment with an anticholinesterase drug. The bulbar, extraocular motor, and shoulder-girdle muscles are involved in nearly all cases. Ptosis may be induced by bright sunlight, emotion, or heat (for example, a shower). A sustained upward gaze will elicit a gradual, slow, downward drift of the eyelids. Weakness is greatest late in the day.[7] Involvement of the masseter muscle may prevent voluntary closing of the jaw, requiring the mandible to be supported by the hand during sitting. Usually sensation and deep-tendon reflexes are normal. Peak incidence is in young adults, but the disease can occur in infancy and childhood. More females have this disease than males.[8]

Willis, in 1672, originally described a woman who "after long hasty or laborious speaking presently she became mute as a fist and cannot bring forth a word."[11] The etiology is thought to be an autoimmune response, possibly a circulating agent that competes with acetylcholine in the motor end-plate. The thymus gland is thought to be the site of the antibody product.

Millichap and Dodge categorized myasthenia gravis in children into three groups, according to the age of onset and the clinical course of the disease[5]: (1) neonatal transient, (2) neonatal persistent, and (3) juvenile myasthenia gravis.

Neonatal Transient Myasthenia Gravis

Approximately 1 in 7 liveborn children of myasthenic mothers shows evidence of the disease at birth. During the first day of life there is a rapid increase in weakness followed by gradual improvement as the maternal antibody is destroyed by the neonate. The infant presents with generalized hypotonia, a poor sucking reflex, a weak cry, life-threatening respiratory weakness, and a weak facial expression.[9] The infant requires urgent treatment followed by observation for at least 1 week. Neostigmine bromide (Prostigmin) is the drug of choice and is given orally. A complete recovery without a relapse generally occurs within 1 to 12 weeks.

Neonatal Persistent Myasthenia Gravis

This type of myasthenia gravis does not differ from myasthenia gravis in the adult. It rarely occurs at birth in children of nonmyasthenic mothers but develops within the first 2 years. Initial symptoms are ophthalmoplegia and ptosis; a more generalized weakness may develop later. The course is more benign but more protracted than in adults. Although the usual course is nonfluctuating and compatible with long survival, an occasional patient dies from respiratory bulbar weakness.

Juvenile Myasthenia Gravis

This form of myasthenia gravis develops after the age of 10 in children of nonmyasthenic mothers and comprises 15% of all types of myasthenia gravis.[3] It is four times more common in girls. Initially, it affects the ocular muscles. Weakness may become restricted to the facial muscles, or it may spread to the extremities where the paresis is greatest proximally and is more evident in the upper extremities. Generalized muscle weakness may develop within 2 years and leads to limitation of physical activity, dysarthria, dysphagia, and diplopia. The disease course is variable with complete spontaneous remission occurring only in those whose weakness is limited to the extraocular motor and facial muscles.

DIAGNOSIS

When a patient presents with a history of muscle weakness that was precipitated by activity or tension, a clinical evaluation for myasthenia gravis is necessary.[1,2] An electromyogram demonstrates amplitude of evoked potentials becoming progressively smaller, especially in the proximal muscles. The diagnosis is confirmed by a positive edrophonium chloride (Tensilon) test. Within the first minute after injection, the patient with myasthenia experiences marked improvement in motor strength and of weak muscles. The cholinergic side-reactions, such as excessive perspiration, salivation, and lacrimation, are absent as opposed to the responses of a normal subject.

Histochemical staining techniques reveal a unique Type 2 focal fibroatrophy and the frequent presence of lymphorrhages. Not all motor units of a given muscle are myasthenic, and those not involved retain their normal histochemical staining properties.

TREATMENT

Prostigmine and abenonium chloride are the drugs of choice. Thymectomy and steroids are reserved for cases in which this drug treatment is ineffective.[6] Curare and gallamine hydrochloride (Flaxedil) are muscle relaxants which are contraindicated should general anesthesia be required. Younger patients, especially girls, benefit more from thymectomies.

The prognosis for children and adolescents is favorable, although occasionally a myasthenic crisis may necessitate the use of a mechanical respirator or the performance of a tracheotomy.[10] Fukuyama reviewed 38 cases of myasthenia gravis in children under the age of 15.[4] Sex distribution was equal. In 14 patients symptoms were evident before age 5, and the majority of symptoms were ocular. Many patients developed bulbar, trunk, and extremity involvement 2 to 4 years after the onset of symptoms. The rate of occurrence was highest in the second and third years of life.

REFERENCES

1. Bowman JR: Myasthenia gravis in young children. Pediatrics 1:472, 1948
2. Eaton LM: Diagnostic test for myasthenia with prostigmin and quinine. Proceedings of the Staff Meetings of the Mayo Clinic 18:230, 1943
3. Fenichel GM: Clinical syndromes of myasthenia in infancy and childhood. Arch Neurol 35:97, 1978
4. Fukuyama Y, Sugiura S, Hirayama Y: Long-term prognosis of myasthenia gravis in infancy and childhood. Advances in Neurological Sciences (Tokyo) 15:884, 1971
5. Millichap JG, Dodge PR: Diagnosis and treatment of myasthenia gravis in infancy, childhood, and adolescence. Neurology 10:1007, 1960
6. Mulder DG, Herrmann C, Buckberg GD: Effect of thymectomy in patients with myasthenia gravis. A sixteen year experience. Am J Surg 128:202, 1974
7. Patten BM: Myasthenia gravis: Review of diagnosis and management. Muscle Nerve 1:190, 1978
8. Simpson JA: Myasthenia gravis and myasthenic syndromes. In Walton JN (ed): Disorders of Voluntary Muscle, ed. 3, p 653. Edinburgh, Churchill Livingstone, 1974
9. Strickroot FL, Schaeffer RL, Bergs HL: Myasthenia gravis occurring in an infant born of a myasthenic mother. JAMA 120:1207, 1942
10. Teng P, Osserman KE: Studies in myasthenia gravis: Neonatal and juvenile types. A report of 21 and a review of 188 cases. Journal of the Mt. Sinai Hospital New York 23:711, 1956
11. Willis T: De Anima Brutorum, p. 404. (Oxford), 1672

Chapter 9

Myelomeningocele

EMBRYOGENESIS OF SPINA BIFIDA

Two major theories have been advanced to explain the development of spinal dysrhaphism. They are: (1) failure of the neural tube (caudal neuropore) to close, and (2) rupture of the normally closed neural tube with resulting damage to the overlying ectoderm and mesoderm.[32,33,65,69] The second theory, which offers a better reason for the spectrum of abnormalities associated with myelomeningocele, can be explained in the following way. The choroid plexus begins secreting cerebrospinal fluid during the fifth week of gestation, but development of the subarachnoid space and foramina of Luschka and Magendie, the normal outlets for cerebrospinal fluid, does not occur until the seventh week of gestation. It is hypothesized that during this 2-week period a relative hydrocephalus and hydromyelia cause increased pressure which possibly is related to the delayed opening of the foramina. The increased pressure may lead to the rupture of the neural tube and escape of the cerebrospinal fluid, which is expressed as a myelomeningocele.

Incidence

Although reports from different areas vary, the worldwide incidence is approximately 1 per 1000 live births.[42,85] The rate of occurrence is influenced by factors such as the mother's social class and the social class in which she was raised. There is an increased incidence of the disease in firstborn infants of young mothers and late-born infants of older mothers.

Genetics

The mode of inheritance for spinal dysrhaphism is not clearly established but appears to be multifactorial. There is considerable risk that the second baby in a family with one affected child may have a neural tube defect. Following the birth of a child with this defect (myelomeningocele or anencephaly), the risk is 1 in 20 for subsequent pregnancies, and if 2 affected children are born, the risk becomes 1 in 2.[44] Environmental modification of these statistics is evident in a study of Irish immigrants in Boston who had a higher rate of myelomeningocele than other ethnic groups in Boston but a lower rate than that found in Ireland.[62]

It is now possible to detect myelomeningocele in a fetus by assay of alpha-fetoprotein in the amniotic fluid.[6] Normally levels of this protein are elevated in the amniotic fluid until the fourteenth week, when they begin to decrease to very low levels. However, in neuroschisis, the production of this protein does not decline. Therefore, by 16 to 18 weeks of gestation, nearly all cases of spinal or cranial dysrhaphism can be detected by bioassay. The diagnosis of myelominingocele is confirmed when there is a positive amniotic assay and a history of a previous child with a neural tube defect.

Natural History

The majority of untreated myelodysplastic infants die within 6 months of birth.[50] However, a significant minority do live longer. Should an untreated infant survive for 2 months, there is a 28% possibility that he will live to be 7 years of age. The emotional, social, and financial factors associated with caring for these patients must be considered. The survivors have considerably greater mental and neurological handicaps than they would have, had they been treated.

Patients with a high-level neurologic loss have the poorest prognosis, both for reasonable life expectancy and for quality of existence. In untreated patients, death in the first 2 years of life usually results from hydrocephalus or intracranial infection.[43,45] Renal failure becomes more prevalent after 1 year of age.

In a study of intensely treated patients, Lorber reported that 80% without hydrocephalus and only 50% with hydrocephalus had intelligence quotients above 80.[52] One third of the survivors were able to walk without orthotic assistance and another 20% were either household or community ambulators with orthotic devices. An additional 20% could be termed therapy ambulators, while the remaining one third were in wheelchairs full time. Fewer than one quarter were continent of urine. Lorber concluded that only 7% of these children had the mental and physical capabilities to be able to compete with their normal peers. Although an additional 20% had normal intelligence, the physical deficits of this group were severe enough to require a sheltered working environment so that the patients could maintain gainful employment.

SELECTION CRITERIA

Lorber identified certain physical findings that correlated with a poor prognosis for survival or a life with severe multi-system defects, including mental retardation.[50,51,52] These physical findings included: (1) paralysis above L3, (2) thoracolumbar or thoracolumbosacral lesions related to the vertebral levels, (3) congenital rigid kyphosis or scoliosis, (4) a grossly enlarged head with a maximum circumference of 2 cm or more above the 90th percentile, related to birth weight, (5) intracerebral birth injuries, and (6) other gross congenital defects. He further stated that infants with serious neurologic deficits and hydrocephalus who develop meningitis or ventriculitis after closure should not have active treatment. Should an untreated child survive 6 months and thrive, the situation would be reviewed and a multi-discipline approach for treatment would be initiated.

DEVELOPMENT OF THE MYELOMENINGOCELE CHILD

Physical Development

Normal child development proceeds through a continuous, orderly sequence of growth.

Hostler stressed that intellectual, motor, and social development is dependent upon the infant's interaction with his environment.[39] When a child's mobility and ability to explore space are limited, the developmental sequence is altered in the areas of gross and fine motor skills, as well as in the areas of cognitive and social accomplishments.

Normal infant–mother bonding is not possible for the myelomeningocele newborn. A continuously-lit hospital incubator provides the infant with a minimum of social interaction, only with parents and hospital staff. A normal 1-month-old infant is able to fix both eyes on light and follow it to the midline, as well as to respond to the sound of a rattle. Because the myelomeningocele infant lacks sufficient social interaction, he or she frequently does not develop these visual and auditory responses. The normal infant acquires new skills which are based upon previously learned activities. However, for the myelomeningocele infant, development during the first few months may be interrupted by prolonged hospitalizations. By 6 months of age these infants may not be able to distinguish family members from friends because of a lack of sufficient interaction with the family. As the child grows older, environmental and functional gaps widen. The myelomeningocele child's movement in space is limited, while the normal child progresses through the stages of crawling, standing, and walking. So that the myelomeningocele child can obtain as normal a developmental sequence as possible, a program has been established at Newington Children's Hospital.[22] It offers the young myelomeningocele child a maximum of supervised sensory and motor stimulation and emphasizes teaching the child to stand and walk at the age when the normal child develops these skills.

Even though contractures can be avoided in the newborn, they may develop if the trunk and lower limbs are not positioned properly. While normal newborns can lie either in the prone or the supine position, the newborn with myelomeningocele must remain in the prone position until the sac closure heals. Trunk posture and lower limb rotation and extension can be controlled either by using a diaper splint (Fig. 9-1), a split mattress (Fig. 9-2), or occasionally an abduction orthosis while the infant is resting.[68] The parents are encouraged to make every effort to achieve infant bonding and no positional devices are used during periods of close physical interaction. During the next several months the normal child develops head control and incorporates ocular righting, tonic labyrinthine, and symmetric tonic neck reflexes as he develops increasing tone of the extensor muscles of the neck, upper extremities, and trunk. These reflexes help the infant to attain head control and can be encouraged in the spinal bifida infant by a vigorous program of sensory and motor stimulation. Activities and games encouraging prone-on-extended elbows and prone-on-extended head positions are repeatedly performed with the brace-free infant. It may be necessary for the infant to wear a trunk-extremity positional orthosis during naps and at night to prevent structural deformity. Toward the end of the first year, the normal child develops

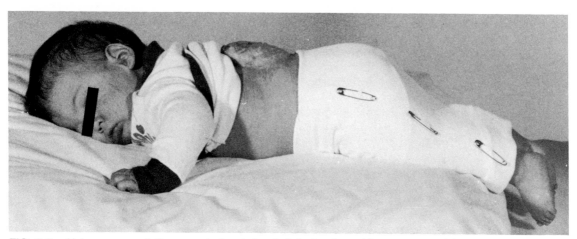

FIG. 9-1. Using a second diaper controls rotation in infants whose hips are not at risk.

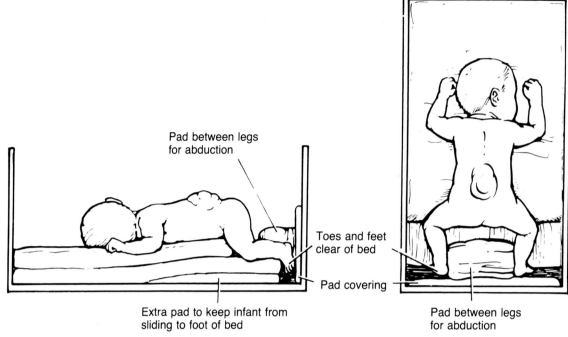

FIG. 9-2. A split mattress and proper positioning ensures hip stability in infants with hips at risk. (Passo SD: Positioning infants with myelomeningocele. Am J Nurs 74:1658, 1974)

righting and equilibrium actions that assist him in sitting. Reciprocal movement replaces gross bilateral patterns. The Newington program for the myelomingocele child continues to emphasize improvement and control of the head, trunk, and upper extremities. A hip hinge is added to the Newington preparatory orthosis (Fig. 9-3). Reciprocal movement is simulated by the use of a crawl-agator or low platform with wheels (Fig. 9-4). Crawling is not permitted because decubiti may develop on the knees and toes of the anesthetic lower limbs.

By age 1 year the normal child is able to stand alone. However, the child with myelomeningocele uses a preliminary standing orthosis which incorporates high-top shoes with clear plastic heels and laces to the toes (Fig. 9-5). An orthosis for trunk control can be combined with these braces and used in conjunction with the standing table to improve the child's upright posture.

By 2 years of age, when the ambulatory potential of the patient can be assessed, the orthopaedist prescribes appropriate trunk and extremity orthoses (Fig. 9-6). As the child progresses from parallel bars to a walker, the therapist helps him to develop a four-point gait. Improvement in ambulation occurs mostly during the preschool years.

Emotional Development

For a normal child, the development of motor skills and the progression from kindergarten through elementary school follow a definite pattern. During these critical years the myelomeningocele patient finds life dominated by a succession of medical and surgical problems and subsequent hospitalizations. These interrupt the sequence of learning and peer interaction at school, thereby fragmenting the child's intellectual and social development.

Adolescence

Adolescence is a time of profound and rapid physical, personal, and social changes. The normal teenager develops ego identity and increasingly relates to others, resulting in more

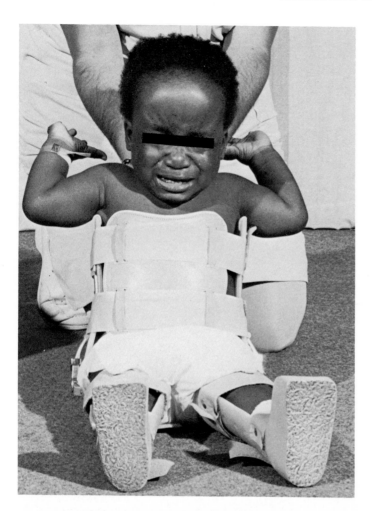

FIG. 9-3. Adding a hip hinge to a preparatory orthosis permits sitting at the expected developmental stage.

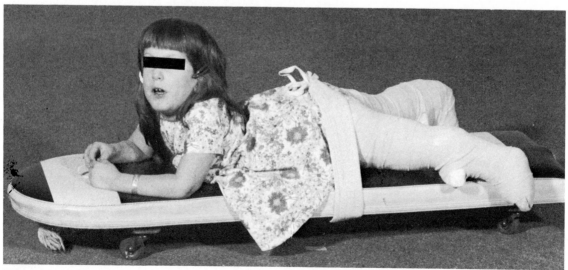

FIG. 9-4. Reciprocal, upper-extremity movement can be accomplished by using this low platform on wheels.

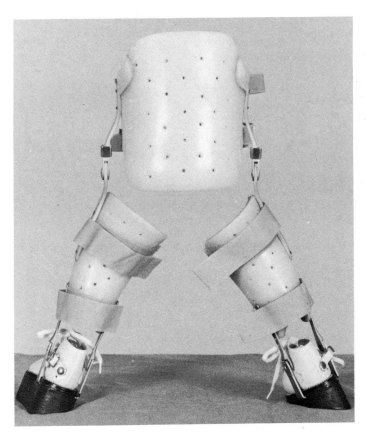

FIG. 9-5. A preliminary standing orthosis permits standing at the expected stage of development.

independence from home. After-school activities, the discovery of the opposite sex, and peer group pressures are important factors in the development of adolescent behavior.

Problems confronting myelomeningocele teenagers are even more complex than these confronting normal teenagers.[38] For the first time they are experiencing a period of uninterrupted education, as medical and orthopaedic problems enter a static phase. Interrelationships with normal peers occur in school, but otherwise opportunites for social and personal development remain limited.[17,18] Typically, myelomeningocele adolescents are still dependent upon parents for assistance in dressing and upon special transportation to and from school. This social isolation adds to the their poor self-image and to the depressed mental state that they may demonstrate. Suicide is considered by over 25% of myelomeningocele teenagers as compared to 7% in the average adolescent population.[73]

Myelomeningocele adolescents face two new physical problems, increasing body weight and height, which may jeopardize the ambulatory ability of some patients. In the Newington experience, 25% of teenage myelomingocele patients walk independently, another 25% walk with crutches part time and use a wheelchair at other times, and 50% select wheelchair ambulation. Patients who combine crutches with wheelchair activity are the best adjusted emotionally and physically. They are able to cope with all forms of architectural barriers, such as stairs or ramps, and are able to go long distances without tiring. They can transfer independently and are capable of handling their own personal hygiene needs. Independent ambulators fatigue over long distances and are more resentful of their handicaps.

Adolescents should be included in the decision-making, rehabilitation process. Usually they are interested in solving problems related to self-care, such as dressing and urinary and bowel care. The stigma of urinary and fecal incontinence is a major contributor to the poor self-image which they have.[17,36]

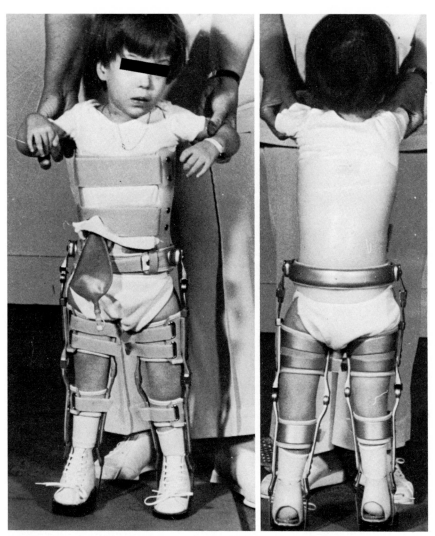

FIG. 9-6. The decision to attach or separate long leg braces from trunk orthosis must be individualized. Note the shoes laced to the toes.

They demonstrate natural instincts for knowledge about sex and the possibilities of marriage.

The adolescent is also interested in developing long-term goals for achieving personal independence. Meaningful vocational rehabilitation should be directed toward job training in professions where there is an established community need. Previous studies have demonstrated that myelomeningocele patients have lower scores in arithmetic and also in visual perception tests, which include spatial ability and manual dexterity.[66] However, they scored well on tests for mechanical comprehension, suggesting that, with careful training, patients not going to college might pursue jobs which require mechanical ability. Since independent mobility is also important to adolescents, they should be encouraged to participate in a driver training program.

The adolescent should be prepared so that when he leaves school, social interaction and maturation will continue.[55] Early reports suggest that these adolescents often leave school and are unemployed.[17] Generally graduates from Newington Children's Hospital High School have selected advanced education. Since they have a need to enter professions in which they can compete with their normal peers, they often have chosen service-oriented fields, such as teaching or hospital administration. It is interesting that these patients, many of whom have above-average intelligence and who are analytical about life, have not pursued the fine arts such as writing, music, or art.

Generally, the first year in college is the first time that these patients have lived away from home and have been totally responsible for their own care. Frequently they develop an ischial decubitis which requires hospitalization (Fig. 9-7). Their ability to cope physically and emotionally with this may determine whether they will be able to complete their formal education and become productive and employed adults.

Patients who have potential employability need strong motivation from the rehabilitation team, particularly from its medical leader.[49] Recognition must be given to the positive social attributes of these patients. They tend to have warm and friendly personalities. Many have normal intelligence and retain excellent upper-extremity function, underlining their potential to be productive in society. Physicians treating these patients must be willing to make a commitment to oversee their total care into adult life. Since society has not developed acceptable social alternatives for the handicapped person, it may become the responsibility of the hospital, and particularly its combined clinic team, to develop a more normal social structure for these patients.

THE CHANGING ROLE OF THE ORTHOPAEDIST

The orthopaedist's objectives for myelomeningocele patients during their first decade of life are directed toward establishing a stable posture and ambulation. Although decisions concerning surgical procedures and mobility goals are discussed with the parents, the surgeon's opinion is generally decisive. However, the teenage patient is intellectually capable of weighing the orthopaedist's recommendations and making a decision as to whether the physician's advice and goals coincide with his own approach to life.

As his surgical role diminishes, the orthopaedist's unique professional and philosophical qualifications as leader of the rehabilitation team emerge. He must be willing to change from the role of surgeon to rehabilitation coordinator. The team must include the adolescent, as well as professional members qualified to cope with long-term emotional, medical, and social problems. The physician must learn to recognize non-orthopaedic problems and work toward developing the concept of total care of the adolescent.

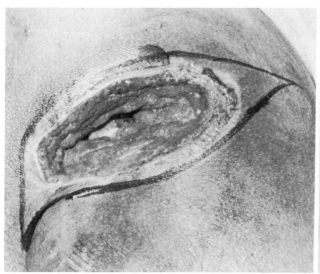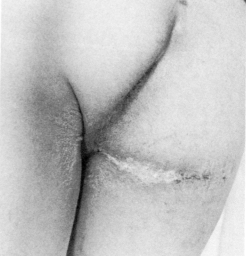

FIG. 9-7. Decubitus resulting from inadvertent deflation of a wheelchair air cushion. Delayed closure was successfully performed after initial debridement.

SPINAL DEFORMITY

The treatment of spinal deformity represents the major orthopaedic challenge in the treatment of myelomenigoccle patients. Spinal curvature can result from: (1) congenital vertebral anomalies secondary to cellular damage of the ventral region of the neural tube, (2) segmental vertebral instability resulting from loss of the posterior elements during the time of fetal hydromyelia and rupture of the neural tube, or (3) progressive extrauterine hydromyelia which leads to progressive axial motor paresis.[35] Paralysis resulting from the neurologic lesion complicates these conditions.

Congenital Scoliosis

Vertebral malformation results when there is a failure of sclerotomal cells to condense and become intervertebral elements.[63] Lateral hemivertebrae originate from one-sided mesenchymal condensation that increases the growth potential of the side of these hemivertebrae. Unilateral failure of vertebral segmentation results in the formation of a one-sided bar with unilateral diminished growth potential (Fig. 9-8).

In addition to spinal deformity associated with myelomeningocele, congenital scoliosis cephalad to the spina bifida is present in 20% of these patients.[10] Since this deformity progresses in a fashion similar to progression of other congenital curves, the goal is to prevent a further increase in the curve by prompt fusion when progession is evident. Allen stresses the need to analyze congential and developmental deformities separately and to make appropriate treatment decisions for each.[2] For example, spinal orthoses can control a paralytic curve which develops in the area of the myelomeningocele, but a localized posterior

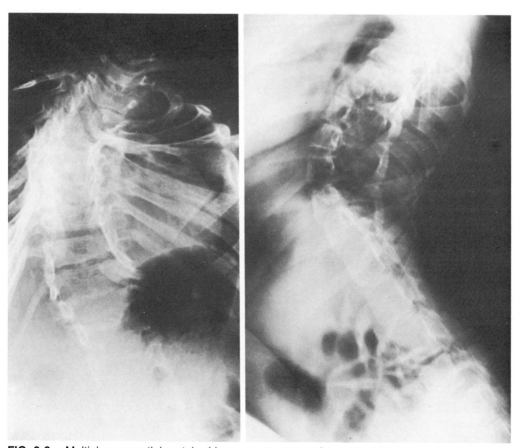

FIG. 9-8. Multiple congential vertebral bars cause progressive congential lordoscoliosis.

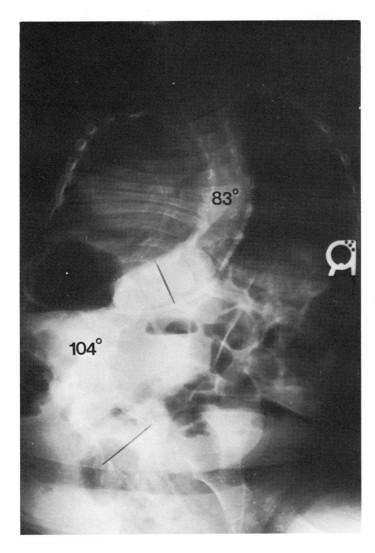

FIG. 9-9. The absence of the neural arches, posterior ligamentous complex, and zygapophyseal joints is compounded by paretic extensor muscles of the trunk.

fusion will be needed for a progressive congential scoliosis. This fusion must be extended to include normal vertebrae cephalad and caudad to the vertebral anomaly.

Developmental Scoliosis

Spinal deformity develops in the area of the rachischisis because of a loss of vertebral stability (Fig. 9-9). This instability results from the absence of the neural arch and facets and concomitant loss of the posterior ligamentous complex. Also, the trunk extensors are not only paretic but lack their neural arch attachment in the area of the myelomeningocele. Thus, the longer the area of rachischisis, the longer the area of combined osseous and soft-tissue deficiency. In Banta's study, 20% of myelomeningocele patients developed significant scoliosis by age 4, and by age 10, all patients with thoracolumbar lesions had significant structural spinal deformity.[3]

Paralytic curves can be expected to progress. Use of a spinal orthosis helps to delay surgery in young patients and allows for normal trunk growth. Patients who are most vulnerable to the early onset of scoliosis are those who will function from a wheelchair in adult life. Thus it is necessary to attain maximum height of the trunk so that these patients can sit comfortably in a wheelchair. Patients whose deformity can be kept under 50° can delay the fusion until near skeletal maturity. In these patients, fusions can be performed successfully in girls ages 10 to 12 and in boys ages 12 to 14. Surgical correction may be indicated at a younger age only when orthotic management has been unsuccessful or progressive pelvic obliquity develops.

Spinal Orthoses

The selection of a specific spinal orthosis depends on the neurologic and functional level of the patient. The patient's motor development, head and trunk balance, spinal and extremity alignment, as well as age and prognosis for survival and ambulation, must be considered. Although the appropriate spinal orthosis may improve function and hold a corrected deformity, it should not be expected to per-

manently correct the deformity by itself. Use of the orthosis limits trunk movement and thus may decrease ambulatory function.

While the absence of sensation is not a contraindication to successful use of an orthosis, it does indicate that the skin should be checked routinely and carefully. Obesity and pelvic obliquity are other factors which limit the brace's effectiveness.

Bunch recommends a modified Milwaukee brace (Fig. 9-10) for young patients with a flexible scoliosis.[9] This orthosis has a long pelvic girdle extending to the lower rib cage and a large thoracic pad, both of which provide additional support. Time in the orthosis is increased gradually, and the patient is checked for skin breakdown.

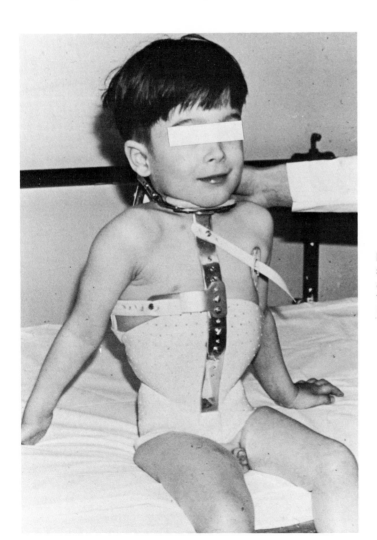

FIG. 9-10. The increased pelvis girdle size enlarges the skin surface area that accepts pressure, thereby decreasing the risk of skin breakdown. (Courtesy of Dr. W. Bunch)

Two variations of spinal orthoses have been developed at Newington Children's Hospital. Both are fabricated over a positive plaster mold taken from a carefully contoured plaster jacket, that was obtained while the patient was in corrective traction. The first type, the total contact jacket, extends from the axillae to the inguinal creases and is used primarily to postpone surgery in the skeletally immature patient.[24] Frequently these patients also use lower-extremity braces, which in some cases can be attached to the spinal orthosis (Fig. 9-11).

The second type, the thoracic suspension orthosis, is a modification of the total contact jacket (Fig. 9-12).[22,24,26] It has a carefully contoured undercut below the anterolateral costal margin and is slightly flared in the thoracic area so that the chest can expand during inhalation. An indentation in the upper abdominal area provides hydraulic resistance to diaphragmatic contracture and thus also facilitates chest expansion. The patient is suspended by a spool and hook mechanism which is attached to a standard wheelchair (Fig. 9-13). The vertical load on the lower spine is reduced by using the lower anterior and lateral thoracic cage as a partial weight-bearing structure and the weight of the suspended pelvis and lower limbs as a corrective distraction force. This allows more correction than could be obtained by using the total contact

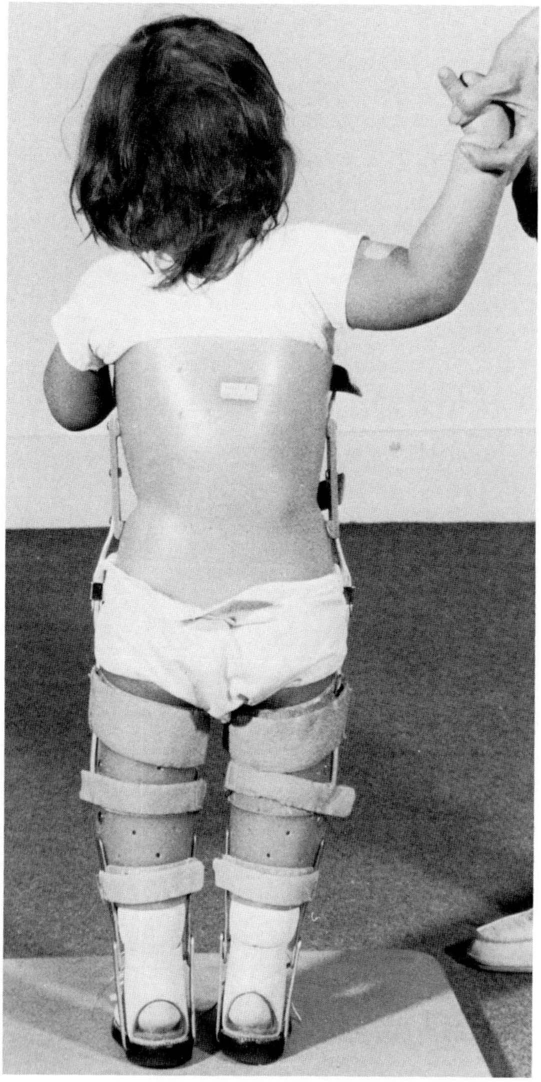

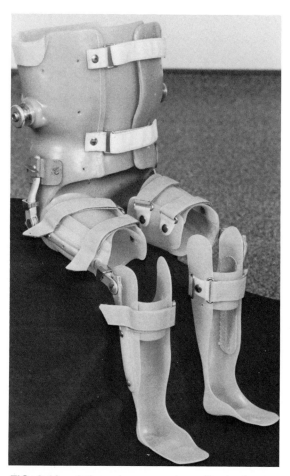

FIG. 9-11. The total-contact orthosis can be contoured to accommodate lumbar kyphosis.

FIG. 9-12. A thoracic suspension orthosis. Accuracy in obtaining the plaster mold, precise orthotic construction and application are requisites for successful use.

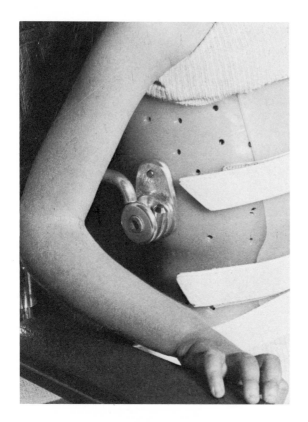

jacket. The compression and shear forces of the orthosis against the thorax must remain below the level of maximum skin tolerance, a level that can be increased with careful progressive wearing.

The reason for using the thoracic suspension orthosis for myelomeningocele patients are to: (1) avoid surgery for patients with high level lesions (Fig. 9-14) or major congenital anomalies (Fig. 9-15) that will not allow them to tolerate surgery, (2) postpone surgical correction of scoliosis or congenital kyphosis in skeletally immature patients with high level lesions, and (3) provide a means of orthotic control for patients who have recurrent ischial pressure sores. It affords increased sitting stability in space and allows for more functional use of the arms.

The initial application of a thoracic suspension orthosis requires hospital admission

FIG. 9-13. The orthotic spindle, seated in a hook attached to the uprights of a standard wheelchair, can easily be raised or lowered.

FIG. 9-14. Adolescents with severe scoliosis and pulmonary compromise require the ongoing use of a thoracic suspension orthosis.

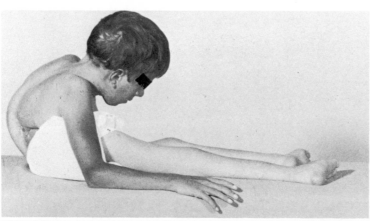

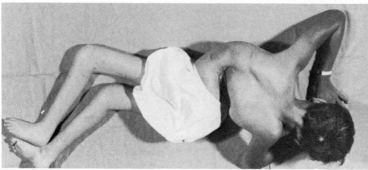

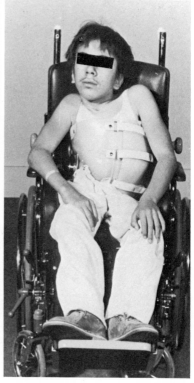

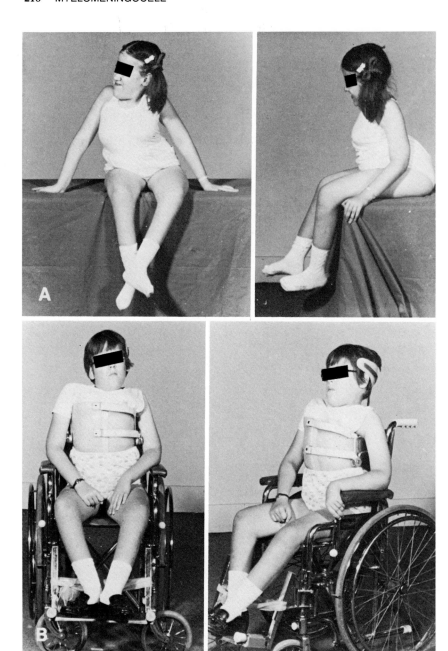

FIG. 9-15. (*A*) Improved position in space is accomplished for an adolescent with congenital thoracic lordoscoliosis and restricted cardiopulmonary function. (*B*) Temporary use of the headrest was required because of functional weakness in the neck flexors.

for a program of progressive wear managed by an experienced team of nurses and orthotists, the physician, and the parents. The patient builds up skin tolerance by wearing the orthosis without suspension for 1 hour. Toler-ance is defined as the disappearance of skin erythema within 20 minutes following re-moval or the orthosis. If it does not disappear, the skin is treated with alcohol followed by an application of tincture of benzoin. Then suspension is begun in the sitting position for 10 minutes every hour and gradually increased until the patient can tolerate suspension for 2 consecutive hours. Initial hospitalization usually lasts 2 to 3 weeks, whereas only 2 to 3 days are needed when repeated orthotic deliveries are made.

After discharge, the patient continues to increase the wearing time in the orthosis and should be able to prolong the time in suspension from 6 to 14 hours per day. This orthosis is not worn at night.

The success or failure of this orthosis depends upon the reliability of the parent or attendant to apply the orthosis, place the patient in suspension, and monitor the skin. If erythema persists for more then 20 minutes after removal of the orthosis, the wearing program must be revised. One of the 25 myelomeningocele patients at Newington Children's Hospital who used the thoracic suspension orthosis developed a full-thickness skin ulcer in an anesthetic area, which required plastic surgical correction. There have been no other significant complications in our experience.

Spinal Fusion

Spinal fusions should be considered when bracing cannot maintain correction of the scoliotic curve below 50°. In addition to arresting progression of a spinal deformity, surgery may be indicated when the curve causes a loss of activity, especially in a functional individual; for fatigue or back pain; and for ischial pressure sores secondary to progressive pelvic obliquity in the nonambulator.

The goals of surgery are to: (1) obtain spinal stability with the head midline, (2) improve ambulatory independence, (3) establish independent sitting balance, thereby freeing the upper extremities for bimanual function, and (4) correct pelvic obliquity and thus relieve excessive skin pressure in the nonambulator.[64] It is recognized that in some rigid curves correction is impossible and spinal stability is the only goal.

The surgeon must decide which type of fusion is most appropriate—posterior, anterior, or a combination; the length of the fusion; and the postoperative management needed until consolidation of the arthrodesis occurs.

POSTERIOR FUSION

Prerequisites for fusion include the presence of posterior elements large enough to provide an osseous bed for application of the autologous bone graft and appropriate instrumentation. Specifications include extending the fusion from the sacrum to two vertebrae above the cephalad end of the curve (Fig. 9-16). Surgical dissection starts in the normal anatomy and proceeds caudally. The normal zygapophyseal joints, as well as the osseocartilaginous laminar bar replacing these joints, are excised and packed with bone. Lateral gutters are created by exposing and decorticating the remaining cortical bone. A generous amount of bone graft is laid over the exposed bony field. To increase the probability of fusion, Bonnett recommends placing autologous bone anterior to the transverse processes.[5] With Harrington instrumentation, which is widely used, the caudal end of the rod is fitted into a large sacral alar hook. Two Harrington rods on the concave side of the curve are recommended. Segmental spinal stabilization may also be used as an alternate method of fixation (Fig. 9-17).[2,54]

Patients with high level paraplegia may benefit from a posterior interbody fusion combined with the standard posterior fusion (Fig. 9-18). A plane of dissection is created between the posterior vertebral body and the posterior longitudinal ligament. The meningeal layers are closed with a continuous suture to prevent leakage of cerebrospinal fluid. The dural sac is then freed up by sharp dissection in a cephalad direction and nerve roots accompanying vessels are ligated at each level until adequate exposure is obtained. This permits visualization and excision of the intervertebral disc contents and the insertion of large amounts of bone graft at the junction of the interbody and posterior fusions.

COMPLICATIONS. The pathoanatomy of the vertebral bodies in the area of the myelomeningocele places the arthrodesis in jeopardy. The goal is to create a long fusion even though there are deficient posterior elements which may compromise the insertion of instrumentation. The rate of pseudarthrosis (Fig. 9-19) is as high as 50% in a series reported by Sriram.[82] He also found that wound infections occurred in cases in which the large myelo-

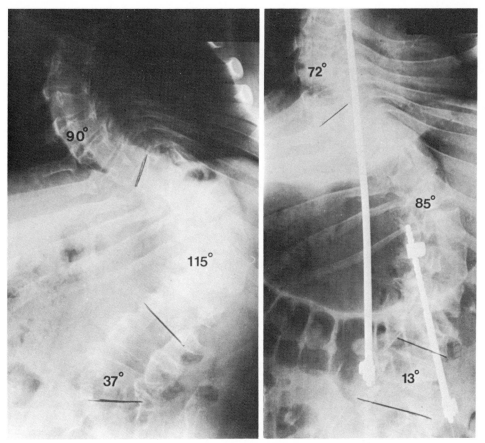

FIG. 9-16. Paralytic neuromuscular curves require spinal fusion extending to the pelvis. The cephalad extension of the rachischisis can be determined by noting the level at which the pedicle shadow no longer overlaps the vertebral body.

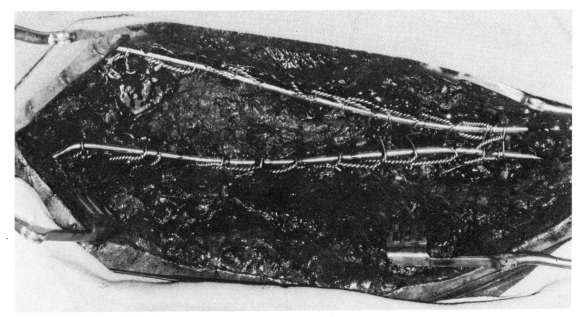

FIG. 9-17. The rudimentary laminae in the area of rachischisis resemble mushrooms and must be individually lassoed before the rod is secured.

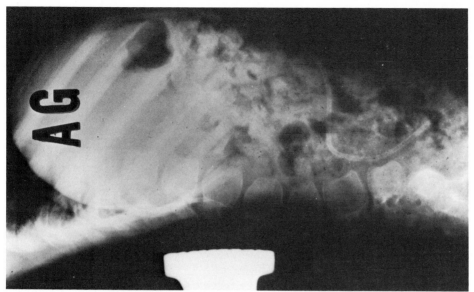

FIG. 9-18. Hyperextension roentgenograms demonstrate flexibility of postural kyphotic deformity and assist in determining whether posterior fusion alone may be indicated.

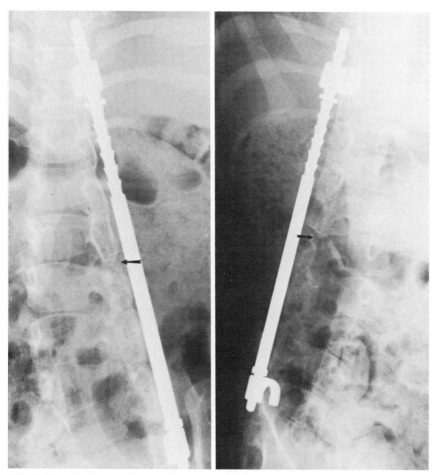

FIG. 9-19. Radiographic pseudarthroses are most prevalent in areas which lack the neural arch.

meningocele sac had been excised or opened and through which cerebrospinal fluid had escaped into the wound.

ANTERIOR FUSION

Indications for anterior fusion are: (1) an intact myelomeningocele sac that needs to be closed to avoid wound infection, (2) marked deficiency of the posterior elements, (3) developmental lordosis, or (4) congenital kyphosis. Since the number of vertebrae that can be exposed by removal of one rib may limit the length of the fusion, two separate incisions may be required. The sacrum is difficult to reach, particularly in patients with lordosis. It is important to completely remove the epiphyseal plates and thoroughly pack the intervertebral spaces with cancellous bone.

Dwyer instrumentation is employed if the size and quality of the vertebral bodies will permit its use. Frequently, anterior fusion is followed 2 weeks later by posterior arthrodesis (Fig. 9-20) in an effort to decrease the incidence of pseudarthrosis.[40] Allen describes a release of the anterior longitudinal ligament plus vertebral fusion without instrumentation followed by use of halo-gravity traction on a circ-o-lectric bed postoperatively.[2]

Congential Lumbar Kyphosis

Congenital lumbar kyphosis is present at birth in 1 of 8 cases of myelomeningocele. Faradic stimulation demonstrates neurologic activity to the L3 to L4 level. The large protruding bony deformity and the wide ecotodermal lesion make closure of the myelomengocele difficult.

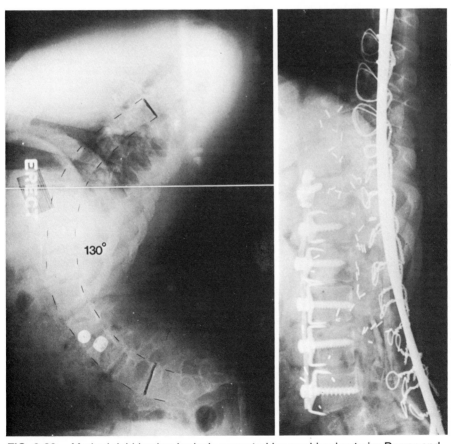

FIG. 9-20. Marked rigid lumbar lordosis corrected by combined anterior Dwyer and posterior spinal segmental stabilization.

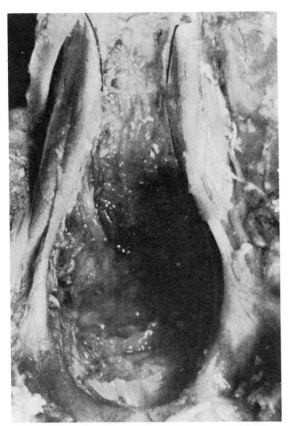

FIG. 9-21. The black silk sutures separate the diaphragmatic crura from the hypertrophied and rotated psoas. The quadratus lumborum is demonstrated on one side. (Drennan JC: The role of muscles in the development of human lumbar kyphosis. Dev Med Child Neurol (Suppl) 22:33, 1970)

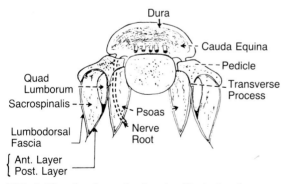

FIG. 9-22. A schematic drawing illustrates the rotation of the psoas muscles and attached transverse processes into the concavity of the kyphos. (Sharrard WJW, Drennan JC: Osteotomy-excision of the spine for lumbar kyphosis in older children with myelomeningocele. J Bone Joint Surg 54B:50, 1972)

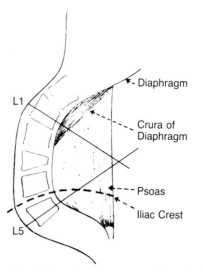

FIG. 9-23. Dual insertion of the diaphragm limits the extent of the kyphos. (Sharrard WJW, Drennan JC: Osteotomy-excision of the spine for lumbar kyphosis in older children with myelomeningocele. J Bone Joint Surg 54B:50, 1972)

PATHOANATOMY OF THE KYPHOS

The kyphos begins in the lower thoracic spine and extends to the sacrum. Thus psoas muscles hypertrophy and rotate into a position anterior to the lumbar spine and become powerful lumbar flexors (Fig. 9-21). The attachment of the psoas muscles to the lumbar transverse processes causes these cartilaginous structures to rotate into the concavity of the curve (Fig. 9-22). The dual insertions of the diaphragm at the thoracolumbar junction and through its crura to the L3 vertebra act as dynamic fixtures for the psoas major and minor muscles to pull against (Fig. 9-23).[23] Failure of the neural arch to develop, limits the posterior attachment of the lumbodorsal fascia to the rudimentary laminae. The attachment of the anterior lumbodorsal fascia to the rotated transverse processes brings the fasciae and the enclosed erector spinae muscles anterior to the pedicles where the muscles become perverted flexors of the spine. Then the deformity becomes fixed.

The abnormal pedicles and laminae are splayed out and displaced anterolaterally by the attached posterior layer of the lumbodorsal fascia. Normal lumbar zygapophyseal joints are not formed. Instead, cartilaginous bridges link the laminae, which later become converted to bone in older children. The effect of this is to create lumbar intervertebral foramina, similar to those in the sacrum, through which nerves pass ventrally into the psoas muscle. Pressure causes wedging of the apical vertebra anteriorly. There is no increase in width of the vertebral bodies in the kyphotic area. The aorta and inferior vena cava follow but do not adhere to the anterior surface of the vertebral bodies.

INDICATIONS FOR SURGERY IN THE NEONATE

Lorber has reported that patients with lumbar kyphosis have a high infant mortality rate and that survivors generally have a lower quality of life than other myelomeningocele patients.[51,52] Primary skin closure of the myelomeningocele may not be possible without limited orthopaedic intervention (Fig. 9-24). This intervention consists of resecting the osseocartilaginous laminar bars bilaterally over the several levels of the kyphos until adequate skin approximation is attained.

TECHNIQUE OF LAMINAR BAR RESECTION[21]

Routine repair fo the myelomeningocele and closure of the dural sac are performed. The dura must be freed up from the posterior as-

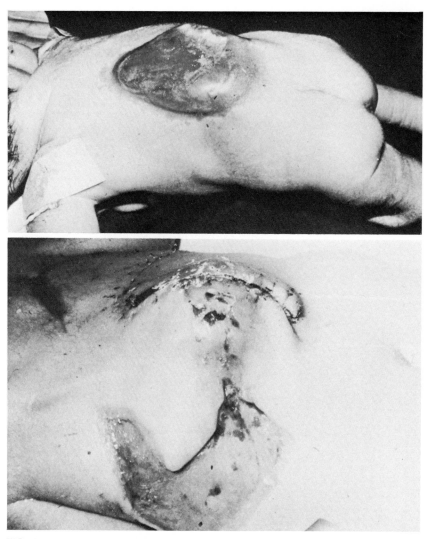

FIG. 9-24. Efforts to obtain full thickness skin coverage at the time of the initial closure are compromised by the rigid kyphotic prominence.

pect of the laminae and vertebral bodies to expose the nerve roots as they leave the underside of the dura and enter the intervertebral foramina (Fig. 9-25). To avoid encountering nerve roots and their accompanying blood vessels, the surgical incision should be made at the caudal aspect of these foramina. When the posterior layer of the lumbodorsal fascia is incised at its attachment to the tip of the lamina, the underlying erector spinae muscles are exposed. After these are stripped from the under surface of the laminar bar, the thick, well-defined, white anterior layer of the lumbodorsal fascia is uncovered. This serves as

an anatomic landmark dividing the area for safe, superficial dissection from the important deeper structures including the nerve roots. A dissector is passed through the foramen lateral to the nerve root and can be visualized as it passes superifically to the well-defined anterior lumbodorsal fascia (Fig. 9-26). A second dissector is used at the next foramen. These two instruments protect the nerve roots and allow the bony segment between the two foramina to be safely removed with a rongeur (Fig. 9-27). The process is repeated at as many levels as necessary to remove a sufficient length of the protruding laminar bar.

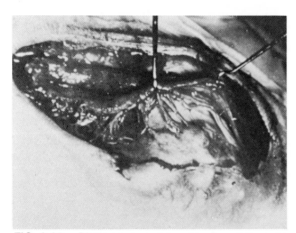 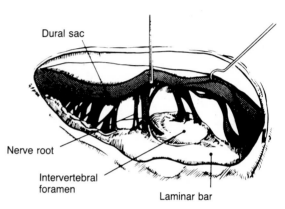

FIG. 9-25. Photograph and line drawing of the kyphos. The plane for dural dissection is established by incising directly to the laminar bar. Note the egress of the nerve roots from the undersurface of the dura and their entrance into the lumber foramina. (Drennan JC: Management of neonatal myelomeningocele. AAOS Instruc Course Lect 25:65, 1976)

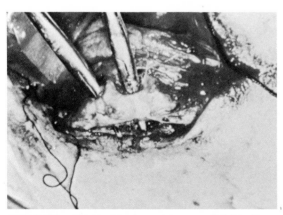 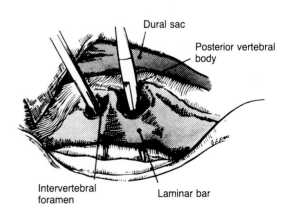

FIG. 9-26. Surgical instruments superficial to the nerve roots afford protection during laminar bar division. (Drennan JC: Management of neonatal myelomeningocele. AAOS Instruc Course Lect 25:65, 1976)

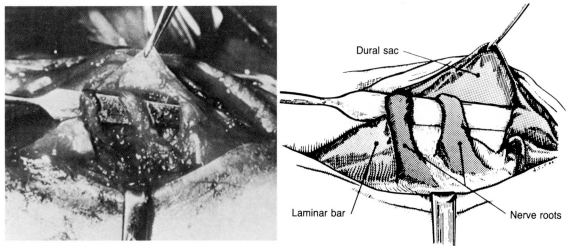

Dural sac

Laminar bar

Nerve roots

FIG. 9-27. Lumbar nerve roots can be visualized clearly after resection of the osseo-cartilaginous laminar bar. (Sharrard WJW: Spinal osteotomy for congenital kyphosis in myelomeningocele. J Bone Joint Surg 50B:466, 1968)

This simple procedure performed bilaterally adds only a few minutes to surgery and in almost all cases reduces the protruding bone so that the skin can be closed.

TECHNIQUE OF SPINAL OSTEOTOMY IN THE NEONATE

Spinal osteotomy is indicated only rarely when resection of the laminar bar is not successful.[21] Since a minority of patients with kyphosis retain lumbar neurologic function, the spinal cord should not be divided as an aid to exposing the vertebrae. Neonatal spinal osteotomy slows down but does not prevent the eventual increase in the kyphotic deformity.

The removal of the laminar bar exposes the nerve roots as they enter the psoas muscle. The psoas and diaphragmatic crura at the apex must be bluntly dissected to allow a malleable retractor to be positioned to protect the abdominal great vessels. A second malleable retractor is used to protect the dura. Small rubber dams retract the bilateral nerve roots both cephalad and caudad to the level of osteotomy. The initial osteotomy, which is performed through the apical vertebra, acts to mobilize the spine for resection of vertebral bodies.[75] Only a segment of an individual vertebral body can be removed at one time through the narrow space between nerve roots (Fig. 9-28). Cancellous apposition is sought after the fragmentary removal of the equiva-

lent of at least 2 vertebral bodies. The child is positioned so that the lower half of his body is hyperextended to juxtapose the cancellous surfaces while the two vertebral segments are depressed. Crossed Kirschner wires are used for fixation. The removed bone is placed anteriorly into the concavity of the curve as a short anterior graft.

Postoperatively, the patient is kept in the prone position, either on an infant Bradford frame or in an isolette with Montgomery straps (wide, adhesive, abdominal slings) until solid fusion is confirmed by roentgenogram.

PROGRESSION OF THE UNTREATED KYPHOSIS

At birth the kyphos extends from the first to the fifth lumbar vertebra and measures greater than 80°. By the end of the third year, the curve can be expected to exceed 120° and will continue to progress (Fig. 9-29). In the upright child, thoracic lordosis develops secondary to the deforming force of upper body weight (Fig. 9-30).[4] Viscera pressing against the remaining attachments of the diaphragm to the thoracic cage cause the ribs to splay. This forces the child to sit with the rib cage resting on the femoral shaft (Fig. 9-31). Also the skin becomes progressively atrophic over the enlarging kyphos. The abdominal muscles, which do not lengthen, further fix the kyphos.

Indications for surgery in the older child are generally chronic or recurrent skin ulcer-

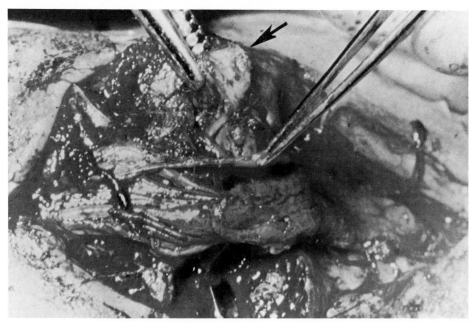

FIG. 9-28. Part of the apical vertebral body is carefully removed between the intact nerve roots.

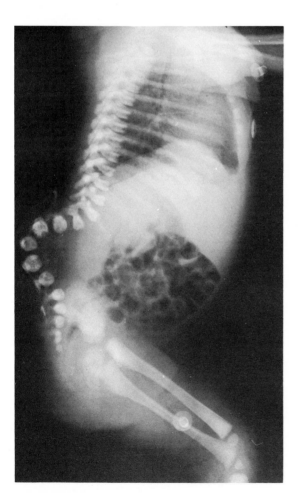

FIG. 9-29. Upper body weight and the occasional retained psoas activity enhance lumbar flexion and progressive kyphosis. Thoracic lordosis is not present in this radiograph of a newborn.

FIG. 9-30. The development of thoracic lordosis complicates orthopaedic management. Both of these structural lateral curves require stabilization.

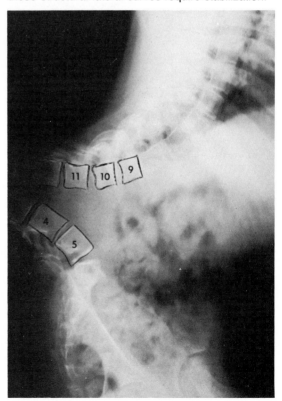

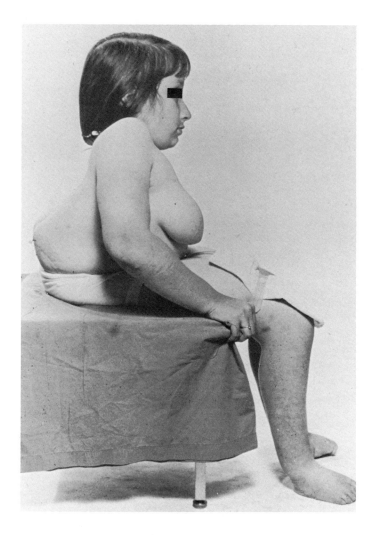

FIG. 9-31. Cosmetic, orthopaedic, and urologic management problems can be identified in this photograph.

ation (Fig. 9-32).[76] Surgery also may be needed to: (1) improve sitting stability, (2) permit use of a spinal orthosis, (3) allow attachment of an abdominal ileostomal bag, or (4) alleviate back pain.

PREOPERATIVE EVALUATION

The majority of authors agree that posterior excision of the kyphos is essential in order to obtain satisfactory realignment of the spine.[53,70,76] The surgeon carefully evaluates anteroposterior and lateral roentgenograms to determine the level of the vertebral ostectomy and the number of vertebrae to be removed. The objective is to decrease the prominence of the bony kyphos and to correct alignment of the pelvis relative to the trunk.

SURGICAL TECHNIQUE

A long transverse incision is extended from the midaxillary line to permit the development of full-thickness skin flaps. By careful, sharp dissection, the attenuated apical skin is separated from the dura. The laminar bar is defined. Then the dura is circumferentially freed up by creating a plane between the posterior aspect of the vertebral body and the posterior longitudinal ligament. The dura is clamped and divided at the caudal aspect of the wound and then mobilized cephalad to obtain complete exposure of the kyphos. Nerve roots and their accompanying spinal vessels are identified and ligated at each level. The procedure used to expose vertebral bodies is similar to that described for correction of kyphosis in the neonate. The progressive devel-

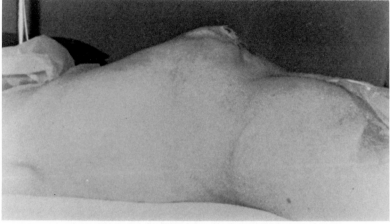

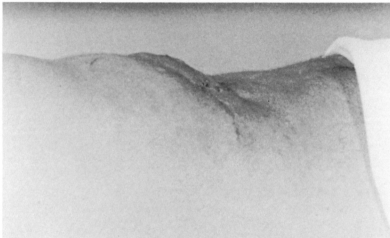

FIG. 9-32. The tenuous lumbar skin coverage in this adolescent is improved following excision of the kyphos combined with anterior and posterior fusion.

opment of fixed thoracolumbar lordosis changes the selection of the vertebrae to be excised. Part of the apical vertebra and one or two vertebrae cephalad to it are removed in a manner to ensure full apposition of cancellous surfaces (Fig. 9-33). Hall recommends that surgery be performed during the second year of life using Harrington compression instrumentation to obtain an anterior and posterior fusion at the time of excision.[34,70] Stabilization is achieved by Harrington compression, using rods with the hooks seated in the foramina, and by using crossed Kirschner wires.

At skeletal maturation, the cartilaginous aspects of the laminar bar are ossified and do not permit adequate apposition of the spine after resection of the vertebral bodies (Fig. 9-34). I recommend excising the bony foraminal roofs and curetting two disc spaces cephalad and caudad to the area of resection. This pro-

cedure mobilizes the adjacent vertebrae and removes the tension from the level of cancellous apposition. The removed bone is cut into wedges that are then placed in the curetted disc spaces. Postoperatively, the patient is maintained in the prone position until solid fusion is confirmed by roentgenogram.

The length of posterior fusion, particularly in the older child, is insufficient and fusion is, biomechanically, under tension. A second-stage anterior fusion is indicated if a kyphos of more than 50° remains after solid posterior fusion can be demonstrated. This can be accomplished with a strut graft spanning the kyphos combined with the inlaid rib graft and careful packing of the excised disc spaces with cancellous bone. The strut graft must extend into the compensatory thoracic lordosis or the lordosis may progress and require subsequent surgery. The patient is immobi-

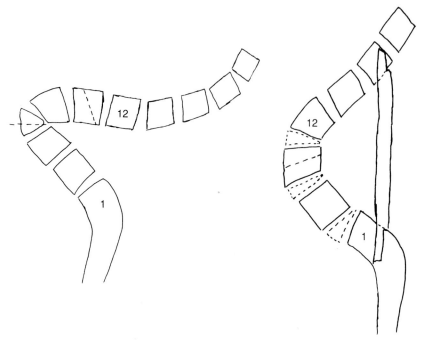

FIG. 9-33. The obliquity of the vertebral osteotomies assures good cancellous bone apposition.

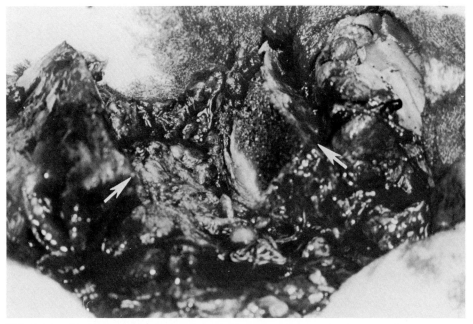

FIG. 9-34. Skeletal maturation creats a rigid kyphos, frequently with poor skin coverage. The fixed deformity will not permit use of the Harrington compression instrumentation, which is recommended for the younger patient.

lized in a two-piece spinal orthosis for a minimum of 1 year following the anterior fusion.

Hemimyelocele

Hemimyelocele is a rare anomaly in which the spinal cord is divided into two sections cephalad to the open mylomeningocele.[28] One-half develops as normal spinal cord within a dural sheath, while the other half develops as a unilateral myelomeningocele. The limb innervated by the intact spinal cord develops normally. The retention of normal unilateral sacral innervation permits normal bladder and bowel function. The affected limb is short. Varying levels of innervation may result in a flail extremity or more commonly a limb with a flexion-adduction contracture at the hip, hyperextension of the knee, and a varus deformity of the foot. The condition is always associated with hemivertebrae and a thoracolumbar or lumbar congenital scoliosis (Fig. 9-35). Since this scoliosis progresses rapidly, a localized posterior fusion is performed early in the first decade of life. Diastematomyelia is frequently associated with the division of the cord and may require excision.

HIP DEFORMITY IN MYELOMENINGOCELE

Muscle imbalance, the primary cause of hip disorders in myelomeningocele, produces abnormal pressure across the immature hip joint. This leads to secondary bony deformity of the proximal femur and acetabulum which in turn may lead to subluxation or dislocation. Adaptive osseous deformity develops only after fixed muscles and soft tissues have been present for a significant lenght of time (Fig. 9-36).[19]

Fetal coxa valga persists due to muscle imbalance and limited weight-bearing. The abnormal mechanical pressure across the growth plate of the proximal femur and lateral acetabulum causes secondary deformity. The acetabulum becomes increasingly deficient in relation to the enlarging femoral head because the pelvis lacks the dynamic muscle force necessary both to rotate the acetabulum and to stimulate its peripheral growth centers.

Goals

Before establishing present and future goals, the level of paralysis and ambulatory poten-

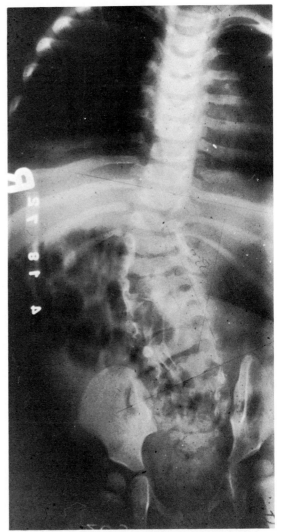

FIG. 9-35. Hemimyelocele is a rare spinal anomaly. Progressive congenital lumbar scoliosis and normal urologic function are common.

tial, as well as other musculoskeletal deformities, must be considered. Anti-gravity strength in the quadriceps muscles is necessary for successful, long-term ambulation.[37] The purpose of surgery is to correct the fixed deformity so that the child can stand with a stable posture. Postoperative morbidity is reduced and rehabilitation is easier when the deformity and muscle imbalance are completely corrected with one operation. Frequently hip surgery can be combined with other corrective procedures.

In the newborn with myelomeningocele,

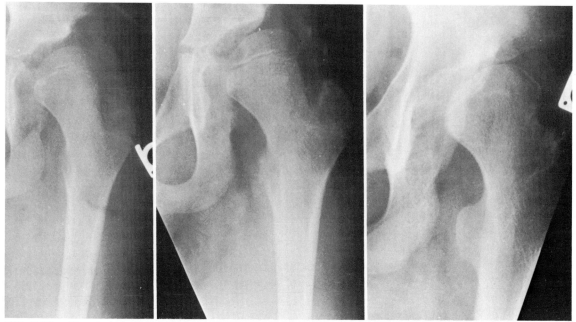

FIG. 9-36. Muscle imbalance resulting from a midlumbar level lesion causes progressive subluxation in this adolescent. Radiographs were obtained at 2-year intervals.

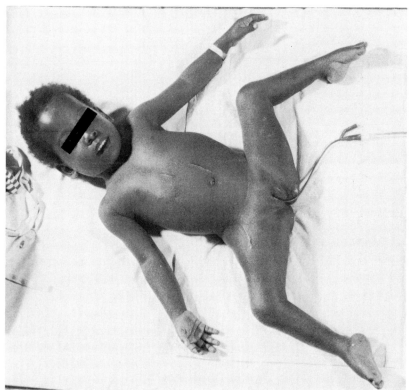

FIG. 9-37. This position allows the iliopsoas to shorten. When the hip is properly aligned, the muscle becomes a dislocating force.

the femoral head and acetabulum usually develop normally. The hip that is dislocated or dislocatable usually can be reduced. The patient may have to lie in the prone position with the hips in abduction during the primary care of the myelomeningocele sac. Before instituting orthotic splints to control abduction and rotation, it may be necessary to correct a fixed deformity with limited soft-tissue surgery.

By 1 year of age the permanent amount of loss of motor power can be determined.[7] The patient's ambulatory potential is apparent by 2 years of age. It may be necessary to perform additional soft-tissue surgery, including tendon transfer, to achieve concentric hip reduction in the young child. Surgical correction of secondary osseous deformity should be delayed until the patient nears 3 years of age. In the older child, paralytic scoliosis and concomitant pelvic obliquity may compromise the end result of treatment of hip dysplasia.

Flail Hip

Patients without innervation below T12 have no active muscles crossing the hip joint. At birth, the hip is usually either in joint or reducible by flexion, a maneuver which eliminates the dislocating effect of the iliopsoas. Subluxation or dislocation may develop in an infant who is allowed to assume a frog-leg posture (Fig. 9-37). When these hips are in flexion, they are stable, but during stance they dislocate anteriorly because the iliopsoas is shortened. Other young children who assume a windblown, recumbent posture place the hip at risk in a fixed position of adduction and internal rotation. Subsequently, by age 3, concomitant suprapelvic obliquity in the form of scoliosis becomes a major problem (Fig. 9-38).

Therefore, emphasis is placed primarily on the prevention of asymmetrical hip deformity in children who will become adult wheelchair ambulators. In infancy a Batchelor-type splint places the hips in the proper abduction and internal rotation position.[56,67] In the young child a trunk-extremity positional orthosis (Fig. 9-3) and physical therapy prevent hip-flexion and fascia-lata contractures. Although the child may attempt to walk by age 2 or 3 with long leg braces with a pelvic band, it is not realistic to expect these patients to maintain long-term ambulation.

Patients who have assumed a frog-leg posture may require radical soft-tissue releases about the hips before a trial with braces can be considered.[58] A lateral incision is made to place the surgical scar in a nondeforming plane. The short lateral rotators, posterior hip capsule, the fascia lata overlying the glutei as well as the psoas, rectus femoris, and tensor fascia lata are released. For 4 weeks postoperatively the patient lies in a prone position on a Bradford frame with the hips held in extension, adduction, and medial rotation.

Despite treatment, marked subluxation or dislocation may develop, which will lead to pelvic obliquity and its sequelae. Even in the young child who has had Ober-type fascial and tendon releases for hip subluxation, deformity will recur unless trunk and extremity orthoses are used immediately after cast removal. The decision to reduce a dislocated hip is made more difficult by the fact that potential loss of motion and recurrence of deformity with growth are recognized complications. Femoral head resection is not indicated because the patient may rapidly develop heterotopic bone with resulting loss of motion (Fig. 9-39) or pelvic obliquity. A child with flail hips is considered a future adult wheelchair ambulator, and loss of flexion sufficient to allow sitting can be catastrophic to long-term function.

The Hip at Risk

Hip instability develops when the flexor–adductor group overpowers the weak abductor–extensor muscles. When the dynamic deforming force is removed or weakened, muscle balance and thus permanent correction are achieved. During the first 18 months of life, braces help to obtain and maintain a concentric reduction. Subluxable and dislocatable hips can be reduced by flexing the hip to decrease iliopsoas tension. Reduction is maintained in infancy by using an abduction orthosis that places the hips in extension and medial and internal rotation, which stretches the iliopsoas to its greatest extent, yet allows motion. A trunk-extremity orthosis with a simple hip hinge can also be locked in a similar position and is introduced at age 1. Soft-tissue contractures are prevented by allowing time out of the orthosis for social stimulation and physical therapy.

During the second year of life when the

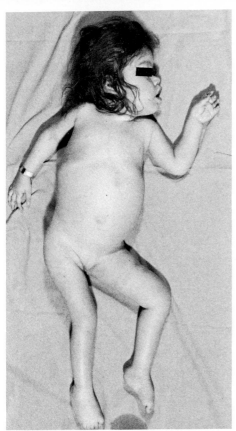

FIG. 9-38. A patient with a thoracic level myelomeningocele. The lumbar scoliosis creates a pelvic obliquity placing the right hip at risk.

FIG. 9-39. Repeated soft-tissue procedures may result in loss of motion. Attempts to regain hip motion through resection of the femoral head result in an iatrogenic arthrodesis. Motion was regained by resection of the proximal one-third of the femur combined with interposition of soft tissue.

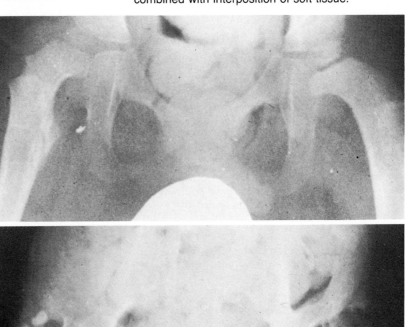

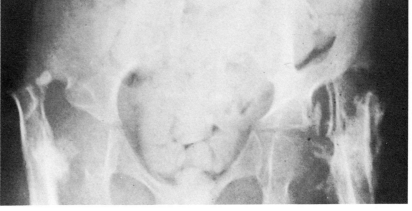

patient begins to stand, additional stress is placed on the hips. Before correcting a persistent instability, an arthrography (Fig. 9-40) is performed to determine femoral head and acetabular development. If a deficiency is demonstrated in patients with antigravity quadriceps strength, an adductor tenotomy and a Mustard iliopsoas transfer combined with capsular resection and plication may be required and can be performed at the same time.[61] Postoperatively, bilateral long leg hip spica casts are used, and physical therapy is begun 4 weeks after surgery. After age 3, correction of bony deformities or the proximal femur may require osteotomies, which are performed bilaterally to avoid creation of limb-length inequality. Acetabuloplasty for dysplasia may be performed at the same time as muscle transfers (Fig. 9-41). The Pemberton osteotomy can be performed in children over 18 months of age.[58] The Chiari osteotomy is indicated for more pronounced acetabular dysplasia and is appropriate after age 4. A teratogenic, hypoplastic, acetabulum, visualized on an arthrogram, is a contraindication to performing established forms of acetabuloplasties. Other soft-tissue procedures include transfer of the adductors to the ischium to counteract recurrent flexion-adduction contractures in patients with L3-5 innervation,

and transfer of the origin of the external oblique to the greater trochanter.[48,84] I have had no personal experience with either of these procedures. They generally are done in combination with other muscle transfers.

The Dislocated Hip

Hip dislocation is most common in the neonate who has a muscle imbalance caused by unopposed hip adductors, iliopsoas, and quadriceps muscles. The iliopsoas blocks reduction by crossing the medial aspect of the hip joint. Imbalanced muscle activity may alter the shape of the proximal femur and result in an increased coxa valga.

After the myelomeningocele sac has been repaired and shunting has been done, closed reduction can be performed when the neonate's hip is flexed and the iliopsoas is relaxes. Recalcitrant hip dislocation in the infant can be corrected by open adductor tenotomy, transfer of the iliopsoas to the anterior hip capsule, and medial hip capsulorraphy.[30] Postoperatively, abduction is accomplished initially with a hip spica cast and later by a trunk-extremity positional orthosis. Patients with strong bilateral quadriceps will benefit from an iliopsoas transfer performed during

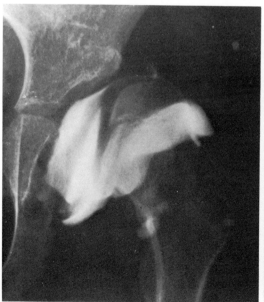 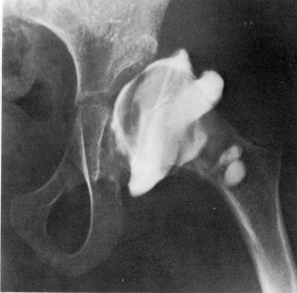

FIG. 9-40. Arthrography is required in the young patient to determine concentricity of reduction and to establish the potential lateral acetabular structure.

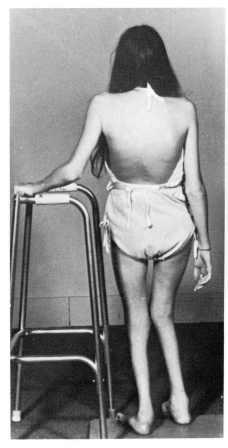
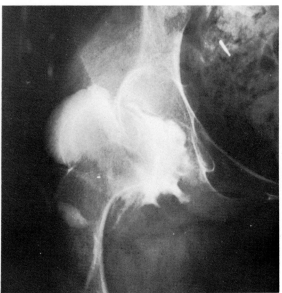

FIG. 9-41. An adolescent with lower level lumbar function whose painful dislocation was corrected by femoral varus osteotomy, Chiari osteotomy, and iliopsoas transfer.

their second year of life. A prerequisite for surgery is antigravity strength of the sartorius and rectus femoris, because they must serve as principle hip flexors following iliopsoas transfer. Muscle balance is achieved by weakening the hip flexors and thus preventing progressive flexion deformity. The Mustard technique, which has the advantage of being technically easier to perform than the Sharrard[8,14,31,61,74] procedure, also retains the viability of the iliacus muscle. The transfer is combined with formal open reduction and resection of the redundant capsule, which is then plicated. A varus osteotomy with femoral shortening may also be required at the time of soft-tissue surgery. Problems associated with iliopsoas transfer have resulted from failing to attain concentric reduction, not recognizing capsular laxity, and underestimating the need for thorough open adductor tenotomy at the time of the muscle balancing procedure.[12,72] The entire hip deformity must be corrected, because partial correction can lead

to recurrence. In patients over 4 years of age, acetabular insufficiency and pelvic obliquity may be encountered. A Heyman shelf arthroplasty may be performed in patients over age 3.[31] The Chiari medial displacement osteotomy provides greater lateral coverage, but the results may be compromised if there is insufficient anteroposterior acetabular development. Canale, however, reports that this procedure improves the quality of gait, corrects pelvic obliquity, and makes bracing easier.[11]

When residual pelvic obliquity persists despite attempts at correction and spinal arthrodesis for scoliosis, an ingenious double-pelvic osteotomy rotates the high-riding acetabulum into a more normal relationship with the femoral head.[46] In this procedure, which was developed by Lindseth, the ilium is divided adjacent to the sacroiliac joint and a trapezoid of bone is removed from the low side and seated in the high-side osteotomy (Fig. 9-42), thereby forcing the high side of the ace-

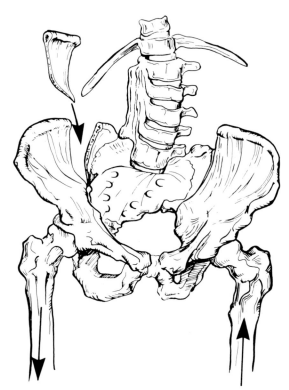

FIG. 9-42. Residual pelvic obliquity can be improved by bilateral posterior iliac osteotomy. (Lindseth RE: Posterior iliac osteotomy for fixed pelvic obliquity. J Bone Joint Surg 60A:17, 1978)

tabulum downward and away from the sacrum.[46]

Reflex Spasticity

Isolated reflex motor activity can be noted in the muscles that are innervated by the sacral segments, particularly the hip external rotators and extensors. Management by transfer or tenotomy has proven unsatisfactory because of a high rate of recurring deformity. Formal anterior sacral rhizotomy has been used successfully in selected patients from Newington Children's Hospital who have no functional lower-extremity motor power. No recurrence has been noted during a 3-year follow-up.

MALALIGNMENT OF THE KNEE IN MYELOMENINGOCELE

Proper knee alignment is essential in walking. Recurrent knee flexion, extension con-

tracture, or angular malalignment jeopardize the ambulatory ability of the child.

Flexion contractures represent the most common problem. There is rarely a fixed deformity at birth, but a contracture may develop later, either because of reflex hamstring activity or because of prolonged use of a wheelchair. Wheelchair patients have a flaccid knee musculature with an associated hip flexion contracture. It is difficult to brace a knee flexion contracture which is greater than 20° (Fig. 9-43A, B, and C). When the deformity exceeds 30°, ambulation is impossible. Deformities greater than 40° can be expected to progress rapidly. Correction of a concomitant hip flexion contracture should be performed when the knee flexion contracture is released. Appropriate orthoses are required to maintain the correction. Lindseth reported 50 patients with knee flexion contractures greater than 10°.[47] Only 5 of these were functional ambulators.

Reflex hamstring activity is most frequently noted in patients with thoracolumbar lesions. The most effective long-term treatment is a formal Eggers' transfer of the offending hamstrings to the femoral condyles. Simple tenotomies can be expected to result in recurrence of the deformity. Sharrard recommends an anterior transfer of the hamstrings to the patella, when the quadriceps is paretic. Abraham noted that the effectiveness of the correction can be correlated with the strength of the quadriceps.[1] A supracondylar extension osteotomy performed through the junction of the metaphysis and diaphysis can be used when patients are near skeletal maturity (Fig. 9-43C). Impacting the smaller diaphyseal shaft into the metaphysis creates a stable situation and permits the use of a long leg cast for immobilization.

Hyperextension due to unopposed quadriceps activity is less common (Fig. 9-44) and rarely requires surgical correction. When there is 40° of knee flexion, a knee–ankle–foot orthosis should be used because of the need to maintain optimal quadriceps function in potential ambulators. Placing the ankle joint component of the orthosis in a few degrees of dorsiflexion causes the knee to assume a position of slight flexion. Formal quadricepsplasty, required in cases with fixed recurvatum, should be performed after the age of 6 months. Lindseth reported that only 3 of

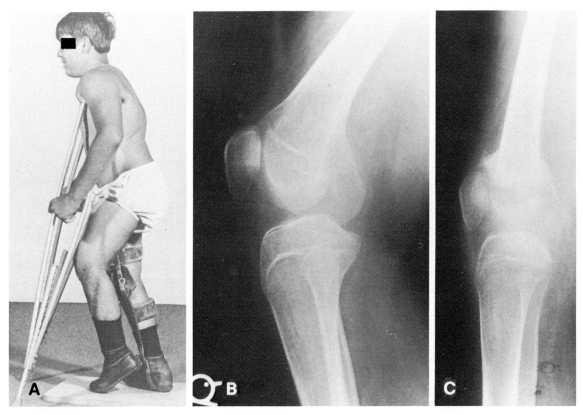

FIG. 9-43. (*A and B*) Progressive knee flexion contracture eventually precluded use of a long leg brace, forcing abandonment of this adolescent's reciprocal four-point gait. (*C*) Extension and impaction of the smaller diaphysis into the metaphysis creates a stable osteotomy.

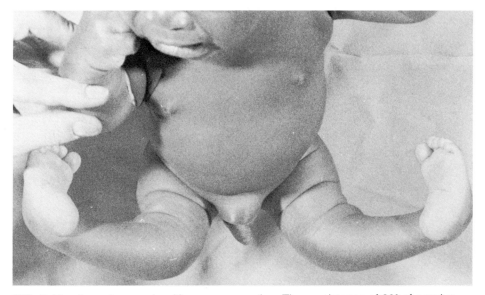

FIG. 9-44. A newborn male with genu recurvation. The persistence of 30° of passive knee flexion permitted this boy to eventually use standard braces in dveloping a reciprocal gait pattern.

16 patients with hyperextension contractures remained functional ambulators.[47]

Congenital dislocated patella also may occur in patients with extension contractures. This problem is detected by a knee arthrogram. Failure to recognize it could lead to the creation of a universal knee joint when passive range-of-motion exercises overstretch the collateral ligaments.

Valgus deformity of the knee in a younger child is generally due to contracture of the iliotibial band in the nonambulator, or may be seen following malalignment of the femur secondary to fracture (Fig. 9-45). When contracture of the iliotibial band is the cause, surgical release of the lateral fascial structures will restore the normal arc of movement to the knee. For malalignment of the femur, a rotational osteotomy may be necessary. Genu valgum may develop in the older ambulatory child when the weight-line passes lateral to the knee joint during stance. The medial knee ligaments become overstretched and eventually oseous deformity is noted. To correct this deformity in adolescents, an impaction type of supracondylar osteotomy has proven satisfactory in my experience.

ANKLE VALGUS

Evaluation of patients with apparent hindfoot valgus must include a weight-bearing, anteroposterior rotentgenogram of the ankle joint. When patients who stand in lower-extremity orthoses transfer the weight-line medial to the axis of the os calcis, medial malleolar skin breakdown and considerable difficulty in orthotic control can be anticipated (Fig. 9-46). Ankle instability may actually increase when the underlying ankle valgus is not recognized, and a subtalar arthrodesis is performed.

Relative shortening of the figula results in a valgus deformity and also is frequently associated with lateral tibial torsion and genu valgum.[57] The shortening occurs most commonly in patients with paralysis of the soleus muscle who have greater than 20° of dorsiflexion. Treatment varies with the age of the child. Dias recommends a tenodesis of the tendo calcaneus to the fibula in patients under age 8.[16] Moore has reported that patients ages 8 to 12 benefit from a reversible epiphysiodesis of the medial distal tibial epiphysis, using staples (Fig. 9-47).[60] A supramalleolar closing wedge osteotomy may be performed in patients who are near skeletal maturation (Fig. 9-48).[79] The latter technique may also correct persistent equinus deformity in the adolescent.

THE FOOT

Most myelomeningocele infants have foot deformities.[77] The extrinsic and intrinsic muscles of the foot and ankle are innervated by the lower lumbar and sacral roots, which are the neurologic levels most commonly involved in myelomeningocele. Muscle imbalance is the primary cause of foot deformity, with intra- and extrauterine positions adapted by the foot often being a secondary cause.

The treatment objective is to obtain plantigrade, braceable feet when the child begins to stand, at about 18 months of age (Fig. 9-49A,B,C).[20] Muscle balance must be obtained to avoid recurrence or development of a secondary iatrogenic deformity.

The feet are small relative to the size of the child and become even more disproportionately diminutive, since foot growth does not parallel the increasing weight and size of the child. The insensate feet therefore have an increased load in relation to their area of weight-bearing. Vasomotor instability, diminished amounts of subcutaneous tissue, as well as increased capsular fibrosis, also make management difficult. Although a high incidence of associated lower-extremity deformities at the hip and knee may make treatment of the foot more difficult, it should not delay the beginning of management.

Failure to achieve a plantigrade position in an anesthetic foot can lead to the development of pressure sores (Fig. 9-50), secondary cellulitis, or osteomyelitis, with the possible need to resect a ray or even amputate the foot.

Ideal management is initiated in the newborn nursery with a series of manipulations and applications of serial plaster casts. The goal is to achieve the maximum possible correction at this time. Treatment consists of manipulating the foot daily to obtain the correction, and applying well-padded casts daily to maintain the correction.

Before manipulating the foot, the distal tibia of the involved extremity is fixed by the orthopaedist's hand and prolonged gentle traction is applied to the forefoot to stretch the small joint capsules. When the larger foot

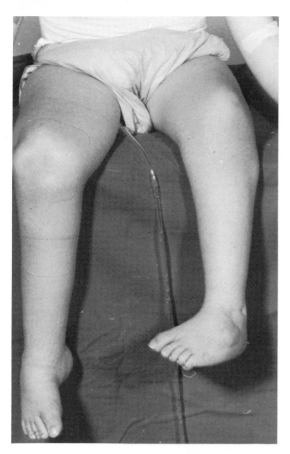

FIG. 9-45. Progressive valgus, following malunion of femoral fracture, places the patella in jeopardy and may result in dislocation. Corrective diaphyseal osteotomy and patellar realignment were performed with the patient retaining 100 degrees' knee flexion. The dynamic inversion of the contralateral foot was corrected by transfer of the tibialis anterior to the heel.

FIG. 9-46. This foot position precludes the lateral longitudinal arch from assuming its rightful share of weight-bearing. Enlarging the varus-producing T-strap keeps skin pressure below the critical level of shearing.

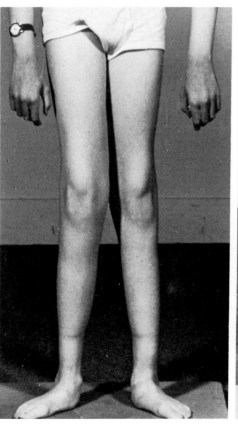

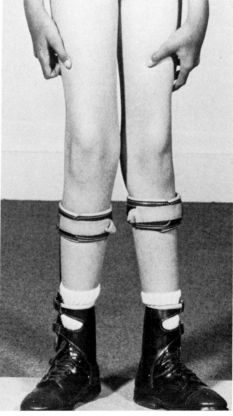

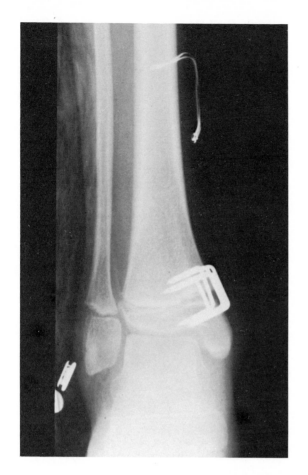

is manipulated, it may be possible to apply traction to the forefoot against the manually-held hindfoot. Careful application of tincture of benzoin and Webril assist in maintaining passive correction. As an example, forefoot correction of an equinovarus deformity can be maintained by passing Webril from the dorsum of the forefoot medially toward and across the plantar surface and encircling the metatarsal heads and toes so as to draw them into pronation and eversion. Similarly, the Webril can be passed up the lateral side of the ankle and lower extremity to assist in holding the correction of the hindfoot varus deformity. The well-padded cast is never used to increase the degree of correction obtained under direct vision. Wedging casts are contraindicated in anesthetic feet. Holding plasters must be used until the foot becomes large enough that a shoe can be worn and an appropriate brace can be used. The original deformity would promptly recur if casting or bracing were abandoned before surgical correction was achieved.

FIG. 9-47. This intermediate age group may benefit from the use of multiple medial staples.

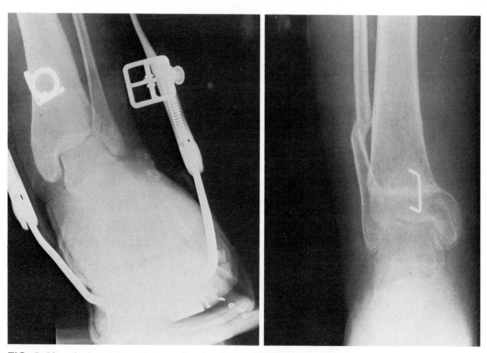

FIG. 9-48. A decubitus ulcer under the first metatarsal head is a common reason for performing the closing supramalleolar wedge osteotomy in adolescents.

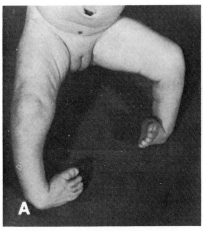
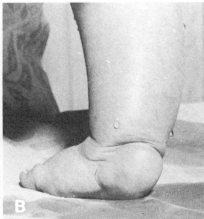
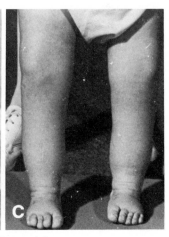

FIG. 9-49. (*A*) Talipes equinovarus foot deformity. (*B*) At 1 year of age following serial casts, sufficient stretching of skin and neurovascular structures permits (*C*) final surgical correction.

In the younger child, foot surgery is limited to soft-tissue procedures, which must be preceded by serial casts. While the foot is in the cast, the soft tissues are stretched to avoid the postoperative compromise of skin viability or neurovascular function. It is technically difficult to perform surgery before the child is 9 months old because of the diminutive size of the osseocartilaginous structures, the narrowness of the joints, and the thickness of the joint capsules. In some cases, tendon lengthenings or tenotomies may need to be done when the capsular ligaments are released. Skin incisions for this radical capsular surgery are closed with an interrupted suture followed by application of a loosely-applied, soft, bulky dressing with a posterior long leg plaster splint. This is used for 2 to 3 days before a well-padded, long leg cast is applied. This cast must extend beyond the visualized anesthetic toes.

The correction of bony deformities is necessary before tendon transfers can be performed. Transfers can be performed to create neuromuscular balance but should be delayed until neurologic function is stabilized, at approximately 1 year of age.[7] Accurate preoperative and faradic evaluation is essential in the selection of the appropriate transfer. The advantage of the transfer, effective removal of an unopposed deforming force, must be balanced against the disadvantage, the loss of original function. Transfers crossing the ankle joint should pass through subcutaneous tissue to avoid becoming adherent to the ankle retinaculum. The extremities are supported in long leg casts for 4 to 5 weeks postoperatively. Then appropriate braces are used.

Foot Surgery in Older Age Groups

Osseous surgery is generally limited to ambulatory patients whose foot length is approaching adult size. These patients require a stable plantigrade foot with good weight distribution between the hindfoot and forefoot during stance and walking (Fig. 9-51). Insensateness and the smallness of the foot, as well as vascular compromise and reflex spasticity, are additional considerations in planning surgical correction. The foot width and length at the conclusion of the surgical correction may determine whether a cosmetically acceptable plastic orthosis can be worn within the shoe or whether more traditional bracing and shoeing will be required. All shoes should have cushioned soles.

Structural bony deformity must be corrected before tendon transfers can be performed. Surgical procedures that do not include arthrodesis may prevent excessive foot shortening and permit joint motion and proprioception. An appropriate calcaneal osteotomy can correct hindfoot calcaneus, varus, or valgus deformity. Metatarsal osteotomies permit correction of most forefoot deformities and may be combined with a calcaneal osteotomy. The limited experience at Newington

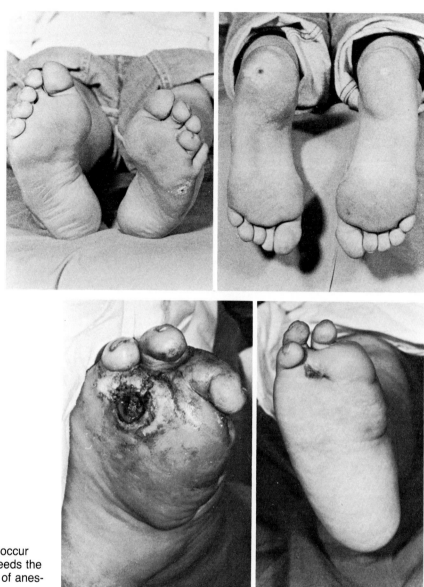

FIG. 9-50. Plantar ulcers occur when the activity level exceeds the weight-bearing capabilities of anesthetic adolescent feet.

Children's Hospital with triple arthrodesis performed for low-level lumbar myelomeningocele patients suggests that satisfactory long-term plantigrade feet can be obtained.

Management of Specific Foot Deformities

EQUINOVARUS DEFORMITY

Equinovarus deformity, the most common foot deformity in these patients, results from an imbalance of the paralyzed dorsiflexors and peroneus muscles and of the active tibialis anterior and posterior muscles (Fig. 9-52A and B).[77,81] This imbalance may cause a contracture of the triceps surae. Beginning in the newborn period, serial manipulations are performed and plaster casts are applied. When the foot is large enough and before surgical correction is performed, a short leg brace, with a T-strap to control the varus, may be used. My surgical method includes capsulotomies of the posterior ankle, subtalar, and talonavicular joints through a posteromedial inci-

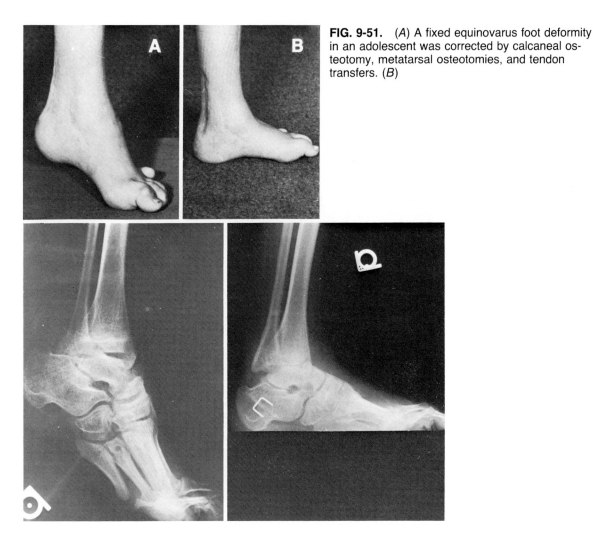

FIG. 9-51. (*A*) A fixed equinovarus foot deformity in an adolescent was corrected by calcaneal osteotomy, metatarsal osteotomies, and tendon transfers. (*B*)

sion. Lengthening of the tendo Achillis, tibialis posterior, and long toe flexor tendons may be required.

The tibialis anterior may be transferred laterally and inserted into the third cuneiform through a separate longitudinal dorsal incision.

Only after muscle balance has been achieved can a talectomy be performed in the 2- to 3-year-old child who has had an ineffective posteromedial release or in a younger patient who has a rigid foot similar to that associated with arthrogryposis.[59] Through an anterolateral approach, the entire bone can be removed as a single structure. A posterior capsulotomy is necessary to allow for satisfactory displacement of the foot. A heel-cord lengthening is performed through a short an-

cillary posterior incision. It is sometimes necessary to remove the navicula in order to achieve sufficient posterior displacement of the foot. Sherk recommends that a roentgenogram be obtained in the operating room to verify the removal of the entire bone.[80] He also noted the need to revise the lateral malleolus in some cases in order to permit the os calcis to seat properly.

EQUINUS DEFORMITY

Equinus deformity can either result in a flail foot because of the forces of gravity or in an extremity that retains unopposed reflex activity of the triceps surae, long toe flexors, and intrinsic muscles.

Paralytic equinus deformity can be pre-

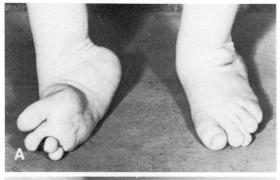

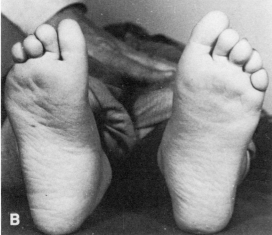

FIG. 9-52. (A) Satisfactory bracing can be accomplished only when the foot can be made plantigrade. (B) Lengthening of the tibialis posterior and lateral transfer of the tibialis anterior accomplish this limited objective.

vented. Repeated manipulations are performed in infants and later, when the child can wear shoes, a brace with a drop-foot lock is used. Although weight-bearing decreases the possibility of recurrence, if a mild to moderate deformity does recur, it can be corrected by carefully stretching the entire foot.

Equinus deformity exceeding 40° may require a percutaneous tenotomy of the tendo Achillis or an open tenotomy of the tendo Achillis and long toe flexor tendon. A supplementary procedure, posterior ankle capsulotomy, and division of the posterior tibial-fibular syndesmosis may need to be done. When the ankle equinus deformity is corrected in a young child, a severe toe flexion contracture may occur. This makes the tips of the toes vulnerable to the development of pressure sores unless the individual long toe flexor tendons

are divided at the level of the proximal phalanx.

Reflex equinus posture is more difficult to manage and recurrences are frequent. Radical excision of the tendo Achillis and tendons of the long toe flexors can be performed during the second year but repeated procedures may be necessary. Later in childhood, plantar denervation, accompanied by the transfer of the long toe flexor tendons through the interosseous membrane to the midline dorsum of the foot, may be required.

EQUINOVALGUS DEFORMITY

Equinovalgus deformity results from overactivity of the peroneus muscles and a shortened tendo Achillis (Fig. 9-53). In the newborn, management is similar to that described for equinovarus deformity, and surgery is delayed until after age 1. Then the peroneus longus is transferred to replace the paretic tibialis posterior. The peroneus longus is divided at the cuboid groove and its distal stump anastomosed to the freed peroneus brevis. A second incision lateral to the tendo Achillis allows the heel cord to be lengthened and the peroneus longus to be advanced into this field. From an incision based over the navicula, a hemostat is passed through the tendon sheath of the tibialis posterior and its tip is palpated above the ankle retinaculum where a short, fourth incision is made. The peroneus longus is passed through a subcutaneous tunnel deep to the tendo Achillis and is guided through the tibialis posterior tunnel into the navicular insertion of that muscle. The transfer is inserted with the foot inverted. The stump of the peroneus longus is attached to the peroneus brevis. After surgery a long leg cast and then a drop-lock brace with a T-strap are used to prevent recurrence of the valgus deformity.

Valgus deformity of the hindfoot may persist in older children. Extra-articular subtalar arthrodesis, described by Dennyson, is the procedure of choice to correct this deformity.[15] He uses cancellous grafts and metallic internal fixation. Both the Grice and Batchelor procedures have a higher rate of nonunion in myelomeningocele feet than in other foot deformities. A medial displacement calcaneal osteotomy may be required to place the heel pad beneath the weight-bearing limb axis for severe residual valgus deformity.

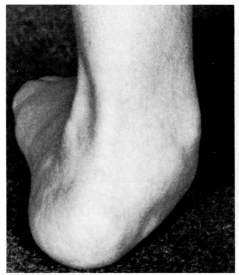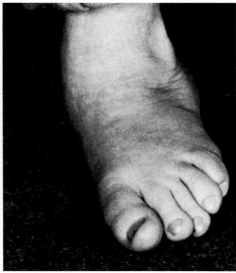

FIG. 9-53. The shortened tendo Achillis can be masked by a lateral calcaneal subluxation.

CALCANEUS DEFORMITY

This uncommon deformity results from unopposed function of the ankle and toe dorsiflexors (Fig. 9-54). The newborn is treated with serial manipulations and casts. Then at 1 year of age transfer of the tibialis anterior and peroneus tertius is performed through the interosseous membrane to the os calcis. Additional tenotomies of the long toe extensors and occasionally capsulotomy of the anterior joint may be necessary. These procedures place the foot in enough plantar flexion so that the transfer can be sutured under tension adequate to retain function. A heel-cord shortening may be required. The segment of the tendo Achillis that remains attached to the os calcis can be sutured to the tendon transfer. Following the use of long leg cast, bracing is required, which limits ankle dorsiflexion to 10° to 15°.

CONGENITAL CONVEX PES VALGUS

This deformity (Fig. 9-55) defies manipulations and casts and thus requires surgical correction. It is caused by strong evertors and dorsiflexors of the foot that overpower the paretic tibialis posterior.[27] A one-stage procedure that combines soft-tissue releases and tendon transfers has given satisfactory long-term results.[13,20]

Since correction will result in redundancy

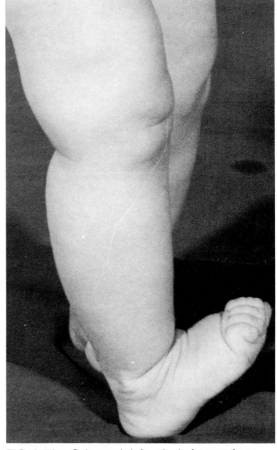

FIG. 9-54. Calcaneal deformity is frequently accompanied by cock-up toe deformities.

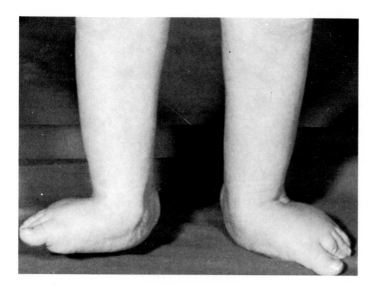

FIG. 9-55. The Persian slipper foot deformity is the result of weakness of the tibialis posterior. Correction requires bony realignment and achievement of muscle balance.

in the medial soft tissues, the majority of the surgery is performed through a posteromedial incision. Capsulotomies of the posterior ankle and anterior and posterior subtalar and talonavicular joints are accomplished. The tibialis anterior is detached for later transfer to the talar neck.[29] Delaying the lengthening of the tendo Achillis until all other soft-tissue correction has been performed permits the surgeon good control of the hindfoot during the capsular surgery. Capsulotomies of the subluxed or dislocated calcaneocuboid joint and the lateral aspect of the subtalar joint can be made through a short lateral incision. The peroneus longus is divided at its cuboid groove, and its distal stump is attached to the freed peroneus brevis. The peroneus longus transfer is performed as previously described for equinovalgus correction. A short dorsal longitudinal incision is made to allow division of the peroneus tertius and long toe extensor tendons. Three Kirschner wires provide fixation. The first pin, drilled from the plantar surface of the foot into the tibia, corrects both equinus and valgus deformities of the hindfoot. Under direct vision, a second pin is passed through the talonavicular joint to correct forefoot eversion, while the third pin, drilled through the calcaneocuboid joint, functions to reduce pronation. A long leg cast is maintained for a minimum of 4 months. Then the patient may resume ambulation with a carefully molded University of California at Berkeley (UC-BL) arch support.[41]

TOE DEFORMITIES

Tenodesis of the flexor hallucis longus to the plantar aspect of the first phalanx affords excellent correction of clawing of the hallux in these children.[78] A Girdlestone–Taylor tendon transfer can be used to correct the lateral clawed toes that develop in children under the age of 10.[83] Adolescents benefit from a Jones operation for clawing of the toes.

AMPUTATION

Amputation should be considered for a foot with precarious skin coverage that resulted from repeated surgical insults or for one with recurrent osteomyelitis and subsequent bone destruction (Fig. 9-56). Problems are particularly common among good walkers whose low-level deficit of motor function enables them to place greater stress on their insensate feet. A carefully performed Syme's amputation and the use of a well-fitted Syme's prosthesis (Fig. 9-57) affords these patients a much more satisfactory level of function than continued desultory efforts at surgical orthotic control of their chronic problem.

FRACTURES

In myelomeningocele patients the tibia and femur are smaller in diameter than those of a normal child. Rális found that the total area of cortical bone, its thickness, number of hav-

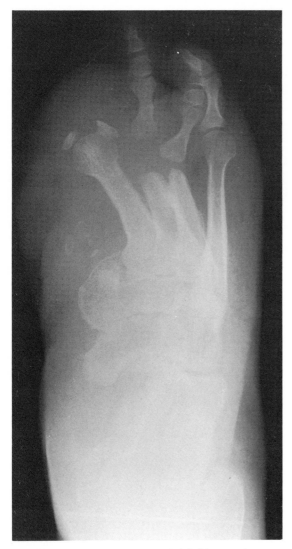

FIG. 9-56. Following repeated debridement for osteomyelitis, there is sufficient loss of forefoot architecture to make long-term weight-bearing of this foot unrealistic. Cosmetic and functional improvement can be obtained by amputation and prosthetic usage.

ing surgery also is associated with an increased incidence of fracture. Fractures also are more common in paralyzed limbs than in extremities that retain active muscle function.

Generally these fractures occur with no history of trauma.[25] Irritability and swelling, redness and warmth of the limb are early signs. The suspected diagnosis is confirmed radiologically. Figure 9-58 demonstrates that the fractures usually occur close to the hip or knee joint.

The remarkable ability of these fractures to heal rapidly (Fig. 9-59) underlines the need for conservative closed methods of treatment. Therefore, relative immobilization is the essential ingredient required for healing. The goal remains to maintain functional alignment and rotation so that the patient's ability to stand and walk with braces is not compromised. There is a great need for individualization in the total care of these patients.

Fractures in infants are uncommon, but if they do occur, treatment is by immobilization with a well-padded plaster cast for 1 to 2 weeks. Fractures near the knee which are satisfactorily aligned may be treated by wrapping the limb with a bulky dressing of sheet wadding or similar material. Fractures in older children are treated in the same way or with a pillow splint. When swelling has diminished, weight-bearing in braces should be permitted as soon as possible. However, if displacement, angulation, or rotation develop with the use of braces, the deformity should be corrected and a well-padded plaster cast considered.

Patients are particularly vulnerable to fracture after cast immobilization has been discontinued. Following any major surgical procedure in the lower extremities which requires a long leg cast, it is recommended that both extremities be placed in a hip spica cast so that standing on a tilt-table is possible. When the cast is removed, special nursing care is necessary. For example, two people are needed to turn the child until sufficient joint motion has returned. Because these children are considered potential walkers, rotational, angular, and longitudinal deformities should be avoided when the fracture has healed. The result should be a well-healed bone in good position so that the child has as much function following the fracture as he had before injury.

ersian systems, and number of large remodeling cavities were diminished.[71] However, the total amount of osteoid tissue in bone was increased. He felt that this delay in mineralization could lead to the softening of new bone matrix, and combined with diminished total bone mass, could be responsible for the frequency of fractures in the metaphyseal and subepiphyseal regions. Disuse atrophy resulting from prolonged immobilization follow-

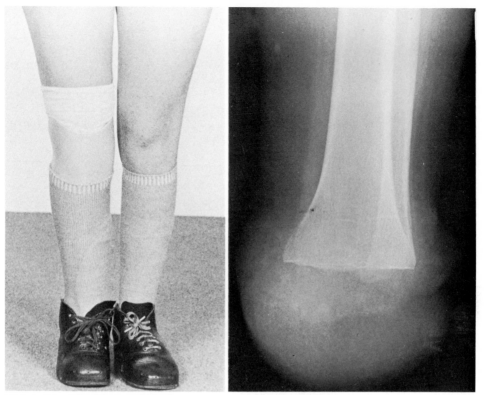

FIG. 9-57. This illustrates the bony stump and prosthetic fitting.

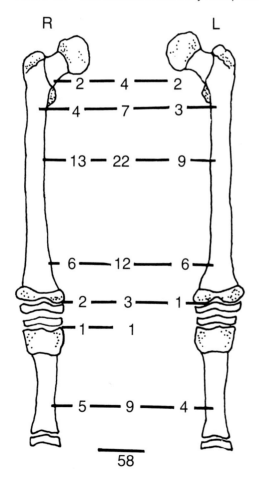

58

FIG. 9-58. Lower extremity fractures. All fractures healed using closed methods of treatment. (Drennan JC, Freehafer AA: Fractures of the lower extremities in paraplegic children. Clin Orthop 77:211, 1971)

OPHTHALMOLOGIC PROBLEMS

Strabismus occurs in one half of myelomeningocele patients and is associated with the presence of hydrocephalus and the ascending level of the spinal lesion. Seventy-one percent of patients with hydrocephalus and thoracic myelomeningocele have strabismus, whereas only 14% of those without hydrocephalus and with a sacral level lesion have strabismus. *Strabismus prevents patients from fusing images from both eyes in the visual cortex. Thus, these patients do not develop normal depth perception and they may have difficulty with ambulation. Severe defects in visual acuity, such as optic atrophy, have diminished because of adequate current shunt management. However, a high frequency of refraction abnormalities, namely astigmatism, are found.

---

*Wheeler MR: Personal communication.

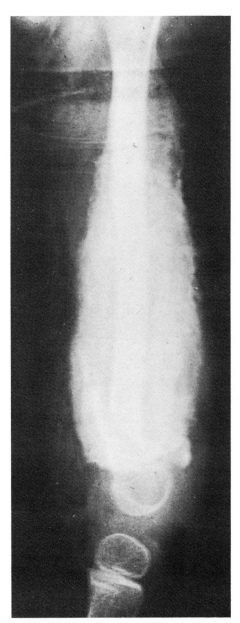

FIG. 9-59. Exuberant callus frequently is noted in the young patient with a long bone fracture.

A special variety of strabismus, A-pattern strabismus, occurs in which the deviation is more divergent when looking down than when looking up. This develops in both convergent and divergent strabismus and is due to over-action of the superior oblique muscles. The A-pattern generally is associated with patients who have difficulty with ambulation.

The eye muscle dysfunction alters attempts at visual fusion as the eyes shift position, since the angle of deviation differs in upward and downward gaze. Early correction by eye muscle surgery and the use of corrective lenses are essential.

REFERENCES

1. Abraham E, Verinder DGR, Sharrard WJW: The treatment of flexion contracture of the knee in myelomeningocele. J Bone Joint Surg 59B:433, 1977
2. Allen BL Jr, Ferguson RL: The operative treatment of myelomeningocele spinal deformity—1979. Orthop Clin North Am 10(4):845, 1979
3. Banta JV: Fifteen year review of myelodysplasia. New Orleans, American Academy of Orthopaedic Surgeons Meeting, 1976
4. Banta, JV, Hamada JS: Natural history of the kyphotic deformity in myelomeningocele. In Proceedings of The Western Orthopedic Association, J Bone Joint Surg 58A:279, 1976
5. Bonnett C, Brown JC, Perry J: Evolution of treatment of paralytic scoliosis at Rancho Los Amigos Hospital. J Bone Joint Surg 57:206, 1975
6. Brock DJ, Sutcliffe RG: Alphafetoprotein in the antenatal diagnosis of anencephaly and spina bifida. Lancet 2:197, 1972
7. Brocklehurst G, Gleave JR, Lewin WS: Early closure of myelomeningocele with especial reference to leg movement. Dev Med Child Neurol [Suppl] 13:51, 1967
8. Broome HL, Basmajian, JV: Survival of iliopsoas muscle after Sharrard procedure. Am J Phys Med 50:301, 1971
9. Bunch WH: The Milwaukee brace in paralytic scoliosis. Clin Orthop 110:63, 1975
10. Bunch WH: Treatment fo the myelomeningocele spine. The American Academy Of Orthopaedic Surgeons Instructional Course Lectures 25:93, 1976
11. Canale TS, Hammond NL III, Cotler JM, Snedden HE: Pelvic displacement osteotomy for chronic hip dislocation in myelodysplasia. J Bone Joint Surg 57A:177, 1975
12. Carroll NC, Sharrard WJW: Long-term follow-up of posterior iliopsoas transplantation for paralytic dislocation of the hip. J Bone Joint Surg 54A:551, 1972
13. Clark MW, D'Ambrosia RD, Ferguson AB Jr: Congenital vertical talus. Treatment by open reduction and navicular excision. J Bone Joint Surg 59A:816, 1977
14. Cruess RL, Turner NS: Paralysis of hip abductor muscles in spina bifida. J Bone Joint Surg 52A:1364, 1970
15. Dennyson WG, Fulford GE: Subtalar arthrodesis by cancellous grafts and metallic internal fixation. J Bone Joint Surg 58B:507, 1976
16. Dias LS: Ankle valgus in children with myelomeningocele. Dev Med Child Neurol 20:627, 1978
17. Dorner S: Adolescents with spina bifida. How they see their situation. Arch Dis Child 51:439, 1976
18. Dorner S: The relationship of physical handicap to stress in families with an adolescent with spina bifida. Dev Med Child Neurol 17:765, 1975

19. Drennan JC: The hip in myelomeningocele. In Katz J, Siffert R, (eds): Diseases of the Hip in Children. Philadelphia, J B Lippincott. 1973

20. Drennan JC: Management of myelomeningocele foot deformities in infancy and early childhood. The American Academy Of Orthopaedic Surgeons Instructional Course Lectures 25:82, 1976

21. Drennan JC: Management of neonatal myelomeningocele. The American Academy Of Orthopaedic Surgeons Instructional Course Lectures 25:65, 1976

22. Drennan JC: Orthotic management of the myelomeningocele spine. Dev Med Child Neurol [Suppl] 37:97, 1976

23. Drennan JC: The role of muscles in the development of human lumbar kyphosis. Dev Med Child Neurol [Suppl] 22:33, 1970

24. Drennan JC: The role of the thoracic suspension orthosis in the management of myelomeningocele spinal deformities. Inter-Clinic Information Bulletin 17(6):5, 1979

25. Drennan JC, Freehafer AA: Fractures of the lower extremities in paraplegic children. Clin Orthop 77:211, 1971

26. Drennan JC, Renshaw TS, Curtis BH: The thoracic suspension orthosis. Clin Orthop 139:33, 1979

27. Drennan JC, Sharrard WJW: The pathological anatomy of convex pes valgus. J Bone Joint Surg 53B:455, 1971

28. Duckworth T, Sharrard WJW, Lister J, Seymour N: Hemimyelocele. Dev Med Child Neurol [Suppl] 16:69, 1968

29. Duckworth T, Smith TWD: the treatment of paralytic convex pes valgus. J Bone Joint Surg 56B:305, 1974

30. Ferguson AB: The medial adductor approach for congenital dislocation of the hip. J Bone Joint Surg 54A:1799, 1972

31. Freehafer AA, Vessely JC, Mack RP: Iliopsoas muscle transfer in the treatment of myelomeningocele patients with paralytic hip deformities. J Bone Joint Surg 54A:1715, 1972

32. Gardner WJ: Myelomeningocele, the result of rupture of the embryonic neural tube. Cleve Clin Q 27:88, 1960

33. Gardner WJ: Myelocele: Rupture of the neural tube? Clin Neurosurg 15:57, 1968

34. Hall JE, Bobechko WP: Advance in the management of spinal deformities in myelodysplasia. Clin Neurosurg 20:164, 1973

35. Hall PV, Campbell RL, Kalsbeck JE: Meningomyelocele and progressive hydromyelia. Progressive paresis in myelodysplasia. J Neurol 43:457, 1975

36. Hayden PW, Davenport SLH, Campbell MH: Adolescents with myelodysplasia: Impact of physical disability on emotional maturation. Pediatrics 64:53, 1979

37. Hoffer MM, Feiwell E, Perry R, Perry J, Bonnett C: Functional ambulation in patients with myelomeningocele. J Bone Joint Surg 55A:137, 1973

38. Hostler SL: The adolescent with myelomeningocele. The American Academy Of Orthopaedic Surgeons Instructional Course Lectures 25:90, 1976

39. Hostler SL: Development of the infant with myelomeningocele. The American Academy of Orthopaedic Surgeons Instructional Course Lectures 25:70, 1976

40. Hull WJ, Moe JN, Winter RB: Spinal deformity in myelomeningocele: natural history, evaluation and treatment. J Bone Joint Surg 56A:1767, 1974

41. Inman VT: UC-BL axis control system and UC-BL shoe insert. Bull Prosthet Res 10:11, 1969

42. Kurland LT: Descriptive epidemiology of selected neurologic and myopathic disorders with particular reference to a survey in Rochester, Minnesota. J Chronic Dis 8:378, 1958

43. Laurence KM: The natural history of spina bifida cystica. Detailed analysis of 407 cases. Arch Dis Child 39:41, 1964

44. Laurence KM: The recurrence risk in spina bifida cystica and anencephaly. Dev Med Child Neurol [Suppl 20]:23, 1969

45. Laurence K, Tew BJ: Natural history of spina bifida cystica and cranium bifidum cysticum. Major central nervous system malformations in South Wales. Arch Dis Child 46:127, 1971

46. Lindseth RE: Posterior iliac osteotomy for fixed pelvic obliquity. J Bone Joint Surg 60A:17, 1978

47. Lindseth RE: Treatment of the lower extremity in children paralyzed by myelomeningocele. The American Academy of Orthopaedic Surgeons Instructional Course Lectures 25:76, 1976

48. London JT, Nichols O: Paralytic dislocation of the hip in myelodysplasia. J Bone Joint Surg 57A:501, 1975

49. Lorber J, Schloss AL: The adolescent with myelomeningocele. Dev Med Child Neurol [Suppl]29:113, 1973

50. Lorber J: Results of treatment of myelomeningocele. Dev Med Child Neurol, 13:279, 1971

51. Lorber J: Spina bifida cystica. Arch Dis Child 47:854, 1972

52. Lorber J: Selective treatment of myelomeningocele: to treat or not to treat: Pediatrics 53:307, 1974

53. Lowe GP, Menelaus MB: The surgical management of kyphosis in older children with myelomeningocele. J Bone Joint Surg 60B:40, 1978

54. Luque ER, Cardoso A: Segmental correction of scoliosis with rigid internal fixation. Preliminary report. Orthopaedic Transactions 1:136, 1977

55. MacKeith R: The feelings and behavior of parents of handicapped children. In Annotations. Dev Med Child Neurol 15:524, 1973

56. McKibben B: Conservative management of paralytic dislocations of the hip in myelomeningocele. J Bone Joint Surg 53B:758, 1971

57. Makin M: Tibio-fibular relationship in paralyzed limbs. J Bone Joint Surg 47B:500, 1965

58. Menelaus MB: The hip in myelomeningocele. Management directed towards a minimum number of operations and a minimum period of immobilization. J Bone Joint Surg 58B:448, 1976

59. Menelaus MB: Talectomy for equinovarus deformity in arthrogryposis and spina bifida. J Bone Joint Surg 53B:468, 1971

60. Moore DW, Raycroft JF, Loyer RE, Paul SW: The treatment of disabling foot and ankle valgus in myelodysplastic children. Presented at the 45th Annual Meeting of the American Academy of Orthopaedic Surgeons, Dallas, February, 1978

61. Mustard WT: A follow-up study of iliopsoas transfer for hip instability. J Bone Joint Surg 41B:289, 1959

62. Naggan L, MacMahon B: Ethnic differences in the

prevalence of anencephaly and spina bifida. N Engl J Med 227:1119, 1967

63. Nogami H, Ingalls TH: Pathogenesis of spinal malformations induced in the embryos of mice. J Bone Joint Surg 49A:1551, 1967

64. O'Brien JP, Dwyer AP, Hodgson AR: paralytic pelvic obliquity . J Bone Joint Surg 57A:626, 1975

65. Padget DH: Spina bifida and embryonic neuroschisis—a causal relationship. Johns Hopkins Med J, 123:233, 1968

66. Parsons JG: Assessments of aptitudes in young people of school-leaving age handicapped by hydrocephalus or spina bifida cystica. Dev Med Child Neurol [Suppl]27:101, 1972

67. Parsons DW, Seddon HJ: The results of operations for disorders of the hip caused by poliomyelitis. J Bone Joint Surg, 50B:266, 1968

68. Passo SD: Positioning infants with myelomeningocele. Am J Nurs 74:1658, 1974

69. Patten BM: Embryological stages in the establishing of myeloschisis with spina bifida. American Journal of Anatomy 93:365, 1953

70. Poitras B, Hall JE: Excision of kyphosis in myelomeningocele. In Meetings and Examinations. J Bone Joint Surg 56A:1767, 1974

71. Ráliŝ ZA, Ráliŝ HM, Randall M, Watkins G, Blake PD: Changes in the shape, ossification and quality of bones from developing paralysed limbs. A clinicopathological and experimental study. In Proceedings and Reports of Universities, Colleges, Councils, and Associations.

72. Reuda J, Carroll NC: Hip instability in patients with myelomeningocele. J Bone Joint Surg 54B:422, 1972

73. Rutter M, Graham P, Chadwick OF, Yule W: Adolescent turmoil: fact or fiction? Journal Of Child Pschology and Psychiatry and Allied Disciplines 17:35, 1976

74. Sharrard WJW: Posterior iliopsoas transplantation in the treatment of paralytic dislocation of the hip. J Bone Joint Surg 46B:426, 1964

75. Sharrard WJW: Spinal osteotomy for congenital kyphosis in myelomeningocele. J Bone Joint Surg 50B:466, 1968

76. Sharrard WJW, Drennan JC: Osteotomy-excision of the spine for lumbar kyphosis in older children with myelomeningocele. J Bone Joint Surg 54B:50, 1972

77. Sharrard WJW, Grosfield I: The management of deformity and paralysis of the foot in myelomeningocele. J Bone Joint Surg 50B:456, 1968

78. Sharrard WJW, Smith TWD: Tenodesis of flexor hallucis longus for paralytic clawing of the hallux in childhood. J Bone Joint Surg 58B:224, 1976

79. Sharrard WJW, Webb J: Supra-malleolar wedge osteotomy of the tibia in children with myelomeningocele. J Bone Joint Surg 56B:458, 1974

80. Sherk HH, Ames MD: Talectomy in the treatment of the myelomeningocele patient. Clin Orthop 110:218, 1975

81. Smith TWD, Duckworth T: The management of deformities of the foot in children with spina bifida. Dev Med Child Neurol [Suppl]37:104, 1976

82. Sriram K, Bobechko WP, Hall JE: Surgical management of spinal deformities in spina bifida. J Bone Joint Surg 54B:666, 1972

83. Taylor RG: The treatment of claw toes by multiple transfers of flexor into extensor tendons. J Bone Joint Surg 33B:539, 1951

84. Thomas CI, Thompson TC, Straub CR: Transplantation of the external oblique muscle for abduction paralysis. J Bone Joint Surg 32A:207, 1950

85. Wallace HM, Baumgartner L, Rich J: Congenital malformations and birth injuries in New York City. Pediatrics 12:525, 1953

Chapter 10

Cerebral Palsy

The orthopaedist has the responsibility to maintain the cerebral palsied patient's position in space and improve mobility as well as to prevent unnecessary deformity and pain. A clear understanding of the neurologic pathophysiology that leads to this syndrome is a prerequisite for accomplishing these goals.[32]

PATHOPHYSIOLOGY OF CEREBRAL PALSY

Feedback Mechanism

The muscle spindle (intrafusal) is an encapsulated structure attached to both ends to normal skeletal muscle (extrafusal). The spindle is responsible for reporting the momentary changes in muscle length and the rate of that change to the central nervous system. Its larger nuclear bag fibers have a central noncontractile segment which contains multiple nuclei. Smaller nuclear chain fibers have similar construction but only a single row of nuclei in its noncontractile segment. Several of these fibers are attached to the contractile ends of the longer nuclear bag fiber.

Muscle spindles are located within the muscle belly and receive their motor innervation from the gamma system. The afferent nerves from the muscle spindle to the spinal cord are classified by the size of the fibers.[72]

Group IA sensory fibers have autogenous excitation. They arise from both types of spindle fibers and when skeletal muscle is stretched they fire rapidly to report the rate of change and then fall off to a slower, steadier rate of firing to report on the change in length. Group IA afferent fibers are also important in the monosynaptic spinal stretch reflex.

Group II sensory fibers arise from the nuclear chain fibers and report only changes in the length of muscle. They are polysynaptic with spinal-cord internuncial cells. The spindle motor nerves are composed of gamma fibers that have plate endings on the contractile ends of both types of intrafusal fibers. The muscle spindle can be excited either by its gamma system or by the contracture of the attached skeletal muscle fibers innervated by the alpha motor system.

The Golgi tendon organ is a stretch receptor located in the inelastic tendinous origins and insertions of muscle and the intermuscular septum. Its only sensory fiber is an afferent Group IB which slowly adapts to increases in tension and acts by polysynaptic connections with internuncial cells to inhibit facilitation at the spinal level. As skeletal muscle contracts to meet the demands of the muscle spindle, there is an increase in tension within the muscle that is continuously monitored by the Golgi tendon organ to prevent the muscle from excessive shortening.

Organization of the Spinal Cord for Reflex Function

Sensory input to the spinal cord from stretch receptors may synapse directly with an anterior-horn motor neuron that completes the spinal stretch reflex. Collaterals from the sensory fibers may also transmit impulses to the cerebellum via the spinal cerebellar tract. Most of the rootlets of these fibers terminate in the internuncial cells which are small, highly excitable nerve cells that outnumber the anterior-horn motor neurons by approximately a 30 to 1 ratio. These cells act as intermediaries in interpreting afferent stimuli that reach the cord from the muscle spindle, and are also the recipient cells for messages from the brain that travel through the reticular system via the cortical spinal tracts. Interpretation for volitional activity of both the supraspinal and peripheral nervous systems can be mediated through these cells. Their vast numbers make possible the myriad of potential combinations and responses to both the gamma and alpha motor systems. The internuncial cells can amplify an incoming signal either by increasing the intensity of local cord response or by spreading the incoming volley more diffusely through the cord, thereby bringing about a more widespread motor reaction. They also serve as a final common pathway for either excitation or inhibition of response at a specific cord level.

Facilitation

The reticular formation is the upward extension of the internuncial cells. Initial stimulation for facilitation begins in the cerebellum and acts via the reticulospinal facilitative mechanism. The reticular formation extends through the entire brain stem, including the subthalamic nuclei and hypothalamus. The vast majority of this formation is facilitative. The stimulation in these areas in animals causes general increase in muscle tone throughout the body. Subluminal cortical input via the pyramidal (facilitative) tracts causes an increase in deep tendon reflexes but the human cerebral cortex does not appear to play any major role in facilitation. It is the brain stem reticular formation that augments the facilitative input that in turn excites the internuncial cells that results in increased spinal reflex activity. The vestibular nucleus and its accompanying vestibulospinal tract are responsible only for the facilitative movement of positioning the head in space.

Inhibition

The inhibitory influence has undergone progressive corticalization during evolution.[32] This enables the human cerebral cortex to override all lower central nervous system pathways. The critical inhibitory areas are: (1) the pre-central motor cortex (area 4), (2) a supplementary motor cortex along the midline, and (3) the pre-motor cortex whose stimulation is responsible only for gross movement (area 6). Area 4 is able to assimilate information from these two areas as well as from the occipital, parietal, and frontal lobes; digest the information and pass it as a coordinated message via the extrapyramidal (inhibitory) system. The progression of the inhibitory control into the neocortex is reflected by the many feedback and collateral circuits present throughout the extrapyramidal tract.

The function of the basal ganglia is limited to motor activity. The ganglia act to inhibit muscle tone throughout the body and thereby significantly contribute to the execution of complex movement and maintenance of posture. Their role in controlling background movement and posture can be illustrated by envisioning a lecturer pointing his index finger at a blackboard. The digital movement is under cortical volitional control but the movement and maintenance of the posture of the shoulder, elbow, and wrist that enables the lecturer to volitionally position his index finger are all strongly influenced by basal ganglion function.

The third inhibitory area is the cerebellum, the great coordinator of activity. Collaterals from the corticospinal tract go to the cerebellum as well as to the internuncial cells and an inhibitory message can be sent from the cerebellar anterior lobe and pyramidal lobules. The reticular inhibitory center located in the infraventral aspect of the brain stem reticular formation assimilates this activity and passes its inhibitory messages to the cord by way of the internuncial cells. This small center has no intrinsic activity but magnifies the impulses it receives from the higher centers.

Spinal Stretch Reflex

The skeletal muscle responds to stretching by prompt contraction, which tends to restore the muscle to its former length. The spinal stretch reflex is fundamental to movement. The reflex is initiated by stretch of the primary receptors of the muscle spindle. The impulse is carried by Group IA fibers which make a monosynaptic connection with an alpha motor neuron in the ventral horn of the spinal cord. The motor neuron stimulation causes 100 to 300 motor units in an individual skeletal muscle to contract. This phase of contraction is followed by a period of reciprocal inhibition during which the muscle cannot contract. Rarely does a single muscle spindle fire. More commonly, for example, when the reflex hammer strikes the patellar tendon placing the quadriceps mechanism under slight stretch, facilitation takes place and a myriad of muscle spindles fire simultaneously, resulting in the visible knee jerk response as the quadriceps contracts.

The elicited response of the neuromuscular system to modification of this spinal reflex by inhibition or facilitation is an essential ingredient in the development of the syndrome of cerebral palsy. As an example, facilitation of the stretch reflex in a muscle group kept under tension results in the development of clonus which persists as long as the tension is maintained.

NORMAL DEVELOPMENT

Brain maturation permits the normal infant an orderly sequence of motor development from apedal through quadripedal to bipedal posture.[17,43] Each new stage is integrated into previous motor patterns.[130] Specific activity develops as muscle groups gain coordination, primitive reflexes become integrated, and equilibrium reactions develop (Table 10-1). Fiorentino has equated maturation of the central nervous system with infant motor development.[45,46] Spinal or brain stem level function limits the patient to prone or supine positioning. Midbrain control permits the child to be quadripedal, allowing crawling or sitting. When cortical maturation is achieved, the infant can become bipedal, has developed equilibrium reactions necessary for protection, and is able to stand and walk.

TABLE 10-1 Normal Motor Milestones

RESPONSE	APPEARS	DISAPPEARS
Automatic Walking	Birth	2-6 wk
Positive Support	Birth	6-8 wk
Galant	Birth	1-2 mo
Rooting	Birth	3-4 mo
Palmar Grasp	Birth	6 mo
Foot Placement*	2 wk	3-4 yr
Moro	Birth	4-6 mo
Landau	6 mo	2½ yr
Parachute	6 mo	Assimilated
Equilibrium	6-8 mo	Assimilated

*May be absent in patients with extensor thrust (spasticity).

DIAGNOSIS OF CEREBRAL PALSY

Cerebral palsy can be defined as a nonprogressive brain disorder occurring before or during birth or during the first years of life up to the age of ten. The syndrome is characterized by insufficient development of postural reflexes, for example, poor head control, as well as prolonged retention of primitive patterns of activity (Table 10-2). Abnormal coordination and muscle patterning result in delayed motor development and impaired patterns of movement.[18,87] Two signs suggesting the diagnosis in infancy are: (1) hyperactive deep-tendon reflexes in a hypertonic or hypotonic child, and (2) the unilateral or bilateral abnormal persistence of neonatal reflexes beyond the time that they should have disappeared or been absorbed into a more sophisticated reflex (Fig. 10-1).[36] Delayed motor milestones, diminished voluntary muscle function, and patterns of voluntary activity result. There may be additional medical problems, for example, epilepsy, drooling, or perceptual difficulties. The incidence remains 1 to 2 per 1,000 in the school age group and 6 to 7 per 100,000 in the newborn population.[68,70,103]

Recent medical advances have dramatically altered the frequency of the clinical types of cerebral palsy.[1,85] Improved management of neonatal hyperbilirubinemia due to Rhesus incompatibility or infection has resulted in fewer basal ganglial insults. This explains why only 12% of patients are presently considered dyskinetic (athetoid) because of lesions in the basal ganglia. Concomitantly, the increasing number of spastic patients can be attributed to the increasing survival of infants born weighing less than 2,500 grams.[94] At present, approximately 75% of newly diagnosed patients can be termed spastic with involvement of the pyramidal and extrapyramidal

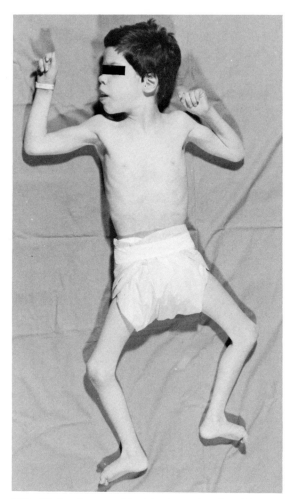

FIG. 10-1. Asymmetrical tonic neck reflex. Note "fencing posture" with occipital extremities in flexion and facial limbs in extension. The reflex is most clearly elicited by voluntary rotation of the head.

systems. Five percent are considered ataxic due to cerebellar dysfunction while another 5% are described as rigid due to diffuse brain damage. Hypotonia and tremors are infrequent major diagnoses.

Types of Cerebral Palsy

TYPE I - SPASTICITY

Spasticity represents a facilitative–inhibitory imbalance due to pyramidal system dysfunction. The spinal stretch reflex is exaggerated when the inhibitory cortical control is reduced. Plantar reflexes are upgoing and the

TABLE 10-2 Persistent Primitive Reflexes That Delay Motor Development

REFLEX	SHOULD DISAPPEAR
Crossed Extension	3-4 mo
Tonic Labryinthine	4 mo
Asymmetrical Tonic Neck	4-6 mo
Symmetrical Tonic Neck	4-6mo
Moro	4-6 mo
Landau	$2\frac{1}{2}$ yr

deep-tendon reflexes become hyperactive. Clonus and tone that increase with muscle group stretching are evident. Patterns of voluntary movement are decreased because of facilitation of certain muscle groups, for example, the adductors combined with a relative inhibition of the abductors. The hypertonicity is greatest in the upper-extremity flexors and lower-limb extensors. Contractures are common (Fig. 10-2) and appear early in the hypertonic groups due to functional, muscle imbalance.

TYPE II - MOTION DISORDER

Dyskinesia results from an insult to the extrapyramidal system and includes patients with athetosis whose primary lesion is in the globus pallidus. Upper-extremity involvement movement is greater than lower-extremity dysfunction and head control may be poor. Labyrinthine and tonic neck reflexes may be prominent. Frequently, asymmetry is noted and gross uncoordinated movements are most visible in the proximal joints. The decrease in posture and tone results in the patient's inability to maintain the body or extremity position in space and accounts for the abnormal involuntary movements which are present only with the patient is awake. Changes in the patient's emotional state may alter muscle tension. Deep-tendon reflexes are decreased and plantar responses are downgoing. Contractures develop late and may be related more to abnormal position than to muscle imbalance.

Dystonia (tension athetosis) can clinically mimic spasticity. However, repeated examinations coupled with relaxation of the patient demonstrate a marked decrease in the apparent hypertonicity. Repeated rapid movement, such as shaking a limb, may also result in decreased tone. Failure to recognize this small group of patients results in serious postoperative problems, which include iatrogenic contractures, particularly following adductor release or heel-cord lengthening.

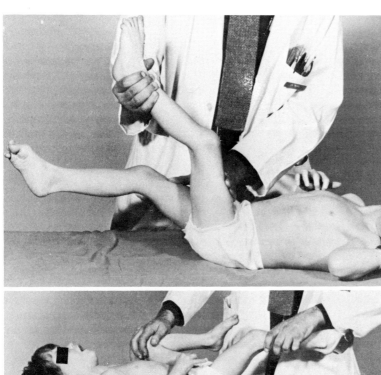
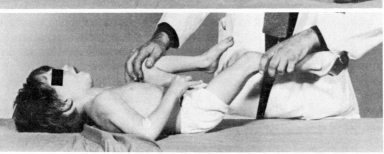

FIG. 10.2. Co-contractures of hip flexors and extensors are common in spastic cerebral palsy and must be recognized in preoperative evaluation. The upper photograph illustrates the Holt method which is preferred for determination of hamstring contractures. While the contralateral limb is held in maximum extension, the ipsilateral hip is flexed to a right angle and the leg then extended. The Thomas test for hip flexion contracture is shown in the lower photograph.

TYPE III - MIXED

Mixed types of cerebral palsy have elements of both the major categories.[60] Motion disorders may be more prominent in the upper extremities and spasticity in the lower extremities. All three forms may have asymmetry in the degree of involvement.

ATAXIA. Ataxic patients have impaired coordination and equilibirum and demonstrate past pointing, a rebound in positioning of an extremity in space to its original position, and nystagmus. The patients frequently are hypotonic, have normal intelligence, and normal deep tendon reflexes. Sitting balance is generally satisfactory.

RIGIDITY. Rigidity differs from spasticity in several important ways. The deep-tendon reflexes are normal. Antigravity muscles, such as plantarflexors and hip adductors, dominate the spastic extremities, whereas the muscles antagonistic to the antigravity muscles are more involved in rigidity. There is plasticity in the extremity, so that when it is positioned in space it tends to retain that position. When a spastic child's lower extremities are abducted, the relative inhibition of the abductors permits the limbs to spring back into an adducted position when the examiner's hands are removed, whereas the limbs of the rigid patient remain in abduction. The terms 'lead pipe' or 'cogwheel' simply infer a clinical description of the two major forms of rigidity.

Geographic Distribution

HEMIPLEGIA

Hemiplegia describes the predominant involvement of one side of the body and may present in infancy with a lack of reciprocal kicking or a tendency for one hand to be fisted. Older infants demonstrate unilateral absence of parachute response, fail to use the upper extremities interchangeably, and may have a delay in unilateral equilibrium reactions. These patients can be expected to ambulate at an average age of 21 months (Fig. 10-3). Abnormal sensory findings may interfere with upper-extremity function. The most common lower-extremity deformity is equinovarus positioning of the ankle and foot (Fig. 10-4).

DIPLEGIA

Spastic diplegia is now the most common type of cerebral palsy and is most frequently associated with prematurity. The neuromuscular imbalance may not become clinically evident until after the age of 6 months when extensor tone creeps into the lower extremities. Reciprocal kicking may not be seen and later motor milestones such as sitting and standing may be delayed. Diplegia implies that the spastic involvement is greater in the lower extremities and is associated with minor motor deficiencies in the upper extremities. Increased femoral anteversion, coxa valga, and hip adduction contractures as well as equinovalgus feet are frequently seen. Esotropia is common.

TOTAL BODY INVOLVEMENT

Total body involvement describes significant four-extremity hyperactivity. Quadriplegics tend to have greater upper-extremity and head-control problems and also tend to be asymmetrical. Ambulation is usually not practical. Root reported that 78 % of patients with total body involvement in his series were confined to a wheelchair.[99] Scoliosis and hip dislocation (Fig. 10-5) are most common in these patients and may jeopardize sitting. Speech, swallowing, and cognitive problems may be noted. Seizures are more common because of the diffuse insult.

Neonatal Reflexes

Specific reflex responses are present at birth in the normal infant but later disappear as they are modified or lost and more sophisticated reflexes develop in the process of central nervous system maturation (Table 10-1). Only after the Moro response has disappeared can the Landau reflex become apparent. The Landau reflex is pathologic if it persists beyond 2 years of age.

The positive-support reflex is gradually absorbed by voluntary control by the ages of 3 to 4 years while the parachute reaction, which becomes visible at 6 months of age, probably persists through life. Patients with persistent obligatory tonic neck reflexes (Fig. 10-1) rarely develop balance and are poor candidates for ambulation.[45,46]

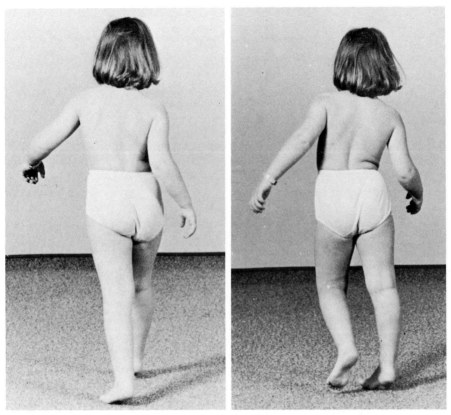

FIG. 10-3. A right hemiplegic gait pattern demonstrates a unilateral Trendelenburg gait because of functional weakness of the hip abductor and extensor muscles of the involved limb. The ipsilateral arm pulls up because of increased flexor spasticity and is an adjunct in the lateral shift of the body mass.

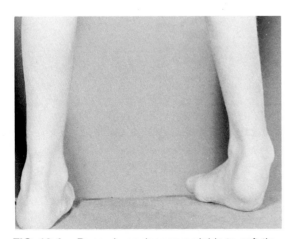

FIG. 10-4. Dynamic equinovarus yields to soft-tissue surgical correction. Fixed deformity of this magnitude frequently requires additional osseous procedures.

Classification Of Goals

MOBILITY[63]

Four types of ambulation can be defined:

1. *Community*—The patient is able to walk indoors and outdoors with or without crutches or braces. Wheelchairs are needed only for long trips in the community.
2. *Household*—Patients are able to walk indoors with the use of crutches or braces but need a wheelchair outside the home.
3. *Physiologic*—Walking is limited to physical therapy sessions and a wheelchair is needed for household and community activities.

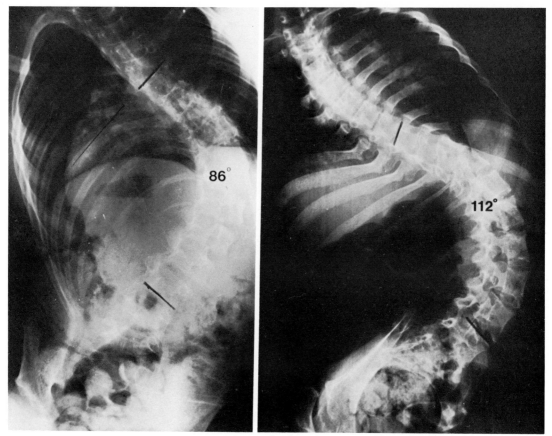

FIG. 10-5. A teenage total-body involved patient demonstrated an increase in neuro-muscular scoliosis over a five-year period. The "high hip" proceeded from subluxation to dislocation as the magnitude of the curve progressed.

4. *Nonambulation*—Patients may be able to stand and transfer but because of lack of balance, require a manually operated or a powered-wheelchair for all mobility.

Nonwalkers can be further classified as:

a. *Independent Sitters*—These patients retain sufficient balance reaction to sit upright without the need for orthotic devices to control the hip or back. They can independently transfer in and out of a wheelchair.

b. *Self-Propped Sitter*—This patient requires support but can maintain sitting balance momentarily. The patient can get in and out of a wheelchair with the assistance of one person and does not need to be lifted.

c. *Propped Sitter*—A propped sitter requires special support to maintain the upright position and needs to be lifted in and out of the wheelchair.[93] Oxygen consumption required for ambulation increases by 50 % for each classification of more motor involvement. This energy consumption may become so great that meaningful activities of daily living may be significantly restricted.

WALKING PROGNOSIS TESTS

Specific reflex responses are normally present at birth (Table 10-1) and later disappear as they are modified or lost when more complex reflexes develop as central nervous system maturation occurs. Bleck used seven primitive and postural reflexes in assessing ambulatory potential in non-ambulatory children over the age of 12 months.[13] These included the asymmetric tonic neck reflex, symmetric tonic neck reflex, neck righting reflex, Moro reflex, parachute reaction, extensor thrust, and foot placement reaction. Presence of one of the first five or absence of one of the last two was recorded as a score of one point. A score of two or more points gave a poor prognosis for walking. A one-point score made prognosis guarded, while a zero score suggested an excellent prognosis for ambulation. He further observed that ambulation ability plateaued by the age of 7 years. Fiorentino noted that patients with persistent obligatory tonic neck reflexes rarely develop balance and are poor candidates for ambulation.[45,46]

Beals proposed a motor quotient for children with spastic diplegia, which is obtained by dividing the chronologic age by the motor age in months at 3 years.[10] This severity index has a potential range of 0 to 36. When the severity index is less than 10, free ambulation is unlikely to occur. Walking is a realistic goal with an index of 10 to 11, and surgery may be directed toward achieving free ambulation. A severity index of 12 to 18 indicates free ambulation is possible, and surgery is performed to improve the quality of walking. The less the motor involvement, the better the functional result. Correction of a fixed deformity did not always result in the correction of a dynamic imbalance. Surgery itself rarely changed the mode of ambulation.

UPPER-EXTREMITY MOTOR PROGNOSIS

Upper limb function is likely to be poor when the patient fails to develop lateralization, limb dominance, or the ability to cross the midline. Deficient sterognostic sensation compromises hand use.[33,129] Beals noted that limitation of intelligence paralleled the upper-limb severity index.[10]

Long-term Rehabilitation Goals

Adult cerebral palsied patients rank communication, performance of activities of daily living, and mobility ahead of walking in their list of goals.[73] The responsible physician should strive for optimal community independence and employment for each patient. O'Reilly found that a child with normal mentality and independence in self-care was most likely to have a favorable adult outcome of treatment.[84] Regular school led to gainful employment, whereas those limited to attending special schools generally functioned only in an adult-sheltered workshop. Twenty-eight percent of cerebral palsied patients were found to have normal intelligence; one third were gainfully employed while an additional third either died or required institutional care as adults. Spastic patients were most likely to have a job. The more severe the intellectual retardation, the lower the capacity for employment.

ORTHOPAEDIC TREATMENT

Orthotics

Orthoses are prescribed to protect a body segment or a joint, prevent deformity, provide stability (Fig. 10-6), and enhance function (Fig. 10-7). Bracing cannot correct a fixed deformity, and failure to recognize this will lead to orthotic failure.[49] Functional deficits that may interfere with bracing include:

1. impaired or absent selective control of motor function;
2. primitive midbrain locomotor patterns which may be only partial voluntary control;
3. primitive reflexes or movements including abnormal stretch reflexes, body position tone, and vestibular tone;
4. dysequilibrium;
5. sensation or body-image deficits or both.

An orthosis is described by the combination of joints it encompasses with the first initial of each controlled joint used in the prescription. A short leg brace becomes an ankle-foot orthosis (AFO), while a long leg brace with a pelvic band is a hip-knee-ankle-foot orthosis (HKAFO).

NIGHT SPLINTING

Sleeping permits reduction of muscle tone and allows an orthosis to place both agonists and

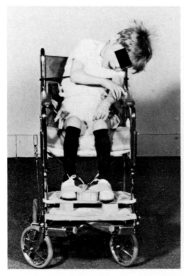
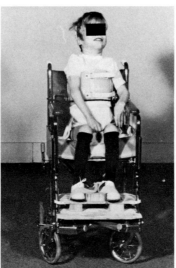
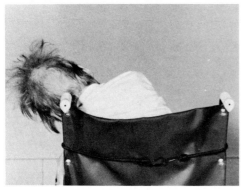
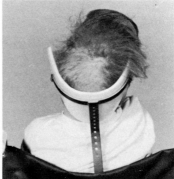

FIG. 10-6. A total-body involved youth with strong tonic neck reflexes and extensor thrust is shown in the left photographs. Functional upright posture is achieved by combining a thoracic suspension orthosis and attached head rest with wheelchair modifications that permit flexion positioning of the lower extremities (*right photographs*).

antagonists under normal muscle tension. Night splinting is particularly helpful in removing excessive stretch from the weaker antagonists.

Small children will accept trunk and lower-extremity abduction orthoses that extend to control the foot. However, older children will no longer tolerate this degree of control and the orthopaedist is forced to either select specific joints to manage or to alternate different types of braces on consecutive nights. For example, bilateral AFOs can be combined with a hip abduction brace.[50] This combination permits flexion–extension of both hips and knees. An orthosis designed to control knee flexion may be used on alternate nights. This

type of splinting is also important in maintaining the surgical correction of fixed deformities in the growing child, particularly in patients with spastic cerebral palsy. Motion disorder patients rarely develop fixed deformities and their need for night splinting is infrequent.

LOWER-EXTREMITY BRACING

ANKLE–FOOT ORTHOSES. Mild hemiplegic or diplegic involvement may be controlled by nighttime use of ankle–foot orthoses. The goal of being brace-free during the day for[9] greater amount of freedom and function serves as a

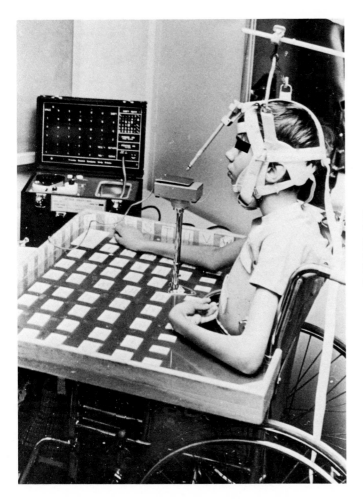

FIG. 10-7. A hypotonic total-body involved adolescent uses a thoracic suspension orthosis and independent cervical suspension to permit use of a head-pointer and electronic communication device.

personal incentive to the patient. Daytime orthotic use may be required when the patient walks with the ankle in either dynamic plantar flexion or varus prepositioning during the swing phase. Dynamic equinus, which prevents the orthosis from keeping the heel down can be controlled by a series of inhibition casts before the brace is employed.[125] A recent study suggests that[9] static triceps-surae contracture is more affected by inhibition casting than by dynamic muscle sensitivity.[86] Similarly, the brace will fail unless[9] triceps-surae contracture is corrected surgically or by a series of corrective casts. These orthoses permit positioning of the foot with zero degree of ankle flexion during the deceleration phase of stance gait immediately following heel-strike.

KNEE–ANKLE–FOOT ORTHOSES. A rehabilitation goal is the transfer of the adolescent with KAFO control into short leg braces if possible, since very few adults retain meaningful ambulation while wearing long leg braces.[31] Changes in bracing should be initially attempted in a physical therapy setting and used in the home and community only after they have been mastered. Older spastic children and adolescents whose overlengthened heel cords have led to a crouch gait may benefit from a correction of knee-flexion contractures either by serial casting or hamstring lengthening. When full knee extension has been achieved, long leg braces with knee joints locked in extension can be temporarily employed. These orthoses markedly hinder patients' efforts at ambulation and ensure the need for upper-extremity crutch use. The patient will initially have one and then the other knee joint unlocked during ambulation. The eventual use of a Saltiel type of

AFO with dynamic knee extension ensures continued adult ambulation (Fig. 10-8).[104] The presence of a hip flexion-contracture is a contraindication to Saltiel bracing and requires correction.

UPPER-EXTREMITY BRACING

Patients who lack posterior equilibrium reaction need upper-extremity balance assists, such as crutches or walkers. The absence of the

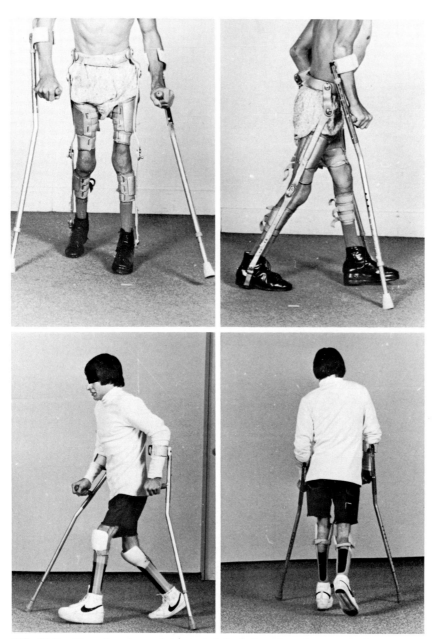

FIG. 10-8. Transfer of an adolescent diplegic from long leg braces with a pelvic band (*upper photos*) to Saltiel ankle–foot orthoses was accomplished over a four-month period. During that time the long leg braces were used for activities of daily living and the Saltiel orthoses limited to therapy ambulation.

posterior equilibrium reaction requires them to lean forward to increase their standing base and this functional need should be recognized when analyzing both orthotic and physical therapy requirements. Attempts at daytime functional bracing of the upper extremity have been disappointing. Night splints which maintain the wrist and hand in a functional position may assist in preventing progressive contractures. The young child with marked lateral balance deficiencies may require a ring walker.

WHEELCHAIRS

Wheelchairs can be classified as either hand-driven or power-driven types. The measurement of the sitting height and the length of segments of the extremities as well as the patient's individual sitting and mobility needs must be considered. Removable hard seats may be required to avoid functional pelvic obliquity that may be associated with hammock seats found in collapsable, portable wheelchairs. Appropriate modifications of foot rests may be necessary to ensure that the feet are maintained in plantigrade, weight-bearing position (Fig. 10-6). Patients with total body involvement or severe motion disorders may require a reclining type of quadriplegic chair with modifications. The width of the wheelchair seat should be wider if it is necessary to employ a spinal orthosis for either positioning in space or controlling a spinal deformity.[22] Dominance of the trunk and lower extremities by tonic neck reflexes or extensor thrust may be controlled by flexing the hips and knees beyond a right angle to change an extensor pattern into a flexor posture. The position of the head and neck in space is important in controlling tonic neck reflexes and may require the use of a cervical sling or custom-made headrest (Fig. 10-9).

TRANSFER DEVICES

Transfer boards and Hoyer lifts are frequently required for the severely involved patient. These become more important as the child grows in both height and weight. Long leg braces may also be necessary in allowing assisted transfer and giving physical relief to the parents. Instruction in transfer techniques is the responsibility of the physical therapist.

SURGERY

Preoperative Planning

Careful patient selection and the establishment of appropriate goals and postoperative management are essential prerequisites for successful surgery. Realistic objectives, for example, household ambulation, must be shared with the family whose role in the rehabilitation program must be established. Prehospital preparation is effective in allaying family and patient psychological upset and in fostering development.[3]

Repeated clinical assessment permits an understanding of the patient's pathphysiology. The potential functional impact of the surgery on other joints is considered. Several modalities permit more precise preoperative analysis. The use of dantrolene sodium (Dantrium) may establish the patient's ability to vertically displace the center of gravity or to change stride length.[47] Task biofeedback sessions may explain why a patient cannot perform a specific task skillfully and permit more realistic goal-setting.

Most surgery is performed for patients who either are ambulatory or who have the potential to walk with or without crutches. Optimally, surgery is performed between ages five to seven years under one general anesthetic. This age permits preoperative gait pattern analysis which now is commonly performed in motion-analysis laboratories.[91] The Newington Children's Hospital's Gait Analysis Laboratory studies include dynamic electromyograms, force plate and computer motion determinations, and video pictures (Fig. 10-10).

Nonambulatory patients with fixed soft-tissue contractures that interfere with function are also surgical candidates. Surgery may also be indicated for the correction of a deformity, for example, hip flexion–adduction contracture causing subluxation, when the soft-tissue contracture could lead to secondary osseous changes or pain due to degenerative joint disease.

The Foot and Ankle

EQUINUS DEFORMITY

Dynamic equinus does not delay standing. The strong extensor thrust may enhance exten-

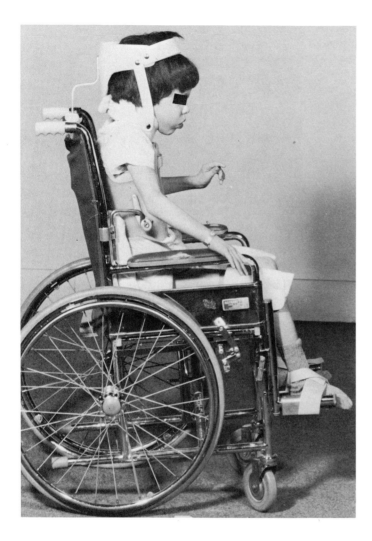

FIG. 10-9. Tonic neck reflexes are obviated by a head control device which permits slight neck flexion. Avoiding pressure over the cervical spine prevents facilitation of the tonic labyrinthine response.

sion of knees, hips, and trunk and removal of this functional trigger may result in an iatrogenic calcaneal quagmire.

Surgery is indicated when the triceps-surae contracture will not permit the foot to be brought to neutral dorsiflexion (Fig. 10-11) when measured with the foot in a varus position, even when the knee is flexed. Lengthening of the gastrosoleus muscles also decreases the exaggerated heel-cord stretch reflex.[6] Excessive correction favors dorsiflexion overactivity and the development of a calcaneal deformity, which is most likely to occur when the heel cord is lengthened in the presence of concomitant untreated hip- and knee-flexion contractures.

A wide spectrum of surgical methods has been advocated in the past 150 years, including a variety of heel-cord lengthening procedures, neurectomy, and gastrocnemius lengthening or origin recession.[4,6,8,40,74,117] Most current authors recommend heel-cord lengthening for equinus contracture.[8,14,115] I prefer a formal Z-lengthening of the heel cord.

TECHNIQUE FOR HEEL-CORD LENGTHENING. Through a medial longitudinal incision, the tendon sheath of the Achilles tendon is identified and incised. The anterior half of the tendon is divided near its insertion. The proximal transverse incision divides the superficial half of the tendon, thereby permitting the residual exposed surface to be covered by the thick subcutaneous fat of the distal calf. A coronal lengthening of the tendon connects these two transverse incisions. In an equinovarus de-

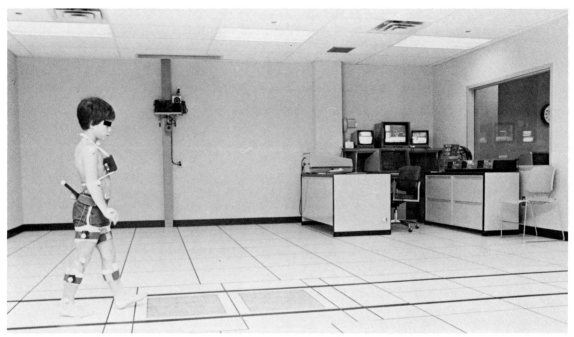

FIG. 10-10. A child about to strike the force plate which measures ground reaction force. An infrared light source is emitted from the camera station (*background*) and is reflected by the markers (*white balls*) which the child wears. The sacral wand measures pelvic rotation and tilt. Electromyographic telemetry is contained in the chest box and obviates the need for dragging a cable which might interfere with the pattern of walking.

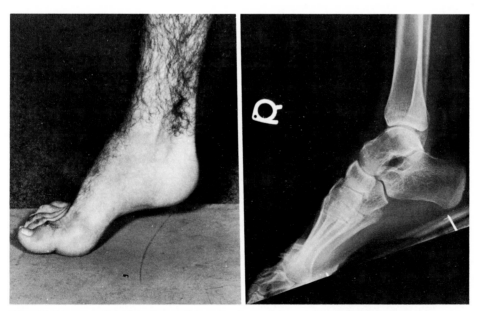

FIG. 10-11. A weight-bearing radiograph of an adolescent hemiplegic with fixed equinus establishes the forefoot as the major area of static deformity. Correction was obtained with intrinsic release.

formity the tendon is lengthened in the sagittal plane and the distal incision is made medially near the insertion into the calcaneus to decrease the invertor activity of the triceps surae. Conversely, when the foot has an equinovalgus deformity, the distal incision is placed laterally.

The foot is manually dorsiflexed to neutral and permitted to passively assume an equinus position while the tendon repair is performed with nonabsorbable mattress sutures. The foot is then passively dorsiflexed to neutral to document that sufficient muscle tension remains and that no excessive dorsiflexion can occur. Postoperatively, a long leg cast is applied with the knee in slight flexion and the foot at a right angle. The cast is worn for five weeks or may be shortened at three weeks to permit knee rehabilitation. An ankle–foot orthosis and regular shoes are then employed. The goal for spastic diplegic and hemiplegic patients is to have them free of braces for daytime activities after 6 months of full-time use of the orthosis. Continuous nighttime splinting is recommended during the growth years. Recurrent equinus contracture occurs in less than 10% of patients.

GASTROCNEMIUS LENGTHENING

Electromyography may permit distinction between gastrocnemius and soleus overactivity.[90] Isolated gastrocnemius phase distortion, or clonus, benefits from gastrocnemius recession. Combined soleus and gastrocnemius overactivity requires a heel-cord lengthening. The gastrocnemius aponeurosis is divided at its junction with the soleus (Fig. 10-12).[4] I have found that this muscle-belly length is variable, which may result in the need for excessive length to the surgical incision. Extensive muscle stripping may also result in scar formation, which may account for the higher recurrence rate with this technique than with either the sliding or Z-lengthening of the heel cord.[116]

SOLEUS NEURECTOMY

Soleus neurectomy, a procedure indicated only in severe functional equinus or clonus is ineffective when the triceps surae have a fixed contracture (Fig. 10-13).[40] Preoperative assessment includes precise identification of the motor nerves to the soleus by means of electrical stimulation with a coated needle and the introduction of 2 ml to 5 ml of procaine, after which the clinical change in gait can be assessed. Dilute procaine blocks the gamma system without abolishing alpha-motor-neuron activity.[110] I prefer formal surgical resection of the motor nerves rather than phenol injection because of nerve rearborization, which frequently occurs several months following alcohol insertion.[92]

EQUINOVARUS DEFORMITY

Equinovarus deformity occurs most commonly in hemiplegics or nonambulatory patients with total body involvement. Serial corrective long leg plaster casts followed by the use of straight-last shoes with a Denis Browne splint set in 15° of external rotation has proven effective in young total-body-involved patients.

Mild fixed equinovarus deformity in the young hemiplegic patient can be controlled by combining an intramuscular lengthening of the tibialis posterior[102] with a heel-cord lengthening. Weak peronei and dorsiflexors may permit secondary forefoot equinus to develop, which can be corrected in the skeletally immature patient by an intrinsic release and posterior tibial lengthening coupled with a staged split anterior tendon transfer (Splatt procedure).[116] Posterior tibial transfer or rerouting procedures are not effective.[11]

Hoffer recommends a split anterior tibial tendon transfer when there is electromyographic demonstration of inappropriate anterior tibial hyperactivity in young patients with spastic hindfoot varus (Fig. 10-14).[65]

TECHNIQUE FOR SPLIT ANTERIOR TIBIAL TENDON TRANSFER. The inital incision is placed over the dorsomedial aspect of the first cuneiform where the insertion of the tibialis anterior tendon is indentified. The tendon frequently has a natural division at its insertion that can be used when the tendon is sharply divided and split with a suture. A second incision is made over the anterior distal leg and a hemostat is passed into the first incision enabling the suture to be drawn into the second wound, while bluntly splitting the tendon. The lateral half of the anterior tibial insertion is then released. A third incision is

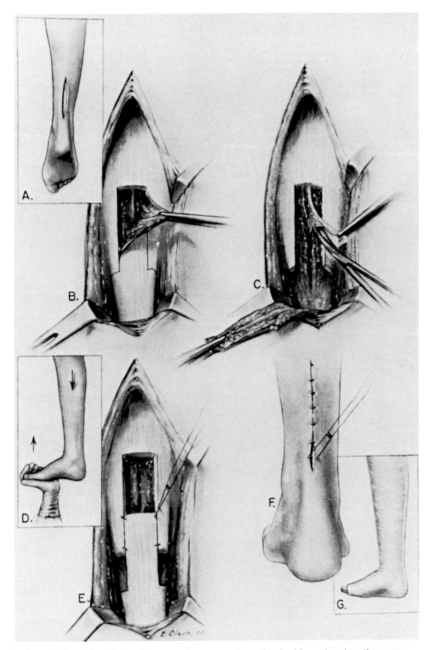

FIG. 10-12. The Baker "tongue-in-groove" method of lengthening the aponeurotic tendon of the gastrocnemius. It is necessary to include dissection of the central aponeurotic tendon of the soleus (*C*). (Baker LD: J Bone Joint Surg 38A:313, 1956)

made over the cuboid and the freed up lateral half of the tendon is passed subcutaneously into a drill hole made in the bone. A Bunnel woven suture is employed and tied over a button in the nonweight-bearing aspect of the medial longitudinal arch. The procedure can be combined with a heel-cord lengthening or a posterior tibial intramuscular lengthening. Postoperative immobilization is continued for 6 weeks. The patient is then transfered to an

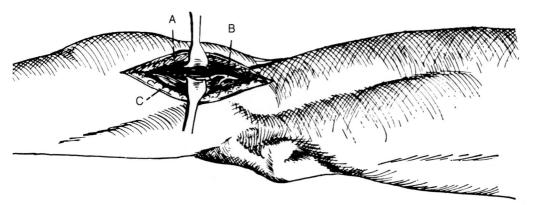

FIG. 10-13. Diagram demonstrating the incision for soleus neurectomy on the lateral side of the leg. *A.* the gastrocnemius muscle, *B.* nerves superficial to the soleus muscle, *C.* the soleus muscle. (Eggers GWN: J Bone Joint Surg 34A:829, 1952)

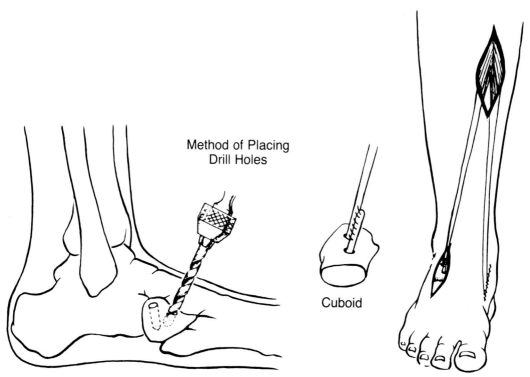

Method of Placing
Drill Holes

Cuboid

FIG. 10-14. Successful use of the Splatt procedure frequently requires a first-stage intrinsic release to correct forefoot equinus. Because of the fragility of immature bone, I prefer to create a tunnel directed toward the non-weight-bearing medial arch and tie the transfer over a felt pad and button. (Hoffer M: Orthop Clin North Am 5:32, 1974)

ankle–foot orthosis. Daytime orthotic control is needed for 6 months. Prolonged use of night splinting is recommended.

EQUINOVALGUS DEFORMITY

Equinovalgus most commonly occurs in ambulatory spastic diplegics or paraplegics. The calcaneus is plantarflexed and everted, and pronation and abduction occur in the mid- and forefoot. Heel-cord lengthening and ankle–foot orthoses may suffice when the valgus is flexible. Tendon surgery is ineffective with fixed deformity and in the growing child a subtalar extra-articular arthrodesis combined with a heel-cord lengthening is the procedure of choice. The complications associated with the Grice method have led Newington Children's Hospital to adopt the Dennyson modification

of the subtalar extra-articular arthrodesis (Fig. 10-15).[28,56]

TECHNIQUE FOR SUBTALAR EXTRA-ARTICULAR ARTHRODESIS.

An Ollier incision extending from the midline of the dorsum of the ankle to the peroneal tendons exposes the contents of the sinus tarsi, which are then freed up and reflected distally. Sharp dissection is required to ensure removal of all soft tissue from the sinus tarsi. A curette is used to decorticate cancellous bone on the medial aspect of the undersurface of the neck of the talus and nonarticular calcaneal surface. Care must be taken not to remove the cortical bone from the lateral aspect of these bones, through which the fixation screw must pass. Blunt dissection between the tendon of the extensor digitorum longus and the anterior tibial neurovascular

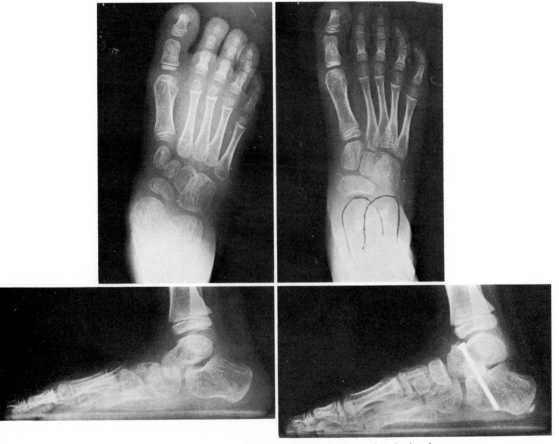

FIG. 10-15. The Princess Margaret Rose modification of the subtalar arthrodesis affords more rigid internal fixation and results in a lower incidence of pseudarthrosis in cerebral palsied patients with equinovarus deformity.

bundle permits exposure of a depression on the superior surface of the talar neck. The calcaneus is held in the corrected position and a Kirschner wire is drilled across this depression through the neck of the talus and into the calcaneus, piercing the infralateral cortex of the calcaneus. A radiograph is obtained to verify reduction and to determine the length of the wood screw. An awl is used to begin a second talar neck site and the screw introduced and advanced until its head bites into the superior surface of the talus before the Kirschner wire is removed. Iliac cancellous chips are then packed into the area of the sinus tarsi and its contents are then reattached. Dennyson permits immediate ambulation in a short leg cast; I prefer to delay ambulation for 6 weeks and continue immobilization until an oblique radiograph demonstrates satisfactory incorporation of the graft into both the talus and calcaneus. Long term use of an ankle–foot orthosis is recommended.

CALCANEAL OSTEOTOMY

A closing wedge calcaneal osteotomy may complement the above soft-tissue procedures when there is an osseous hindfoot varus deformity.[38,118]

TECHNIQUE FOR CALCANEAL OSTEOTOMY.

Through a lateral incision approximately one-half inch below the peroneal tendons, the lateral aspect of the calcaneus is exposed subperiosteally. Posterior stripping is carried out in front of the tendo Achillis and the intrin-

sics and plantar fascia are removed from the inferior calcaneus. A wedge of the os calcis is removed, which has a lateral base not exceeding one-fourth inch in diameter. An awl is placed in the distal fragment to assist in bony approximation, which is maintained by use of a staple.

BUNIONS

Painful hallux valgus develops as a secondary deformity in spastic ambulatory patients with severe equinovalgus feet (Fig. 10-16). The overactive peroneus longus everts the hindfoot and forefoot. This shifts the peroneal sheath origin of the adductor hallucis proximally and laterally, thereby enhancing its mechanical advantage. The great toe pronates and moves laterally because of excessive weight-bearing on its medial and inferior surfaces. The McKeever metatarsophalangeal arthrodesis has proven to be the most effective method of treatment (Fig. 10-17).[80,96]

HAMMER TOES

Hammer toes (Fig. 10-18) may also develop, requiring flexor tenotomies, interphalangeal fusions, and transfers of the extensor tendons into the metatarsal heads.

TRIPLE ARTHRODESIS

Triple arthrodesis is reserved for patients who are nearing skeletal maturity.[42,67] Attempts to correct severe deformity by bony surgery alone,

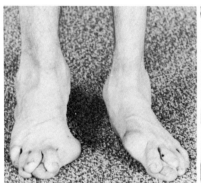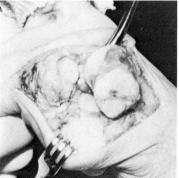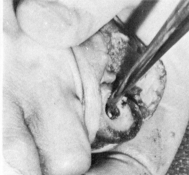

FIG. 10-16. (*Left*) Photographs of symptomatic bunions in an ambulatory adult patient; (*Middle*) degenerative changes in the metatarsal head are shown; (*Right*) the proximal phalanx must be curetted into the shape of a cone to receive the remodeled metatarsal head.

may lead to excessive shortening of the foot in length and height, which creates problems in regard to wearing shoes. Banks recommends preliminary correction of equinus by heel-cord lengthening.[8] He limits the triple arthrodesis to the correction of valgus or varus deformity. I prefer the use of staples in both the calcaneocuboid and talonavicular joints in cerebral palsied patients.

CALCANEAL DEFORMITY

A calcaneal deformity results from the surgical overlengthening of the heel cord (Fig. 10-19). It is most appropriately managed by correcting proximal joint-flexion deformities. Long-term use of a rigid ankle–foot orthosis is required. Secondary adaptive changes in the immature ankle mortice may require correc-

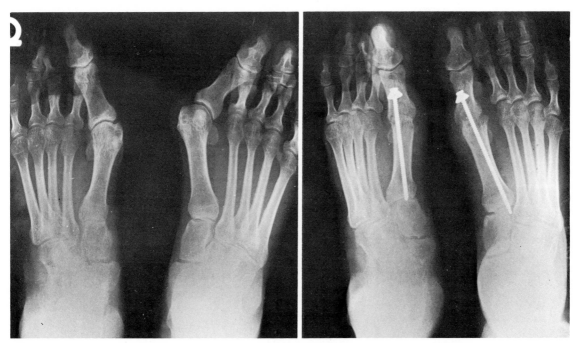

FIG. 10-17. Radiographs demonstrate successful bilateral McKeever metatarsophalangeal arthrodeses.

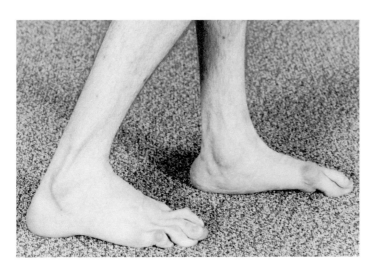

FIG. 10-18. Painful hammer toes may limit ambulatory activities.

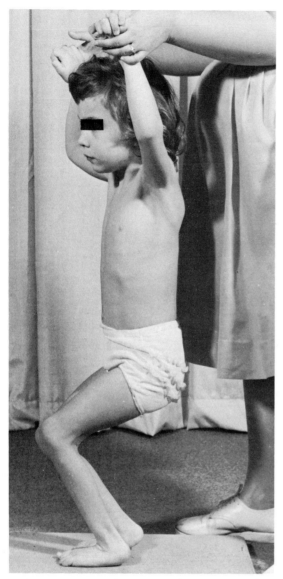

FIG. 10-19. Heel-cord lengthening in the face of unrecognized hip- and knee-flexion contractures results in an overlengthened heel cord and an increase in crouch gait.

tion through a supramalleolar osteotomy performed near skeletal maturity.

The Knee

FLEXION DEFORMITY

Flexion is the most common spastic knee deformity.[95] It may be associated with a crouch stance that includes hip-flexion and equinus

contracture, or it may present as an isolated deformity resulting from spastic contracted hamstrings (Fig. 10-20). Tight hamstrings also may be responsible for shortening the stride length and may cause a functional sitting kyphosis resulting from posterior tilting of the pelvis.

The degree of contracture can be measured by the traditional straight-leg-raising technique. Greater accuracy is achieved by initially flexing the hip to a right angle and then passively extending the knee joint (Fig. 10-2).[66] The measured popliteal angle represents the angular deficit from passive full extension.

Surgical correction is indicated when there is a knee-flexion deformity greater than 15° during stance phase. Greater deformity requires a significant increase in the quadriceps force necessary for upright stance. Surgery performed to improve function is delayed until ambulation has been established with or without crutches. Associated hip and ankle contractures should be corrected simultaneously to prevent secondary iatrogenic deformities, such as increased lumbar lordosis.

Preoperative assessment should include gait analysis. Electromyograms may demonstrate prolonged hamstring activity throughout stance phase and may even extend into swing phase.[127]

Bleck noted that many diplegic patients have active contractions of both the quadriceps and hamstrings, which balance each other and prevent clinical deformity.[16]

Foster recommends a trial with preoperative casts to isolate the dominant element of the crouch gait.[48] Patients who achieve an erect stance with cylinder casts, benefit from hamstring lengthening since the knee is the dominant joint. Erect posture with a short leg cast would indicate the need for correction of an equinus deformity by heel-cord lengthening. When either type of cast forces the patient to lean the trunk forward, iliopsoas recession would also be recommended.

SURGICAL PROCEDURES. I prefer Z-lengthening of the hamstrings to a simple tenotomy in order to ensure preservation of flexor power. In young children, generally only medial hamstrings require lengthening.[41] Medial and lateral hamstrings surgery may be indicated in older patients with chronic contracture when the electromyogram demonstrates the

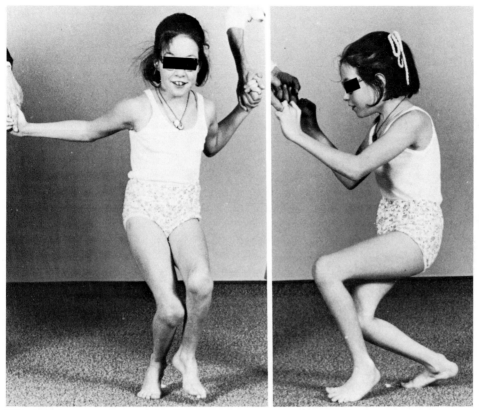

FIG. 10-20. Spastic contracted hamstrings lead to marked knee-flexion contractures and the need for the adjacent joints to accommodate themselves to the isolated knee deformity.

absence of quadriceps spasticity. Semimembranosus may also require lengthening by an aponeurotomy performed in the popliteal space at a point sufficiently proximal from its tibial insertion to ensure muscular continuity. A posterior capsulotomy is not indicated, although occasionally the contracted posterior retinaculum requires division to permit improved quadriceps function. The use of serial well-padded, opening wedging casts in the immediately postoperative period may provide additional correction. Transplantation of the hamstring tendons into the femoral condyles to assist in the extension of the hip has proven ineffective and may result in increased lumbar lordosis in the presence of a fixed hip-flexion contracture.[39] Excessive hamstring lengthening can result in genu recurvatum and can be avoided by erring on the side of conservatism when considering the amount of hamstring surgery to be performed.

When surgery is limited to the knee, postoperative use of cylinder casts permits early weight-bearing. These casts can be bivalved at 3 weeks postoperatively, and a determination made by the physical therapist and orthopaedist on the need for interim knee orthoses. Initial use of KAFO braces may be required while the quadriceps regain antigravity strength and voluntary control. Ambulation is begun in the therapy setting with the knee joints locked. Later, ambulation is possible with the knee joints unlocked and, eventually, an ankle–foot orthosis of a Saltiel type (Fig. 10-8) can be used to augment weak quadriceps function. This rehabilitation program may require 6 months of intensive physical therapy.

PATELLA ALTA. Patella alta may also be associated with knee-flexion contracture.[75] A lateral radiograph obtained with the knee flexed 30° illustrates the length of the patella and its ligament. Patella alta is present when

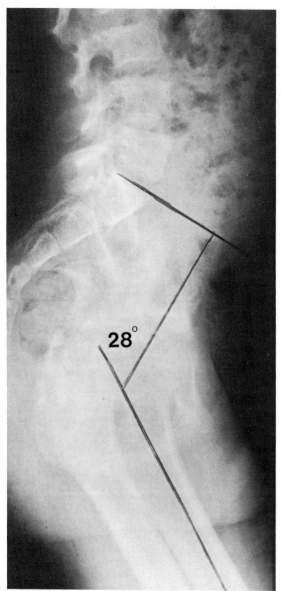

28°

FIG. 10-21. Sacrofemoral angle is determined on a standing lateral radiograph of the lumbar spine, pelvis, and proximal femoral shaft. A line is drawn along the top of the sacrum to measure the degree of pelvic inclination. A second line is made along the shaft of the femur. The angle formed by the intersection of the two lines is termed the sacrofemoral angle and in normal persons measures 45° to 65°.

companied by considerable risk of developing chondromalacia patellae because of the incompatibility of the patellar articular surface with the opposing femoral articular cartilage.[24] Bleck combines patellar tendon advancement with hamstring lengthening in patients whose epiphyses have closed.[14]

GENU VALGUM

Proximal tibial osteotomy may be required when genu valgum and external tibial rotation develop in ambulatory patients with shortened strides who have contracted adductors and hamstrings. Simple tibial external rotation is more readily managed by a supramalleolar osteotomy, which may also permit the correction of a secondary valgus deformity of the ankle joint.

HYPEREXTENSION DEFORMITY

Hyperextension deformity results from spastic quadriceps activity, which places the center of gravity in front of the knee and ankle joint.[35] Electromyography demonstrates continuous activity of the rectus femoris and vastus musculature throughout gait. Iliopsoas recession combined with a rectus femoris tenotomy corrects knee hyperextension and hip-flexion contractures, and also permits the reduction of lumbar lordosis.

The second cause of hyperextension is limited control of ankle plantarflexion, which halts the forward progression of the tibia in early stance if calf muscles are weak or later in stance if the calf muscles are strong.[119] Rosenthal has employed a fixed ankle below-knee orthosis designed to maintain the ankle in 5° of dorsiflexion when there is sufficient quadriceps strength to prevent uncontrolled knee flexion.[100] Weakening of the triceps surae would also benefit this latter cause of recurvatum. Uncontrolled hyperextension during growth may result in adaptive depression of the anterior tibial articular surface and overgrowth of the posterior tibial condyle. Proximal tibial osteotomy may be indicated to correct this secondary deformity.

The Hip

PREOPERATIVE ASSESSMENT

CLINICAL. Functional hip and knee muscle imbalance determines the gait pattern in

the ratio of the length exceeds 1 to 1.25. Correction of knee-flexion contracture creates quadriceps functional insufficiency and may lead to a recurrence of the contracture. Patellar tendon-advancement procedures are ac-

cerebral palsy, with iliopsoas overactivity evident in most patients. Those dominated by spastic hamstrings demonstrate hip flexion and internal rotation combined with knee flexion and a decreased lumbar lordosis, which permits the center of gravity to be centered over the feet. The group with spastic quadriceps demonstrates hip flexion and marked internal rotation with hyperextended knees and an increase in lumbar lordosis. Hip internal rotation and flexion deformity without knee abnormalities result when neither the quadriceps or hamstrings spasticity predominates.

RADIOLOGY. Bleck has developed a method of measuring fixed hip-flexion contracture using a standing lateral radiograph of the lumbar spine, pelvis, and proximal femur.[16] The relationship of the pelvis to the femur is constant in all groups with hip-flexion contractures as long as the patient stands erect. The sacrofemoral angle is created by the intersection of one line drawn along the top of the sacrum with a second line parallel to the femoral shaft (Fig. 10-21). The normal range for the angle is 45° to 65°, while a hip-flexion deformity demonstrates an angle of less than 45°.

GAIT ANALYSIS. Simon studied the interrelationship of the trunk, pelvis, and limb by gait analysis, which included motion studies, electromyograms, and force plate analysis and was able to isolate three patterns that differed in pelvic, femoral, and consequent hip motion.[120] The first type demonstrated a relatively normal pattern of both the pelvic and femoral components of hip motion but with delays in the rate of progression related to out-of-phase muscle activity. The second type exhibited disruption of the normal directional pattern of hip rotation due to abnormal movement of the trunk and pelvis in addition to abnormal electromyographic activity. The third type showed a relatively fixed relationship between the trunk, pelvis, and femur that severely limited rotational movement. The ability to distinguish between the apparent and actual hip-joint rotation may explain why the outcome of derotational hip surgery may be less satisfactory than soft-tissue surgery, which is directed toward correction of the muscle imbalance.[89]

Hip surgery should be delayed until independent gait has been achieved unless there is evidence of a secondary structural deformity, for example, hip subluxation. The initial primary dynamic muscle imbalance can lead to soft-tissue contracture and eventual bony deformity unless corrected. Functional surgery is most effective when performed on patients between the ages of 4 and 8 years. The increasing complexity of salvage surgery in older patients combined with the patients' psycho-social conflicts frequently diminishes the value of later efforts at correction. Hip surgery can be combined with other lower-extremity joint procedures.

ADDUCTION DEFORMITY

Adductor spasticity may cause diminished standing balance with a narrow-based or scissoring gait coupled with a shortened stride.[7] Sharrard has recommended adductor tenotomy in patients whose abduction of each hip is limited to 20° with or without the presence of scissoring.[113] Nonambulatory patients with limited range of motion and problems with perineal care or radiographic evidence of hip subluxation may undergo isolated tenotomies of the adductors and iliopsoas through a medial approach.[110,114]

TECHNIQUE FOR ADDUCTOR TENOTOMY. A transverse incision is made over the prominent adductor longus tendon approximately 1 cm distal to the inguinal crease. The scanty fat is swept away, exposing Camper's fascia, which is incised longitudinally over the visible tendon of the origin of the adductor longus. This muscle is circumferentially freed up with a McDonald dissector and then divided through its tendinous origin by electrocautery. The hip is abducted with the knee in extension to facilitate location of the gracilis, which is similarly isolated and divided. The anterior portion of the adductor magnus may also require tenotomy. A small amount of additional correction can be obtained by bluntly spreading the fascicles of the adductor brevis with a hemostat. Myotomy of the brevis or pectineus is rarely required. The procedure is done bilaterally when both lower extremities demonstrate spasticity. I reserve anterior branch obturator neurectomy for patients with progressive neurologic diseases such as progressive leukodystrophy or measles encephalopathy.[55] Perry recommends an electromyogram for ambulatory patients, to assist the physician in making the decision as to whether the gracilis and medial hamstring tenotomies should be combined with the adductor release.[89]

Postoperatively, long leg casts with an abductor bar holding each hip in 30° to 40° of abduction is employed. Marked spasticity and asymmetrical involvement may, postoperatively, lead to one hip assuming a position of 0° abduction while the other hip is widely abducted. This positional problem can be managed by extending the plaster immobilization upward to include the pelvis. Following 10 to 14 days of immobilization, hydrotherapy and active abduction in extension exercises and a gradual resumption of ambulation are permitted.[7] Indefinite use of a nighttime hip-abduction orthosis is recommended.

ADDUCTOR TRANSFER. Transfer of the adductor origin to the ischium has been reported to improve gait, increase hip abduction and stability.[26,57,124] The adductors are converted from accessory hip flexors to accessory extensors by transferring them posterior to the instant center of the hip joint. Guggenheim recommends the transfer be performed for diplegic patients with ambulatory potential before adaptive bony changes develop in the proximal femur and acetabulum.[58] This technically-demanding procedure has limited application for most patients with cerebral palsy.

HIP-FLEXION DEFORMITY

Surgical correction is recommended for hip-flexion contractures of greater than 20°. Bleck has identified the iliopsoas as the primary cause of this deformity.[12,16] He recommends iliopsoas recession for ambulatory patients with hip-flexion contractures and either a flexed-knee gait pattern due to spastic hamstrings or a hyperextended-knee gait pattern due to spastic quadriceps. Iliopsoas recession is most effective in spastic diplegic patients who have either a marked abnormality in gait pattern or conditions favorable for ambulation, and who have a hip flexion contracture greater than 15° and a sacrofemoral radiologic angle under 45°. Surgery is generally performed on patients between the ages of 5 and 7 years and may be combined with the other lower-extremity surgery. Iliop-

soas tenotomy is reserved for nonambulatory patients.

TECHNIQUE OF ILIOPSOAS RECESSION. Employing an anterior incision, the sartorius and lateral femoral cutaneous nerve are retracted laterally. The rectus femoris origin is identified and the femoral nerve bluntly freed from the iliac muscle and retracted medially. The iliacus is dissected from the anterior hip capsule. External rotation and flexion of the hip permits isolation of the psoas tendon, which is divided at the lesser trochanter and sutured to the exposed anterolateral hip capsule at the base of the femoral neck (Fig. 10-22). Patients whose hip flexion is accompanied by a hyperextended-knee deformity also require the release of the rectus femoris origin through the same incision.

Postoperatively, the patient should stay in bed for 3 weeks and be permitted to raise the trunk 30° to 40° for meals. During this time, active physical therapy for hip extensors, abductors, and external rotators is initiated. Postoperative cylinder casts are used only if additional hamstring surgery is performed. After the 3 weeks, gait training is begun in the parallel bars with advancement to crutches or a walker.

HIP-FLEXION INTERNAL ROTATION DEFORMITY

Iliopsoas recession and femoral derotational osteotomy may be required in patients over age 6 who have a pronounced internal rotation gait. An examination with the patient in the prone position and the patient's hips in extension demonstrates a passive range of motion of 80° to 90° of internal rotation with less than 15° of external rotation. At Newington Children's Hospital, patients under age 8 are managed by a supracondylar derotational osteotomy with crossed Kirschner-wire fixation (Fig. 10-23). A subtrochanteric derotational osteotomy is indicated in children above the age of 8. A 90° angle compression nail (ASIF) (Fig. 10-24) can be used either through a lateral approach or through the posterior incision recommended by Root.[99] Postoperative management includes 3 weeks of bedrest followed by the use of crutches with weight kept off the operated extremity for an additional 5 weeks.

Compensatory external tibial torsion may

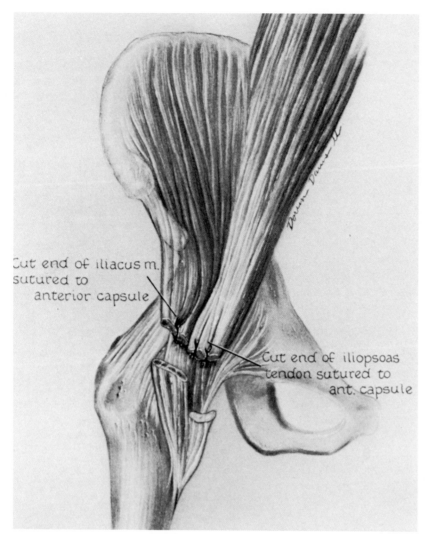

Cut end of iliacus m.
sutured to
anterior capsule

Cut end of iliopsoas
tendon sutured to
ant. capsule

FIG. 10-22. A blunt dissection of the iliacus permits exposure of the anterior hip capsule. The iliopsoas tendon is sutured near the base of the femoral neck on the anterolateral aspect of the joint capsule with heavy nonabsorbable sutures. (Bleck EE: J Bone Joint Surg 53A:1479, 1971)

become more evident following correction of the internal rotation of the femur and may lead to the development of a Chaplinesque gait pattern. I prefer to correct the tibial deformity by means of a supramalleolar derotational osteotomy, which may also permit correction of any elements of structural ankle valgus.

HIP-EXTENSION DEFORMITY

The rare patient who walks with a grotesque gait with marked truncal rotation because of functional hip extension ankylosis can benefit from proximal hamstring release.[112] These patients are unable to flex their hips, and straight leg raising is less then 30°. They cannot climb stairs. Because they sit with their hips in full extension, they develop a marked functional kyphosis and may present with a chief complaint of mid-dorsal back pain, since that is the only area of the spine that comes in contact with the back of the chair. A proximal hamstring release is not indicated when there is a significant co-contracture of hip and knee flexors, because this will lead to a prompt

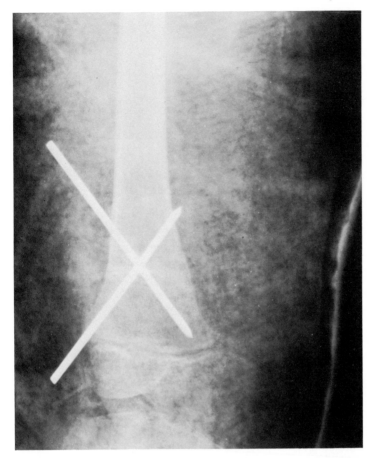

FIG. 10-23. A crossed Kirschner wire fixation along with plaster immobilization can be used for distal femoral derotational osteotomy in patients under eight years.

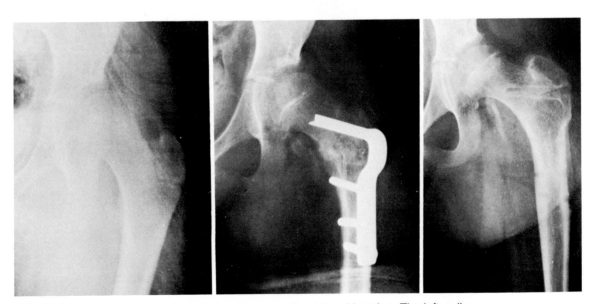

FIG. 10-24. An eleven-year-old diplegic with progressive hip subluxation. The left radiograph demonstrates preoperative hip subluxation. This was corrected by means of a 90° angle compression nail (ASIF). The right radiograph demonstrates the end result following removal of the nail.

increase in the patient's crouch gait.[34] Careful patient selection is mandatory when considering this rarely indicated procedure.

TECHNIQUE FOR PROXIMAL HAMSTRING RELEASE. A longitudinal incision is made through the gluteal cleft. The fibers of the gluteus maximus are swept superiorly, exposing the origin of the hamstrings from the ischial tuberosity as well as from the sciatic nerve. The origin is freed up circumferentially and the hamstring released through their short tendinous origin. Postoperative sitting with the knees in extension is encouraged during 2 weeks of bedrest. Gait training is then resumed and is generally accompanied by a significant improvement in the patient's function, for example, the ability to climb stairs. Straight leg raising postoperatively, can be accomplished to greater than 60°.

HIP SUBLUXATION

Spasticity in the iliopsoas and adductor muscles initiates lateral displacement of the femoral head. Subluxation can first be demonstrated seen on a routine anteroposterior roentgenogram as a break in Shenton's line (Fig. 10-25). Serial measurements of the acetabular index in younger patients, as well as the CE angle of Wiberg, are additional important radiographic criteria. Excessive pressure on the outer acetabular margin may prevent or distort normal acetabular development and eventually lead to acetabular dysplasia.[2,9,30]

Muscle-balancing procedures in ambulatory patients under age 6 include combined anterior tenotomy and iliopsoas recession. Nonambulatory patients in this age group are managed by adductor and iliopsoas tenotomy. Older patients require a subtrochanteric derotational varus osteotomy coupled with an iliopsoas recession. Actual coxa valga can be demonstrated by an anteroposterior roentgenogram with the hips in maximum internal rotation to negate the apparent valga due to the associated femoral anteversion (Fig. 10-26). A closing varus wedge osteotomy should not decrease the neck shaft angle below 125° (Fig. 10-27) and is performed when the true neck shaft angle exceeds 145°. Varus alignment of less than 115° may cause functional abductor weakness and may result in limb length inequality when the surgery is performed unilaterally. Fixation with a 90° angle

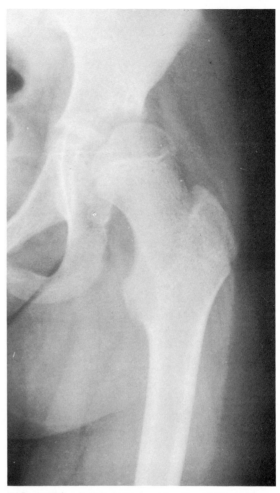

FIG. 10-25. Initial radiographic sign of hip subluxation is a break in Shenton's line. The normal arc that extends from the obturator foramen toward the femoral calcar is interrupted as the proximal femur begins to migrate superiorly and laterally.

compression nail (ASIF) is preferred for internal fixation.

Results of acetabular reconstruction are inconsistent. Correction when the patient is older than 4 years of age may be obtained with a Chiari osteotomy.[25] Both the Steel and Sutherland innominate osteotomies may alternatively be used in patients whose ischiae have fully ossified.[122,126] Painful subluxation in an ambulatory adult may require total hip replacement (Fig. 10-28).[27]

HIP DISLOCATION

Hip dislocation occurs most frequently in the nonambulatory total-body involved patient and

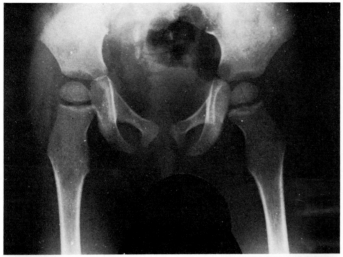

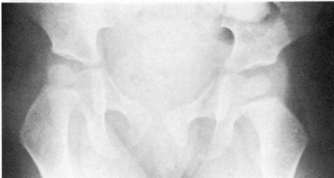

FIG. 10-26. Apparent coxa valga on a neutral rotation radiograph (*upper*) is decreased when the same patient is examined with the hip in internal rotation (*lower*). The actual degree of coxa valga can be more accurately determined by the second method.

is a result of iliopsoas and adductor spasticity associated with excessive femoral anteversion and acetabular dysplasia.[61,76,83,105,111,128] Samilson reported that 90% of dislocated hips occurred in this type of patient with 7 years as the mean age for the dislocation.[105] Fixed flexion–adduction contractures accompanying hip dislocation may lead to formidable problems in caring for the total-body involved patient. Weight distribution through the buttocks and thighs becomes asymmetrical and may lead to the development of ischial or trochanteric bursitis or to the development of pressure ulcers. Pelvic obliquity may threaten sitting balance and has been implicated in the development of scoliosis. Peroneal hygiene may become a serious nursing problem. Posterior dislocation creates unequal sitting thigh lengths, which may require special wheelchair seat modifications. Pain may accompany hip dislocation in older patients with total-body involvement or dystonia. A vicious

cycle is initiated with the pain leading to increased muscle spasm, which further increases the pain. This pattern may be aggravated by attempted movement.

TREATMENT. Prevention remains the preferred method of management. Total-body involved patients under 7 years of age with hip subluxation can be managed by bilateral adductor and iliopsoas tenotomies performed through a medial approach.[121] Plaster abduction immobilization for 2 weeks followed by resumption of sitting in a wheelchair with an abduction platform wedge is recommended.

Orthopaedic management of hip dislocation is difficult. Soft-tissue surgery by itself is inadequate.[23,27,99] Femoral head and neck resection usually results in increased pain as the resected end of the femur is forced against the ilium by the spastic muscles. Castle recommends resection of the proximal third of the femur combined with construction of a

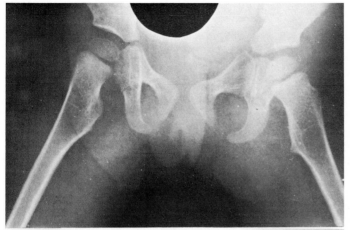

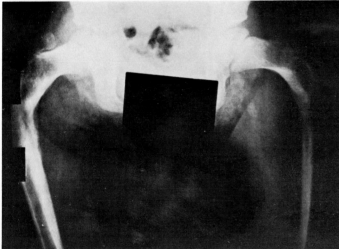

FIG. 10-27. The longitudinal growth of long bones is influenced by pressure applied to the epiphyseal growth plate. Forces parallel to the direction of the epiphyseal growth plate act to inhibit growth. The correction of the coxa valga (*upper radiograph*) has not remodeled five years after bilateral femoral varus osteotomies because the growth plate has been made perpendicular and subject to abnormal pressure forces.

capsular flap across the acetabulum and suturing of the quadriceps muscle around the resected end of the femur for relief of pain and ease of peroneal care in the severely mentally and physically retarded patient.[23]

Relocation of the femoral head may be indicated. An adductor tenotomy and iliopsoas tenotomies are performed through a medial approach, a hip joint capsulorraphy and pelvic osteotomy through an anterior exposure, and a subtrochanteric femoral shortening and varus derotational osteotomy through a lateral incision. The Chiari osteotomy has had the widest application for acetabular dysplasia, although both the Sutherland and Steel innominate osteotomies also have been used.

Hip arthrodesis and total hip replacement are reserved for the skeletally-mature patient with hip pain. Arthrodesis is indicated for the nonambulatory total-body involved patient with pain both in sitting and in recumbency. Root recommends that the hip be fused in a comfortable sitting position with 45° of flexion and 15° of abduction and neutral rotation.[98]

The Upper Extremity

The inability to replace sensory or fine motor-control deficiencies limits upper-extremity surgery to only 4% of the cerebral palsy population. Successful management requires thorough preoperative and postoperative planning as well as repeated assessment of the function of the hand.[53,107] Persistence of tonic neck reflexes and the absence of a parachute reaction beyond 9 months of age interferes with functional improvement after surgery.

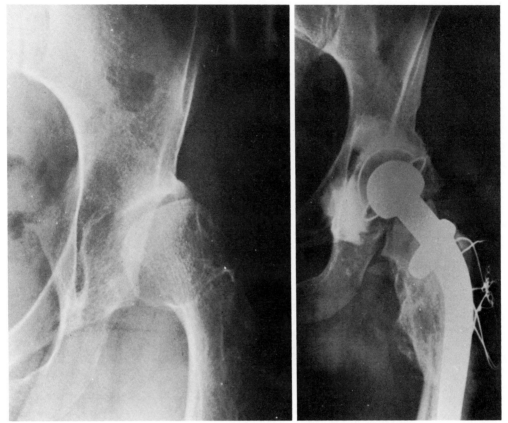

FIG. 10-28. Painful subluxation may require total joint replacement in the adult patient. (Radiographs courtesy of Dr. R. Sirkin.)

The ideal candidate for upper extremity surgery has spastic hemiplegia, is intelligent and well-motivated with a rudimentary pattern of grasp and release, has reasonable hand sensitivity, is older than 6 years of age and able to cooperate with the postoperative rehabilitation program. Surgery is most commonly performed in the hemiplegic patient to improve the helping hand in the performance of activities of daily living, increase the speed of hand and forearm movement and coordination, or to produce a better cosmetic appearance. Hemiplegics benefit most from improvement in grasp and release performance. Patients with total-body involvement may note improvement in two-handed activities of daily living despite limited hand and finger function. Many of these patients will also use nighttime splinting with the wrist in extension, fingers in almost complete extension, and the thumb out of the palm in order to prevent development of fixed contractures. Upper-extremity surgery in motor disorders is rarely indicated because the results are unpredictable, and positioning of the hand in space is limited.

PHYSICAL EXAMINATION

Upper-limb positon is determined by flexor or extensor hypertonicity. The pattern of arm extension synergy includes shoulder protraction, arm adduction and internal rotation, elbow extension, forearm pronation, wrist extension and ulnar deviation, and finger flexion. Arm flexor synergy demonstrates shoulder retraction, arm abduction and external rotation, elbow flexion, forearm supination, wrist flexion and radial deviation, and finger extension. The use of plaster immobilization may break up these dominant patterns and assist the orthopaedist in isolating the dominant muscle group and its overflow effect on the contiguous joints. Passive range of motion of all upper-extremity joints should be measured and the presence of hypotonia or spasticity determined.

MOTOR TESTING. Formal muscle evaluation can be performed with older patients whereas observation of a young child during play may yield a more meaningful assessment of the child's motor function. The pattern of grasp and release should be studied while the patient holds both a large and a small object. Functional testing and analysis by an occupational therapist may be important. Dynamic electromyographic assessment is beneficial when tendon transfers or tenotomies are being considered.[88,109]

SENSORY EVALUATION. Stereognosis, two-point discrimination, and proprioception, as well as the ability to position and control the limb in space, are important clinical determinants. Astereognosis may interfere with function but is not a contraindication to surgery.[129] Goldner recommends that the patient be examined with both the patient's hands overhead and the patient's eyes closed.[51,52] The examiner then places objects in each of the patient's hands while asking him to identify the objects.

THE SHOULDER

Shoulder internal rotation during gait magnifies residual elbow flexion. Mild deformities can be corrected by a physical therapy program designed to strengthen the external rotators and stretch the pectoral muscles (Fig. 10-29). Occasionally, more severe internal rotation requires a humeral derotational osteotomy in order to improve hand position and function.

THE ELBOW

Loss of more than 30° of full elbow extension may interfere with the use of crutches or a walker. Mital recommends lengthening the biceps brachii combined with excision of the lacertus fibrosus and aponeurotomy of the brachialis (Fig. 10-30).[81,82] Patients with excessive dystonic elbow flexion may also be functionally disabled. The use of a 1% lido-

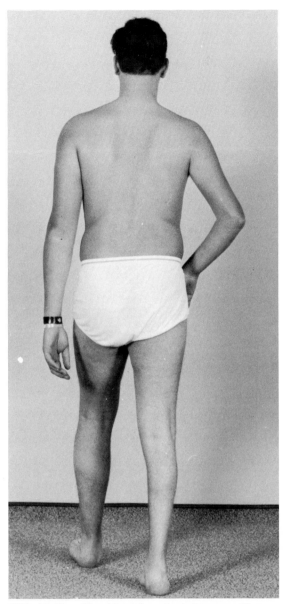

FIG. 10-29. Shoulder internal rotation magnifies a 30° elbow-flexion conracture. Physical therapy stressing both shoulder range-of-motion and active exericses for external rotator and extensor muscles is recommended for problems of this magnitude.

caine solution to perform a musculocutaneous nerve block decreases biceps brachii tone and permits both assessment of the improved elbow range of motion and demonstration that the brachioradialis strength is sufficient to permit elbow flexion against gravity. Patients meeting these criteria benefit from an open

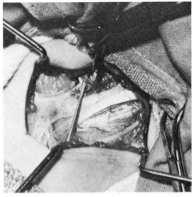
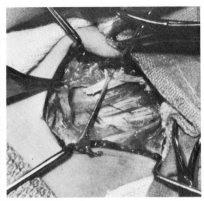
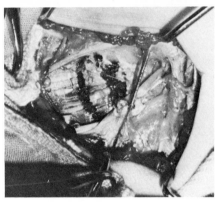

FIG. 10-30. An elbow-flexion contracture can be corrected by soft-tissue procedures. The left operative photograph demonstrates the contents of the antecubital fossa. The middle photograph shows a forceps holding the Z-lengthened tendon of the biceps brachii. Note that the lacertus fibrosis has also been excised. Aponeurotomy of the brachialis completes the procedure (*right photograph*).

motor neurectomy of the musculocutaneous nerve.

THE FOREARM

Patients with severe flexion contractures of the hand and wrist have limited effective hand function because of the stretched extensor and reduced flexor excursions. Severe elbow-flexion deformity coupled with forearm pronation can be corrected by the Inglis release of the flexor–pronator origin.[69] Improvement of hand control and the ability to place and use the hand in a functional position are the most impressive results of this operation. Inglis recommends lengthening the tendons at the musculotendinous junction when flexion contracture is limited to one or two muscles.

TECHNIQUE FOR RELEASE OF THE FLEXOR–PRONATOR ORIGIN. The incision is made over the medial epicondyle extending from 2 inches above the epicondyle to the midpoint of the forearm over the ulna. The ulnar nerve is identified and the nerve supply to the flexor

carpi ulnaris and flexor digitorum profoundus is preserved. After elevating the ulnar nerve from its groove, the origins of the flexor carpi ulnaris and flexor digitorum profundus are released from the subcutaneous border of the ulna. The dissection begins distally and continues proximally along the ulna and interosseous membrane. The ulnar nerve is replaced in the groove and the entire flexor–pronator mass is divided at its origin for the medial part of the humeral epicondyle. The median nerve can then be visualized as it passes through the pronator teres. It may also be necessary to release the radial origin of the flexor sublimis, lacertus fibrosus, and the fascia of the brachialis muscle. The ulnar nerve is then

FIG. 10-31. *A.* Initial incision is shown. The tendon is divided and the ulnar nerve is exposed in the insert. *B.* The second incision is demonstrated with the muscle being freed in a proximal direction. *C.* The third incision exposes extensor carpi radialis longus. *D.* The technique of transfer insertion is shown. (Green WT: Surg Gynec Obstet 75:337, 1942)

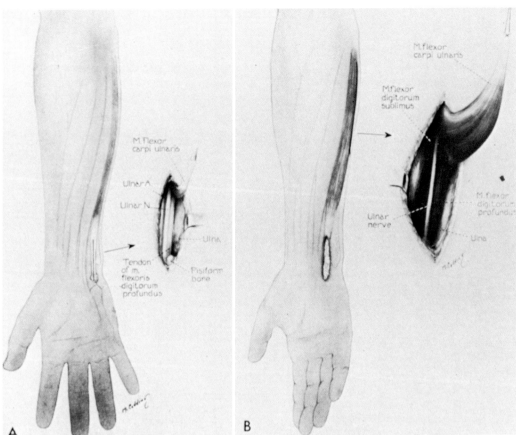

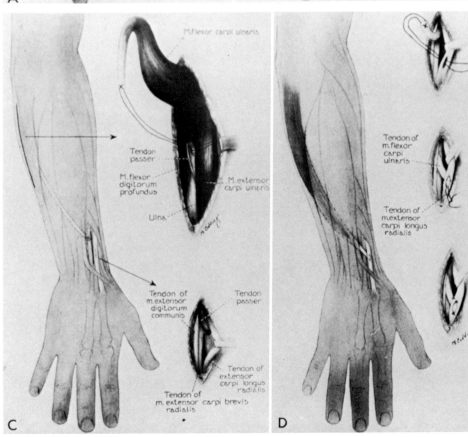

transplanted anteriorly. The bony prominence of the upper condyle may require resection. Postoperatively, the patient is placed in a long arm dressing with the arm in supination and the wrist and fingers in a neutral position for 3 weeks. The patient is then placed in functional hand splints, which are used day and night.

THE WRIST

When the wrist can be corrected passively but assumes the flexed position during grasp, flexor carpi ulnaris transfer is preferred (Fig. 10-31). Green stressed that a prerequisite for this procedure is excellent finger control.[54] He noted that the ability to extend the wrist and maintain it is fundamental to finger function. He pointed out that wrist motion, supination and pronation compliment hand function and these movements are lost with a wrist fusion. The transfer can be attached either to the extensor carpi radialis brevis insertion or, when additional supination is required, to the insertion of the extensor carpi radialis longus. Perry recommends the dynamic electromyographic evaluation of the flexor carpi ulnaris when considering tendon transfer.[88] Demonstrated activity during grasp would suggest transfer to the extensor carpi radialis brevis to assist wrist dorsiflexion, whereas activity during release indicates that the transfer would be more appropriately placed in the extensor digitorum communis. Continuous electromyographic activity during both grasp and release is an indication for lengthening of the tendon.

TECHNIQUE FOR CARPI ULNARIS TRANSFER. The flexor carpi ulnaris is transferred around the medial side of the ulna to be inserted on the dorsum of the wrist. A distal incision allows the tendon to be detached from the pisiform and sharp dissection is carried proximally along its ulnar origin. A more proximal incision over the muscle belly permits the muscle to be freed until it can pass in a straight line from its origin to its dorsal insertion. The neurovascular supply enters in the proximal third of the muscle and limits the proximal dissection. The intermuscular septum is excised at the medial edge of the ulna at a suitable level. To permit transferring the muscle to the dorsal forearm, the tendon is sutured with the forearm in full supination

and 45° of wrist dorsiflexion. A long arm cast is applied, which is bivalved, and an active exercise program is initiated over the next 6 weeks.

WRIST ARTHRODESIS. Wrist fusion is rarely indicated. Arthrodesis can be considered only after a short arm cast application has determined finger extension power in the corrected position. It is imperative that the orthopaedist determine the need for wrist flexion or extension as well as stability in grasp and release activities. Wrist fusion is more commonly indicated for cosmetic reasons in the face of a severe fixed deformity or when generalized muscle control is so limited that even limited functional active flexion–extension of the fingers cannot be accomplished. Surgery should be delayed until the patient is over 12 years of age to avoid embarrassment of the distal radial growth plate.

THUMB-IN-PALM DEFORMITY

This difficult problem arises from the weakness of the thumb extensors and abductors in the presence of strong flexors. This deformity blocks entry or placement of objects into the palm and prevents the thumb from participating in grasp or pinch. The thumb contracture is frequently associated with forearm pronation and finger and wrist flexion. A persistent spasm of adductor pollicis, first dorsal interosseous, flexor pollicis brevis, and adductor pollicis brevis results in overstretching of their antagonists and leads to the position where the thumb is acutely flexed into the palm and comes to lie under the flexed fingers.

TECHNIQUE FOR MYOTOMY[77]. A tenotomy of the adductor pollicis is performed through an incision at the level of the palmar crease at the base of the thenar eminence. The flexor tendons of the ulnar four fingers are retracted towards the ulna together with the neurovascular bundles, thus exposing the adductor pollicis. The adductor pollicis, flexor pollicis brevis, and the distal two thirds of abductor pollicis brevis are released through this incision (Fig. 10-32). The first dorsal interosseous is divided near the first metacarpus. Additional tendon surgery to augment abduction of the first metacarpus in extension of the

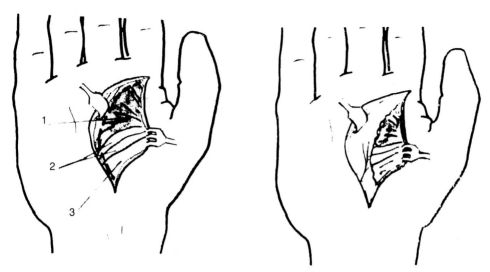

FIG. 10-32. Myotomy of the adductor pollicis permits release of the first metacarpus and does not allow hyperextension of the metacarpophalangeal joint that sometimes occurs with adductor pollicis tenotomy. (Matev I: J Bone Joint Surg 45B:703, 1963)

proximal phalanx can be performed through a separate dorsoradial incision. The operation has the advantage of not permitting hyperextension of the metacarpophalangeal joint of the thumb.

THUMB ARTHRODESIS

Goldner recommends fusion of the metacarpophalangeal joint of the thumb when there is evidence of hypermobility and instability of this joint in older children.[51]

Spinal Deformity

Neuromuscular scoliosis is seen most frequently in nonambulatory total-body involved patients, particularly those requiring institutional care.[5,97,108] Scoliosis that develops in a borderline ambulator may threaten the loss of walking ability. Thoracolumbar curves are most common and are also most likely to progress.[106] Curves that exceed 25° should be managed by a total-contact orthosis. A Milwaukee brace with an enlarged neck ring may be indicated in the rare patient with a high thoracic scoliosis and a history of grand mal seizures. The use of a Risser cast to gain partial correction of the scoliosis before application of a spinal orthosis is frequently used. Rang recently described a

program of special seating which is useful for the profoundly handicapped child with cerebral palsy.[93]

Scoliosis which exceeds 50° despite orthotic intervention, is most appropriately managed by spinal fusion. Preoperative supine bend roentgenograms are important in determining curve flexibility and the length of the fusion. The presence of abnormal posturing or fixed lower-extremity contractures may complicate postoperative management and lead to a decision to use either halo-skeletal traction or to perform preliminary release of the lower-extremity contractures.[15]

A significant rate of complications with isolated posterior fusion with Harrington instrumentation or anterior spinal fusions with Dwyer instrumentation have been reported.[37,59] A more effective technique employs preliminary halo-skeletal traction followed by a first-stage anterior spinal fusion with Dwyer instrumentation followed by a second-stage posterior spinal fusion with Harrington instrumentation.[19] The posterior fusion should extend to the sacrum when the scoliosis extends into the pelvis (Fig. 10-33). Prompt postoperative immobilization in a spinal orthosis is necessary for 1 year. Posterior spinal fusion with segmental spinal instrumentation avoids the need for postoperative immobilization and is my method of choice.

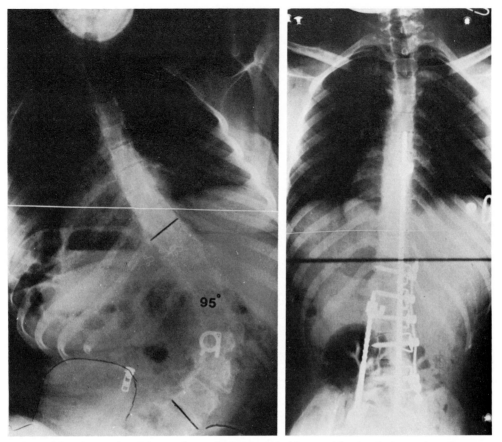

FIG. 10-33. A spastic adolescent's scoliosis corrected by combined anterior and posterior spinal fusion. Spinal segmental instrumentation may alternatively be used.

Fractures

Fractures occur most commonly in the total-body involved bedridden patient in association with grand mal seizures during which the patient falls or receives a direct blow, *e.g.,* striking the siderail of the bed. Contracture or fixed hip dislocation also increases the incidence of fractures in bedridden patients. Dent reported fractures which result in osteomalacia in patients using anticonvulsant medications.[29]

Management of the fractures must be individualized.[123] Internal fixation may be appropriate for ambulatory patients. Rosenthal reported fractures of the patella due to excessive tension in the quadriceps mechanism, usually in the presence of a flexion contracture.[71,101] He recommends the initial use of a plaster cylinder or a night brace to hold the knee in extension. Should this be unsuccess-

ful, a hamstring release to correct the flexion deformity followed by plaster immobilization may be required. Total-body involved patients may benefit from a spica cast that has been modified to accommodate coexistent contractures in contiguous joints. McIvor noted that malunions are frequent but with osseous union the patient's functional status is generally restored to the prefracture state.[79]

Spinal Deformity Associated with Juvenile Spinal-Cord Injury

Scoliosis, kyphosis, or lordosis may develop secondary to spinal-cord injury in young patients without radiologic evidence of a related fracture or dislocation (Fig. 10-34). The pediatric spine has sufficient elasticity to be able to withstand considerable traction and torsion, while the spinal cord itself is lacerated

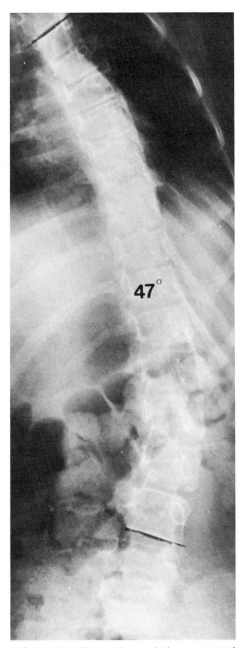

47°

FIG. 10-34. The major period or progression of spinal deformity is the adolescent years with the rate of deformity decreasing as osseous maturity is achieved. This radiograph of a twelve-year-old quadriplegic demonstrates a typical long thoraco-lumbar scoliosis.

by the same amount of force. All girls under 13 years of age and all boys under 15 years of age with cervical or thoracic injuries will develop significant spinal deformity with pelvic obliquity.[21] The introduction of spinal orthoses when the potential for spinal deformity exists has the advantage of restoring sitting balance and frees the patient's upper extremities for activities of daily living. Posterior spinal fusion with Harrington instrumentation was associated with a high incidence of postoperative complications. Thus, authors currently recommend either a combined anterior and posterior spinal fusion or the use of spinal segmental instrumentation.[21,44,78]

Head-Injured Children

Several important characteristics separate this group from newborn patients with the syndrome of cerebral palsy. Since developmental milestones had been achieved prior to the cerebral insult, the attending physician can no longer rely on the primitive reflexes as reliable prognostic or therapeutic aids. There may be considerable fluctuation in spasticity during the first year after head injury during which time dynamic extremity deformities are appropriately managed by plaster casts and positioning.[64] Reconstructive procedures should be delayed until at least 1 year after the head injury.

Long-term neuromuscular disabilities result from residual significant spasticity or ataxia or both. These problems are related to the depth and duration of coma and not to the patient's age at the time of injury. Hoffer has defined coma as[62]:

Level 1—the patient is normal in terms of cognition and recording ongoing events.

Level 2—the patient is semi-comatose, unable to record ongoing events, and lacking recall.

Level 3—the patient is even more comatose and responds only to noxious stimuli, but in a purposeful manner.

Level 4—the patient is in a deep coma and responds only in a very diffuse way to the most noxious of stimuli.

Level 5—the patient is in a deep coma and is unresponsive. Head-injured children who reach level 2 by 6 weeks after injury will probably develop independent selfcare and ambulation. When this level is reached by 12 weeks, partial dependence is a probable result. When level 3 or deeper coma persists for longer than 3 months, the patient is likely to be totally dependent.

The most common lower-extremity surgery includes heel-cord lengthening and toe-flexor releases. A split anterior tendon transfer may be required for a dynamic heel varus. The more severely involved patients with more significant coma may require major lower-extremity joint releases. Phenol blocks to the upper-extremity motor nerves are effective in preventing the development of contractures when they are performed within 6 months of head injury before a fixed deformity develops.[20]

Anoxic patients are much more severely involved than the head-injured group. Patients in a deep coma for more than 1 week have a poor prognosis.[60] Acquired mental retardation and communication problems compound efforts at rehabilitation. A minority of these patients regain ambulation. Painful early hip dislocation may develop, which can be successfully treated by early soft-tissue releases.

REFERENCES

1. Adams MM, Marks JS, Gustafson J, Oakley GP: Rh hemolytic disease of the newborn: Using incidence observations to evaluate the use of Rh immune globulin. American Journal of Public Health 71:1031-1035, 1981
2. Arkin AM, Katz JF: The effects of pressure on epiphyseal growth. J Bone Joint Surg 38A:1056, 1956
3. Atkins DM: Evaluation of a preadmission preparation program: Goals clarification as the first step. Child Health Care 10:48, 1981
4. Baker LD, Hill LM: Foot alignment in the cerebral palsy patient. J Bone Joint Surg 46A:1, 1964
5. Balmer GA, MacEwen GD: The incidence and treatment of scoliosis in cerebral palsy. J Bone Joint Surg 52B:134, 1970
6. Banks HH: The foot and ankle in cerebral palsy. In Samilson RL (ed): Orthopaedic Aspects of Cerebral Palsy. Philadelphia, JB Lippincott, 1975
7. Banks HH, Green WT: Adductor myotomy and obturator neurectomy for correction of the hip in cerebral palsy. J Bone Joint Surg 42A:111, 1960
8. Banks HH, Green WT: Correction of equinus deformity in cerebral palsy. J Bone Joint Surg 40A:1359, 1958
9. Beals RK: Developmental changes in the femur and acetabulum in spastic paraplegia and diplegia. Dev Med Child Neurol 11:303, 1969
10. Beals RK: Spastic paraplegia and diplegia: An evaluation of non-surgical and surgical factors influencing the prognosis for ambulation. J Bone Joint Surg 48A:827, 1966
11. Bisla RS, Louis HJ, Albano P: Transfer of the tibialis posterior tendon in cerebral palsy. J Bone Joint Surg 58A:497, 1976
12. Bleck EE: The hip in cerebral palsy. Orthop Clin North Am 11:79, 1980
13. Bleck EE; Locomotor prognosis in cerebral palsy. Dev Med Child Neurol 17:18, 1975
14. Bleck EE: Orthopaedic Management of Cerebral Palsy, p 187. Philadelphia, W B Saunders, 1979
15. Bleck EE: Spinal and pelvic deformities in cerebral palsy. In Samilson RL (ed): Orthopaedic Aspects of Cerebral Palsy. Philadelphia, JB Lippincott, 1975
16. Bleck EE: Surgical management of spastic flexion deformities of the hip with special reference to iliopsoas recession. J Bone Joint Surg 53A:1468, 1971
17. Bobath K: The motor deficit in patients with cerebral palsy. Clinics in Developmental Medicine, No. 23, Philadelphia, JB Lippincott, 1966
18. Bobath K, Bobath B: An assessment of motor handicap of children with cerebral palsy and their response to treatment. Occupational Therapy Journal 27:1, 1958
19. Bonnett C, Brown JC, and Grow T: Thoracolumbar scoliosis in cerebral palsy. J Bone Joint Surg 58A:328, 1976
20. Braun RM, Hoffer MM, Mooney V, McKeever J, Roper B: Phenol nerve block in the treatment of acquired spastic hemiplegia in the upper limb. J Bone Joint Surg 55A:580, 1973
21. Campbell J, Bonnett C: Spinal cord injury in children. Clin Orthop 112:114, 1975
22. Carlson JM, Winter R: The "Gillette" sitting support orthosis. orthotics and Prosthetics 32:35, 1978
23. Castle ME, Schneider C: Proximal femoral resection-interposition arthroplasty. J Bone Joint Surg 60A:1051, 1978
24. Chandler FA: Re-establishment of normal leverage of patella in knee flexion deformity in spastic paralysis. Surg Gynecol Obstet 57:523, 1933
25. Chiari K: Medial displacement osteotomy of the pelvis. Clin Orthop 98:55, 1974
26. Couch WH, DeRosa GP, Throop FB: Thigh adductor transfer for spastic cerebral palsy. Dev Med Child Neurol 19:343, 1977
27. Cristofaro R, Koffman M, Woodward R, Baxter S: Treatment of the totally involved cerebral palsy problem sitter. Paper presented at the annual meeting of the American Academy for Cerebral Palsy and Developmental Medicine, Atlanta, 1977
28. Dennyson WG, Fulford, R: Subtalar arthrodesis by cancellous grafts and metallic fixation. J Bone Joint Surg 58B:507, 1976
29. Dent CE: Osteomalacia with long-term anticonvulsant therapy and epilepsy. Brit Med J, 4:69, 1970
30. Drennan JC: The hip in myelomeningocele. In Katz JF, Siffert RA (eds): Disorders of the Hip in Children. Philadelphia, J B Lippincott, 1983
31. Drennan JC: Current status of bioengineering. Instructional course presented at the annual meeting of the American Academy for Cerebral Palsy and Developmental Medicine, Detroit, 1981

32. Drennan JC: Pathophysiology of cerebral palsy. Paper presented to the Canadian Orthopaedic Association, Quebec, 1975

33. Drennan JC: The upper extremity in cerebral palsy. Instructional course presented at the annual meeting of the American Academy for Cerebral Palsy and Developmental Medicine, Toronto, 1978

34. Drummond DS, Rogala F, Templeton J, Cruess R: Proximal hamstring release for knee flexion and crouched posture in cerebral palsy. J Bone Joint Surg 56A:1598, 1974

35. Duncan WR: Release of rectus femoris in spastic children. J Bone Joint Surg 37A:634, 1955

36. Dubowitz V: The Floppy Infant, 2nd ed Clinics in Developmental Medicine, Philadelphia, No. 76, J B Lippincott, 1980

37. Dwyer AF: Experience of anterior correction of scoliosis. Clin Orthop 93:191, 1973

38. Dwyer FC: Osteotomy of the calcaneum for pes cavus. Bone Joint Surg 41B:80, 1959

39. Eggers GWN: Transplantation of hamstring tendons to femoral condyles in order to improve hip extension and to decrease knee flexion in cerebral spastic paralysis. J Bone Joint Surg 34A:827, 1952

40. Eggers GWN, Evans EB: Surgery in cerebral palsy. J Bone Joint Surg 45A:1275, 1963

41. Evans EB: The knee in cerebral palsy. In Samilson RL (ed): Orthopaedic Aspects of Cerebral Palsy. Philadelphia, J B Lippincott, 1975

42. Evans EB: The status of surgery of the lower extremities in cerebral palsy. Clin Orthop 47:127, 1966

43. Fay T: Neuromuscular reflex therapy for spastic disorders. J Fla Med Assoc 44:1234, 1958

44. Ferguson RL, Allen BL: Segmental spinal instrumentation for routine scoliotic curve. Contemporary Orthopaedics 2:450, 1980

45. Fiorentino MR: Reflex Testing Methods for Evaluating Central Nervous System Development. 2nd ed, Springfield, Il, Charles C Thomas, 1973

46. Fiorentino MR: A Basis for Sensorimotor Development—Normal and Abnormal. The Influence of Primitive, Postural Reflexes on the Development and Distribution of Tone. Springfield, Il, Charles C Thomas, 1981

47. Ford LF, Bleck EE, Collins FJ, Stevick D: Efficacy of dantrolene sodium in the treatment of spastic cerebral palsy. Dev Med Child Neurol 18:770, 1976

48. Foster RS, Munger DH: Evaluation of crouch gait due to spastic cerebral palsy. Paper presented at the annual meeting of the American Academy for Cerebral Palsy and Developmental Medicine, Atlanta, 1977

49. Gage JR, Drennan JC: Orthotics in cerebral palsy. In Thompson GL (ed): Comprehensive Management of Cerebral Palsy. New York, Grune & Stratton, In Press 1982

50. Garrett AL, Lister M, Drennan J: New concept in bracing for cerebral palsy. Journal Of The American Physical Therapy Association 46:728, 1966

51. Goldner JL: The upper extremity in cerebral palsy. In Samilson RL (ed): Orthopaedic Aspects of Cerebral Palsy. Philadelphia, J B Lippincott, 1976

52. Goldner JL: Upper extremity reconstructive surgery in cerebral palsy or similar conditions. The American Academy Of Orthopaedic Surgeons Instructional Course Lectures. American Academy of Orthopaedic Surgeons, XVIII:169, St Louis, C V Mosby, 1961

53. Goldner JL: Upper extremity tendon transfer in cerebral palsy. Orthop Clin North Am 5:389, 1974

54. Green WT: Tendon transplantation of the flexor carpi ulnaris for pronation-flexion deformity of the wrist. Surg Gynec Obstet 75:337, 1942

55. Gregg N: Further observations on congenital defects in infants following maternal rubella. Transactions Of The Ophthalmological Society Of Australia 4:119, 1946

56. Grice DS: Extra-articular arthrodesis of the subtalar joint for correction of paralytic flat feet in children. J Bone Joint Surg 34A:927, 1952

57. Griffin PP, Wheelhouse WW, Shievi R: The adductor transfer for adductor spasticity: A Clinical and electromyographical gait analysis. Orthop Trans 1:76, 1977

58. Guggenheim J: The hip adductor transfer in cerebral palsy. Paper presented at the annual meeting of the American Academy for Cerebral Palsy and Developmental Medicine, Detroit, 1981

59. Harrington PR: Treatment of scoliosis correction and internal fixation by spine instrumentation. J Bone Joint Surg 44A:591, 1962

60. Hoffer MM: Basic considerations and classification of cerebral palsy. Instructional Course Lectures. American Academy of Orthopaedic Surgeons, XXV:96, C V Mosby, 1976

61. Hoffer MM, Abraham E, Nickel V: Salvage surgery at the hip to improve sitting posture of mentally retarded, severely disabled children with cerebral palsy. Dev Med Child Neurol 14:51, 1972

62. Hoffer MM, Brink J: Orthopaedic management of acquired cerebrospasticity in childhood. Clin Orthop 110:244, 1975

63. Hoffer MM, Feiwell E, Perry R, Perry J, Bonnett C: Functional ambulation in patients with myelomeningocele. J Bone Joint Surg 55A:137, 1973

64. Hoffer MM, Garrett A, Brink J, Perry J, Hale W, Nickel V: The orthopaedic management of brain-injured children. J Bone Joint Surg 53A:567, 1971

65. Hoffer MM, Reswig JA, Garrett AM, Perry J: The split anterior tibial tendon transfer in treatment of spastic varus of the hindfoot in childhood. Orthop Clin North Am 5:31, 1974

66. Hold KS: Assessment of Cerebral Palsy. p 214. London, Lloyd–Luke, 1965

67. Horstmann HM, Eilert RE: Triple arthrodesis in cerebral palsy. Paper presented at the annual meeting of the American Academy of Orthopaedic Surgeons, Las Vegas, 1977

68. Illingworth RS: Recent Advances in Cerebral Palsy. Boston, Little, Brown & Co, 1958

69. Inglis AE, Cooper W: Release of flexor-pronator origin for flexion deformities of the hand and wrist in spastic paralysis: A study of eighteen cases. J Bone and Joint Surg 48A:847, 1966

70. Jones MH: Differential diagnosis and natural history of the cerebral palsy. In Samilson RL (ed): Orthopaedic Aspects of Cerebral Palsy. Philadelphia, J B Lippincott, 1975

71. Kaye JJ, Freiberger RH: Fragmentation of the lower

pole of the patella in spastic lower extremities. Radiology 101:97, 1971

72. Khalili AA, Benton JG: A physiologic approach to the evaluation and management of spasticity with procaine and phenol nerve block. Clin Orthop 47:97, 1966

73. LeBlanc M: Quoted In Bleck EE, Orthopaedic Management of Cerebral Palsy. p 87. Philadelphia, W B Saunders, 1979

74. Little WJ: On the influence of abnormal parturition, difficult labours, premature birth and asphyxia neonatorum on the mental and physical condition of the child, especially in relation to deformities. Transactions Of The Obstetrical Society of London 3:293, 1862

75. Lotman DB: Knee flexion deformity and patella alta in spastic cerebral palsy. Dev Med Child Neurol 18:315, 1976

76. Magilligan DJ: Calculations of the angle of anteversion by means of horizontal lateral roentgenography. J Bone Joint Surg 38A:1231, 1956

77. Matev I: Surgical treatment of spastic "thumb-in-palm" deformity. J Bone and Joint Surg +5B:703, 1963

78. Mayfield JK, Erkkila JC, Winter RB: Spine deformity subsequent to acquired spinal cord injury. J Bone Joint Surg 63A:1401, 1981

79. McIvor W, Samilson RL: Fracture in patients with cerebral palsy. J Bone and Joint Surg 48A:858, 1966

80. McKeever DC: Arthrodesis of the first metatarsophalangeal joint for hallux valgus, hallux rigidus and metatarsus primus varus. J Bone and Joint Surg 34A:129, 1952

81. Mital MA: Flexion contractures and involuntary flexor bias in the upper extremities at elbows—Its surgical management. In Proceedings of the American Academy of Orthopaedic Surgeons, J Bone and Joint Surg 57A:1031, 1975

82. Mital MA: Flexion contractures and involuntary bias in upper extremities at the elbow: Its surgical management (abstr). Dev Med Child Neurol 19:116, 1977

83. O'Brien JJ, Sirkin RB: The natural history of the dislocated hip in cerebral palsy. Paper presented at the annual meeting of the American Academy for Cerebral Palsy and Development Medicine, Atlanta, 1977

84. O'Reilly DE: Care of the cerebral palsied: Outcome of the past and needs of the future. Dev Med Child Neurol 17:141, 1975

85. O'Reilly DE, Walentynowicz JE: Etiological factors in cerebral palsy: An historical review. Dev Med Child Neurol 23:633, 1981

86. Otis JC, Root L, Pamilla JR, Kroll MA: Effect of inhibitory casting on spastic plantarflexors. Presented to the Pediatric Orthopaedic Society, Palm Beach, 1981

87. Perlstein MA, Barnett HE: Nature and recognition of cerebral palsy in infancy. JAMA 148:1389, 1952

88. Perry J, Hoffer MM: Preoperative and postoperative dynamic electromyography as an aid in planning tendon transfers in children with cerebral palsy. J Bone Joint Surg 59A:531, 1977

89. Perry J, Hoffer MM, Antonelli D, Lewis G, Greenberg R: Electromyography before and after surgery for hip deformity. J Bone Joint Surg 58A:201, 1976

90. Perry J, Hoffer M, Giovan P, Greenberg R: Gait analysis of the triceps surae in cerebral palsy. J Bone Joint Surg 56A:511, 1974

91. Perry J: The cerebral palsy gait. In Samilson RL (ed): Orthopaedic Aspects of Cerebral Palsy. Philadelphia, J B Lippincott, 1975

92. Phelps WM: Long-term results of orthopaedic surgery in cerebral palsy. J Bone Joint Surg 39A:53, 1957

93. Rang M, Douglas G, Bennet GC, Koreska J: Seating for children with cerebral palsy. Journal Of Pediatric Orthopedics 1:279, 1981

94. Rawlings G, Reynolds EOR, Stewart A, Strang LB: Changing prognosis for infants of very low birthweight. Lancet 1:516, 1971

95. Reimers J: Contracture of the hamstrings in spastic cerebral palsy. A study of three methods of operative correction J Bone Joint Surg 56B:102, 1974

96. Renshaw TR, Sirkin RB, Drennan JC: The management of hallux valgus in cerebral palsy. Dev Med Child Neurol 21:202, 1979

97. Robson D: The prevalence of scoliosis in adolescents and young adults with cerebral palsy. Dev Med Child Neurol 10:447, 1968

98. Root L: Total hip replacement in cerebral palsy. Paper presented at the annual meeting of the American Academy for Cerebral Palsy and Developmental Medicine, Atlanta, 1977

99. Root L: The totally involved cerebral palsy patient. Instructional Course Lecture, American Academy of Orthopaedic Surgeons, Las Vegas, 1977

100. Rosenthal RK: A fixed-ankle below-the-knee orthosis for the management of genu recurvatum in spastic cerebral palsy. J Bone Joint Surg 57A:545, 1975

101. Rosenthal RK, Levine DB: Fragmentation of the distal pole of the patella in spastic cerebral palsy. J Bone Joint Surg 59A:934, 1977

102. Ruda R, Frost HM: Cerebral palsy. Spastic varus and forefoot adductus, treated by intramuscular posterior tibial tendon lengthening. Clin Orthop 79:61, 1971

103. Rutter M, Graham P, Yule W: A neuropsychiatric study in childhood. Clinics in Developmental Medicine, Nos. 35/36, Philadelphia, J B Lippincott, 1972

104. Saltiel J: A one-piece laminated knee locking short leg brace. Orthotics and Prosthetics 23(2):69, 1969

105. Samilson RL: Dislocation and subluxation of the hip in cerebral palsy. J Bone Joint Surg 54A:863, 1972

106. Samilson RL: Orthopaedic surgery of the hips and spine in retarded cerebral palsy patients. Orthop Clin North Am 12:83, 1981

107. Samilson RL: Surgery of the upper limbs in cerebral palsy. Dev Med Child Neurol 9:109, 1967

108. Samilson RL, Bechard R: Scoliosis in cerebral palsy. Current Practice in Orthopaedic Surgery, St. Louis, C V Mosby, 1973

109. Samilson RL, Morris JM: Surgical improvement of the cerebral palsied upper limb: Electromyographic studies and results in 128 operations. J Bone Joint Surg, 46A:1203-1216, 1964

110. Samilson RL, Carson J, James P, Raney F: Results and complications of adductor tenotomy and obturator neurectomy in cerebral palsy. Clin Orthop 54:61, 1967

111. Samilson RL, Tsou P, Aamoth G, Green WM: Dislocation and subluxation of the hip in cerebral palsy.

Pathogenesis, natural history and management. J Bone Joint Surg 54A:863, 1972

112. Seymour N, Sharrard WJW: Bilateral proximal release of the hamstrings in cerebral palsy. J Bone Joint Surg 50B:274, 1968

113. Sharrard WJW: The hip in cerebral palsy. In Samilson RL (ed): Orthopaedic Aspects of Cerebral Palsy. Philadelphia, J B Lippincott, 1975

114. Sharrard WJW, Allen JMH, Heaney SH, Prendiville Q: Surgical prophylaxis of subluxation and dislocation of the hip in cerebral palsy. J Bone Joint Surg 57B:160, 1975

115. Sharrard WJW, Bernstein S: Equinus deformity in cerebral palsy. J Bone Joint Surg 54B:272, 1972

116. Sherman FC, Westin GW: Plantar release in the correction of deformities of the foot in childhood. J Bone Joint Surg 63A:1382, 1981

117. Silfverskiöld N: Reduction of the uncrossed two-joint muscles of the leg to one-joint muscles in spastic conditions. Acta Chir Scand 56:315, 1923-24

118. Silver CM, Simon SD, Spindell E, Eichtman HM, Scala M: Calcaneal osteotomy for valgus and varus deformities of the foot in cerebral palsy. J Bone Joint Surg 49A:232, 1967

119. Simon SR, Deutsch SD, Rosenthal RK: Genu recurvatum in spastic cerebral palsy. Preliminary report. Orthopaedic Transactions 1:75, 1977

120. Simon S: The pathophysiology of internal rotation gait. Paper presented to the Pediatric Orthopaedic Society, Palm Beach, 1981

121. Smith ET: Hip dislocation in cerebral palsy. Dev Med Child Neurol 11:291, 1969

122. Steel HH: Triple osteotomy of the innominate bone. J Bone Joint Surg 55A:343, 1973

123. Stein RE, Stelling FH: Stress fracture of the calcaneus in a child with cerebral palsy. J Bone Joint Surg 59A:131, 1977

124. Stephenson CT, Donavan MM: Transfer of hip adductor origins to the ischium in spastic cerebral palsy. Dev Med Child Neurol 13:247, 1971

125. Sussman MD, Cusick B: Preliminary report: The role of short-leg, tone-reducing casts as an adjunct to physical therapy of patients with cerebral palsy. Johns Hopkins Med J 145:112, 1979

126. Sutherland DH, Greenfield R: Double innominate osteotomy. J Bone Surg 59A:1082, 1977

127. Sutherland DH, Schottstaedt ER, Larsen LJ, Ashley RK, Callander JN, James PM: Clinical and electromyographic study of seven spastic children with internal rotation gait. J Bone Joint Surg 51A:1070, 1969

128. Tachdjian MO, Minear WL: Hip dislocation in cerebral palsy. J Bone Joint Surg 38A:1358, 1956

129. Tachdjian MO, Minear WL: Sensory disturbances in the hands of children with cerebral palsy. J Bone Joint Surg 40A:85, 1958

130. Wright T, Nicholson J: Physiotherapy for the spastic child: An evaluation. Dev Med Child Neurol 15:146, 1973

Index